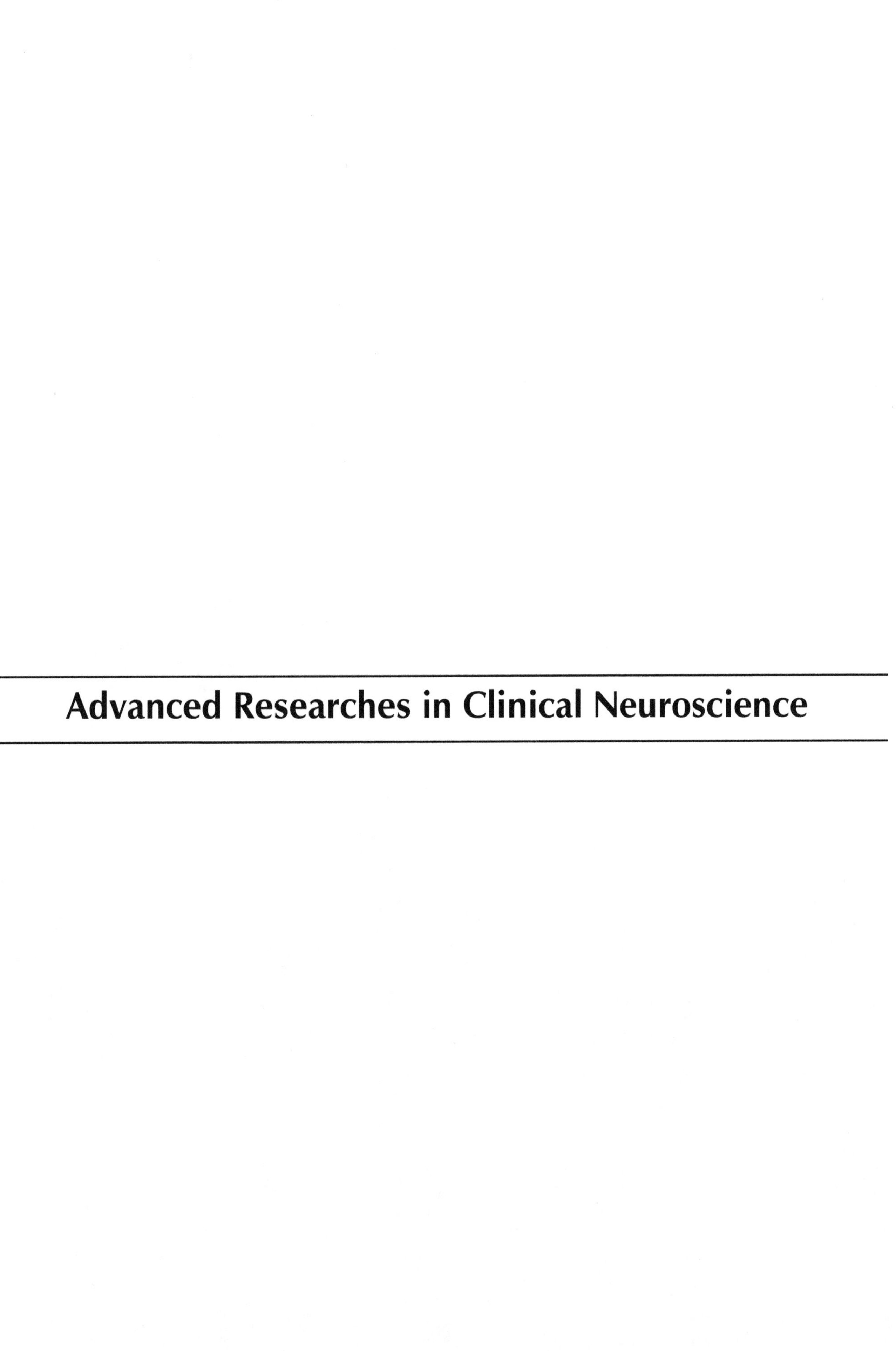

Advanced Researches in Clinical Neuroscience

Advanced Researches in Clinical Neuroscience

Editor: Conelth Dickerson

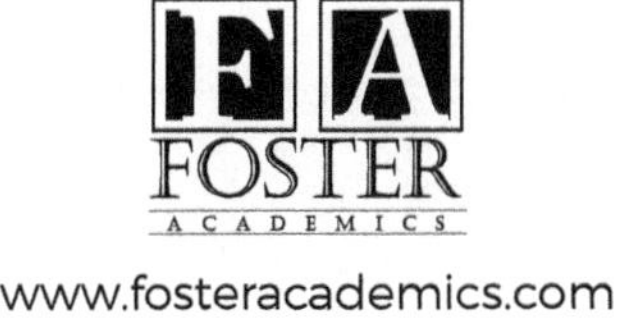

www.fosteracademics.com

www.fosteracademics.com

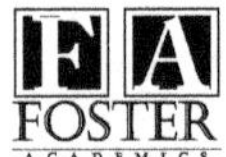

Cataloging-in-Publication Data

Advanced researches in clinical neuroscience / edited by Conelth Dickerson.
p. cm.
Includes bibliographical references and index.
ISBN 978-1-63242-715-1
1. Neurosciences. 2. Nervous system--Diseases. 3. Neurology. I. Dickerson, Conelth.
RC341 .A38 2019
612.8--dc23

Foster Academics,
118-35 Queens Blvd., Suite 400,
Forest Hills, NY 11375, USA

ISBN 978-1-63242-715-1 (Hardback)

Contents

Preface

Clinical neuroscience is a field of neuroscience that strives to develop an understanding of the underlying mechanisms of diseases and disorders of the brain and the central nervous system. Some of these disorders are Alzheimer's disease, Huntington's disease, multiple sclerosis, addiction, Parkinson's disease, autism, bipolar disorder, etc. The diagnosis and treatment of such disorders are within the scope of this field. Other medical specialties which use neuroscientific principles are neuroradiology, neuropathology, anesthesiology, rehabilitation medicine, etc. Psychiatrists, clinical psychologists and neurologists are some of the professionals trained in clinical neuroscience. This book brings forth some of the most innovative concepts and elucidates the unexplored aspects of clinical neuroscience. Some of the diverse topics covered in this book address the advanced researches in this domain. In this book, using case studies and examples, constant effort has been made to make the understanding of the difficult concepts, as easy and informative as possible for the readers.

The researches compiled throughout the book are authentic and of high quality, combining several disciplines and from very diverse regions from around the world. Drawing on the contributions of many researchers from diverse countries, the book's objective is to provide the readers with the latest achievements in the area of research. This book will surely be a source of knowledge to all interested and researching the field.

In the end, I would like to express my deep sense of gratitude to all the authors for meeting the set deadlines in completing and submitting their research chapters. I would also like to thank the publisher for the support offered to us throughout the course of the book. Finally, I extend my sincere thanks to my family for being a constant source of inspiration and encouragement.

Editor

1

The Magnetic Acoustic Change Complex and Mismatch Field: A Comparison of Neurophysiological Measures of Auditory Discrimination

Shu Hui Yau [1,2,3], **Fabrice Bardy** [4,5], **Paul F Sowman** [1,2] **and Jon Brock** [1,2,6] *

[1] ARC Centre of Excellence in Cognition and its Disorders, Australia;
[2] Department of Cognitive Science, Macquarie University, NSW, Australia;
[3] Graduate School of Education, University of Bristol, United Kingdom;
[4] HEARing Co-operative Research Centre, VIC, Australia;
[5] National Acoustic Laboratories, NSW, Australia;
[6] Department of Psychology, Macquarie University, NSW, Australia

* **Correspondence:** jon.brock@mq.edu.au

Abstract: The Acoustic Change Complex (ACC), a P1-N1-P2-like event-related response to changes in a continuous sound, has been suggested as a reliable, objective, and efficient test of auditory discrimination. We used magnetoencephalography to compare the magnetic ACC (mACC) to the more widely used mismatch field (MMF). Brain responses of 14 adults were recorded during mACC and MMF paradigms involving the same pitch and vowel changes in a synthetic vowel sound. Analyses of peak amplitudes revealed a significant interaction between stimulus and paradigm: for the MMF, the response was greater for vowel changes than for pitch changes, whereas, for the mACC, the pattern was reversed. A similar interaction was observed for the signal to noise ratio and single-trial analysis of individual participants' responses showed that the MMF to Pitch changes was elicited less consistently than the other three responses. Results support the view that the ACC/mACC is a robust and efficient measure of simple auditory discrimination, particularly when researchers or clinicians are interested in the responses of individual listeners. However, the differential sensitivity of the two paradigms to the same acoustic changes indicates that the mACC and MMF are indices of different aspects of auditory processing and should, therefore, be seen as complementary rather than competing neurophysiological measures.

Keywords: Acoustic change complex; auditory discrimination; magnetoencephalography; mismatch field; mismatch negativity

1. Introduction

The ability to discriminate between different sounds is a basic prerequisite for spoken language perception [1]. However, poor performance on behavioural tests of auditory discrimination need not necessarily indicate a perceptual impairment. This is especially true in populations such as young children, or individuals with neurodevelopmental or degenerative conditions, for whom poor attention or task understanding might impact adversely upon performance. For this reason, researchers have increasingly made use of electroencephalography (EEG) and magnetoencephalography (MEG) to passively measure event-related cortical responses to changes in auditory stimuli, taking the presence and magnitude of the elicited brain response as an index of perceptual discrimination.

The majority of these studies have employed an oddball paradigm, in which participants hear a sequence of discrete sounds composed of frequent "standards" and rare "deviants" that differ along a single stimulus dimension. The Mismatch Negativity (MMN) or its magnetic counterpart, the Mismatch Field (MMF), is calculated by subtracting the brain response to the standard from the response to the deviant sound [2,3]. The amplitude of the MMN has been found to correlate with performance on behavioural discrimination tasks [4–7]. However, a number of researchers have questioned the reliability of the paradigm, noting that the MMN response is not always elicited, even for easily discriminable stimuli [6,8–12]. A less commonly used alternative is the acoustic change paradigm in which participants hear a continuous auditory stimulus containing a discrete change in, for example, pitch. This elicits a P1-N1-P2 evoked potential referred to as the Acoustic Change Complex (ACC) [13–15]. Like the MMN, the ACC is correlated with behavioural measures of intensity and frequency change [13,16,17] and has good test-retest reliability [15,16].

Surprisingly, only one study to date has directly compared the MMN and the ACC. Using EEG, Martin and Boothroyd [14] elicited an ACC response by presenting participants with 790 ms stimuli that transitioned at their midpoint from a complex tone to spectrally matched noise (or back again). The MMN was elicited using 150 ms tones and noise bursts as standards and deviants. Martin and Boothroyd reported that the ACC response was 2.5 times larger than the equivalent MMN. Moreover, every participant produced an ACC response that was clearly visible and identifiable.

The current investigation extended Martin and Boothroyd's study in two directions. First, rather than tones and noises, we employed linguistically relevant stimuli. Specifically, participants heard semi-synthesized vowel sounds with changes in either pitch (fundamental frequency) or vowel identity (formant frequencies). Second, rather than EEG, we used MEG to measure the MMF and the magnetic ACC (henceforth mACC). As a research tool, MEG has a number of advantages over EEG, particularly for studies of child and clinical populations. Set-up is quick and straightforward and does not involve scalp-scratching or physical contact with the sensors [18,19]. Moreover, MEG has higher spatial resolution, allowing for more accurate source reconstruction and clearer resolution of hemispheric differences [20,21]. However, because MEG is mostly sensitive to cortical sources oriented tangentially to the surface, it does not always provide a superior signal to EEG.

Participants were tested in two 15-minute sessions, once with an MMF paradigm using pitch- and vowel-changes in semi-synthesized speech, and once using a mACC paradigm with the same stimulus changes. We compared the amplitude and signal to noise ratio (SNR) of the MMF and mACC, and objectively determined whether a reliable response could be obtained for each individual participant. In this way, we aimed to determine whether the ACC advantage identified by Martin and Boothroyd extended to MEG and to linguistically-relevant acoustic changes.

2. Materials and Method

2.1. Subjects

Seventeen participants were tested, but three were excluded due to (a) movement of the head-position cap during recording; (b) missing event triggers; and (c) excessive noise in the source waveforms. The final sample included 14 participants, aged 19–40 years (mean = 29.02, SD = 8.71). Thirteen of the fourteen participants were right-handed according to the Edinburgh Handedness Inventory [22]. Participants had a mean score of 11.9 (SD = 2.9) on the Matrices subtest of the Wechsler Adult Intelligence Scale [23]—a measure of nonverbal IQ (population mean = 10, SD = 3). None of the participants reported any history of neurological abnormalities or hearing impairment and hearing threshold was in normal range (<20 dB HL) at frequencies 0.25, 0.5, 1, 2, 4, 8 kHz for all subjects. Written consent was obtained from all participants and procedures were approved by the Macquarie University Human Research Ethics Committee. Participants received monetary compensation for taking part in the study.

2.2. Stimuli

Three synthesized speech vowels were generated in Praat [24] based on source-filter theory. The standard sound (e_{low}) was a synthesized /e/ vowel sound. The pitch deviant (e_{high}) differed from the standard in its fundamental frequency, whereas the vowel deviant (u_{low}) had the same fundamental frequency as e_{low}, but differed in the second and third formats, making an /u/ sound. Table 1 shows the frequency composition of the three sounds.

Table 1. Formant Frequencies (in Hertz) for the three stimuli.

	e_{high}	e_{low}	u_{low}
F0	138	125	125
F1	280	280	280
F2	2620	2620	920
F3	3380	3380	2200

For the MMF paradigm (Figure 1, upper panel), the stimuli were each 75 ms in duration (including 10 ms ramp on and off). Each sequence contained 86% standards (e_{low}), 7% pitch deviants (e_{high}) and 7% vowel deviants (u_{low}) in a pseudo-random order. Within each sequence, at least the first ten sounds were standard sounds in order to create a memory trace and at least two standard sounds were presented between deviants. Stimulus onset asynchrony (SOA) was jittered uniformly between 450–550 ms. Stimuli were presented in three blocks, each lasting 5 minutes, resulting in 1600 trials including 112 pitch deviants and 112 vowel deviants.

For the mACC paradigm (Figure 1, lower panel), a single continuous sound sequence was created, consisting of five units of sound, each of 1500 ms. To prevent audible clicks whilst maintaining as much as possible a constant stimulus amplitude, each stimulus was windowed with a 10 ms rise-fall ramp and the stimuli were concatenated with 5 ms of overlap. Each sound sequence (total duration 7500 ms) was separated by a 1500 ms silence. The order of the sounds in each sequence was: e_{low}, e_{high}, e_{low}, u_{low}, e_{low}. A total of 96 sequences were presented across three 5 minute blocks, so participants heard 96 onset responses, 96 pitch changes (e_{low} to e_{high}), and 96 vowel changes (e_{low} to u_{low}). mACC responses were also elicited by the e_{high} to e_{low} and u_{low} to e_{low} changes but these were not analysed as corresponding changes were not present in the MMF paradigm.

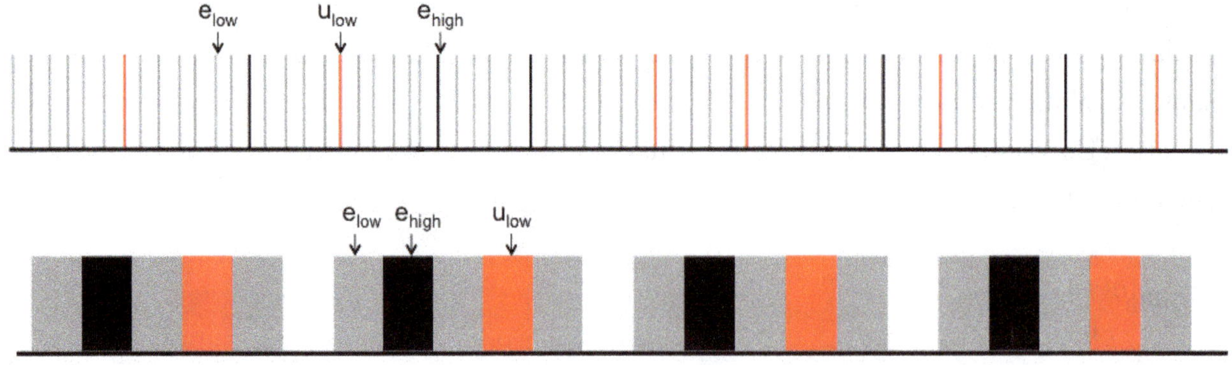

Figure 1. Schematic representation of the MMF (above) and mACC (below) paradigms.

2.3. MEG recording

All MEG testing was performed at the KIT-Macquarie Brain Research Laboratory. Neuromagnetic data were recorded at 1000 Hz using 160-channel whole cortex MEG (Model PQ1160R-N2, KIT, Kanazawa, Japan). The MEG system consists of 160 coaxial first-order gradiometers with a 50 mm baseline [25,26]. During the recording, participants lay on a comfortable bed inside the magnetically shielded room and watched a silent DVD of their choice projected on the ceiling to keep them occupied and awake. They were told to ignore the sounds, give their full attention to the movie, and keep still throughout.

Prior to MEG recording, five marker coils were placed on an elasticised cap on the participant's head, and their positions and the participant's head shape were measured with a pen digitiser (Polhemus Fastrack, Colchester, VT). Head position was measured with the marker coils before and after each MEG recording. Participants were monitored for head movements via a video camera placed inside the magnetically shielded room. Participants who exceeded head-movement of 5 mm (pre- and post-marker coil measurement, as pre-processed in MEG160) were excluded from further analyses.

The mACC and MMF were acquired in two separate acquisition blocks, each with 3 blocks of sounds. Order of testing was randomized across participants. All sound sequences were presented binaurally using MATLAB software at 75dB SPL via pneumatic tubes and custom insert earphones. The stimulus delivery system has a relatively flat frequency response between 500 and 8 kHz and an approximate 10 dB/octave roll-off for frequencies below 500 Hz [27].

2.4. MEG data analysis

MEG data were analysed using the SPM12 M/EEG analysis suite [28] and custom MATLAB scripts. The initial processing steps were as follows: (i) downsample to 250 Hz; (ii) high pass filter at 0.1 Hz; (iii) bandstop filter between 49 and 51 Hz; (iv) low pass filter at 30 Hz; (v) epoch between −100 and 400 ms (from either the onset of the response or the change in the stimulus); (vi) baseline correct between −100 and 0 ms. At this point, we computed the "single trial" MMF by subtracting the response to the preceding standard (predeviant) from the deviant response [29]. Next, for all conditions, we performed robust averaging [30], which down-weights extreme values, thereby minimizing the influence of artefacts. We then re-applied the 30Hz low pass filter to remove any high frequency noise introduced by robust averaging and calculated the global field power (see Figure 2) which provides an overall measure of scalp field strength at each time point [31].

The mACC and MMF responses were extracted from virtual sensors placed in the vicinity of bilateral auditory cortex using a single sphere forward model. Bilateral dipoles were fitted to the M100 response to the onset of the sequence (mACC) or the standard stimulus (MMF), operationalized as the peak in the global field power between 52 and 152 milliseconds. Dipoles were placed in left and right auditory cortex (MNI coordinates: [40 −21 9]; [−40 −21 9]) then fitted by allowing them to orient freely and move within a gaussian centred at this location with standard deviation 10 mm. Next we used the dipole solution as a spatial filter to extract single-trial epoched "virtual sensor" data from the bilateral auditory cortices. Source waveforms for each hemisphere and condition were calculated by robust averaging of the single-trial waveforms followed by 30 Hz low-pass filtering (see Figure 3).

Statistical analyses of the waveforms were performed in R (R Markdown detailing each step of the analyses is available at http://rpubs.com/JonBrock/242837). From each hemisphere, paradigm, and condition, we determined the peak amplitude (maximum for the mACC and minimum for the MMF as these have opposite polarities) within a 100 ms window centred on the peak in the corresponding grand mean global field power. We calculated the SNR by dividing the root mean square of the response post stimulus onset (i.e., 0 to 400 ms) by the root mean square of the response during the baseline period (−100 to 0 ms). Amplitude and SNR measures were subjected to analysis of variance (ANOVA) with Paradigm (mACC vs MMF), Stimulus (Pitch vs Vowel) and Hemisphere (Left vs Right) as repeated measures.

We also performed single-trial analysis of each waveform to determine whether there was a statistically reliable response for each participant. We conducted a one-sample (mACC or MMF vs zero) non-parametric test implemented using the "std_stat" function of the EEGlab toolbox [32] applied to the single trial data for the epoch−100 –400 ms. We ran 1000 permutations and set statistical significance at a p-value of 0.01, false discovery rate corrected.

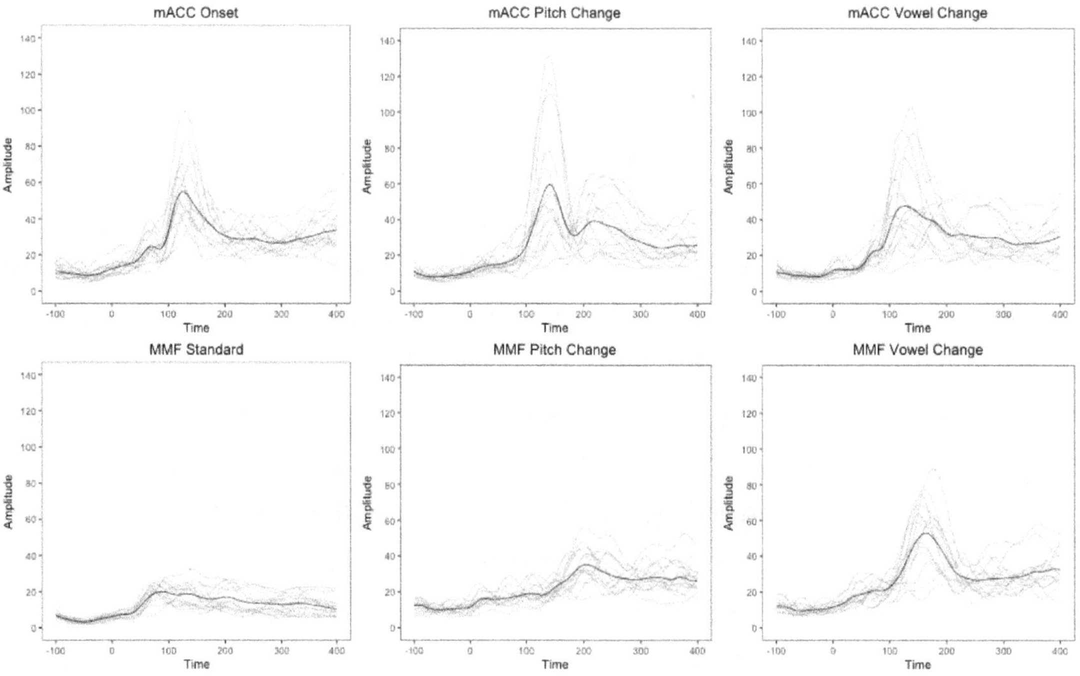

Figure 2. Global field power waveforms for the mACC and MMF paradigms. Grey lines show the responses for individual subjects. Black lines show the mean of all subjects.

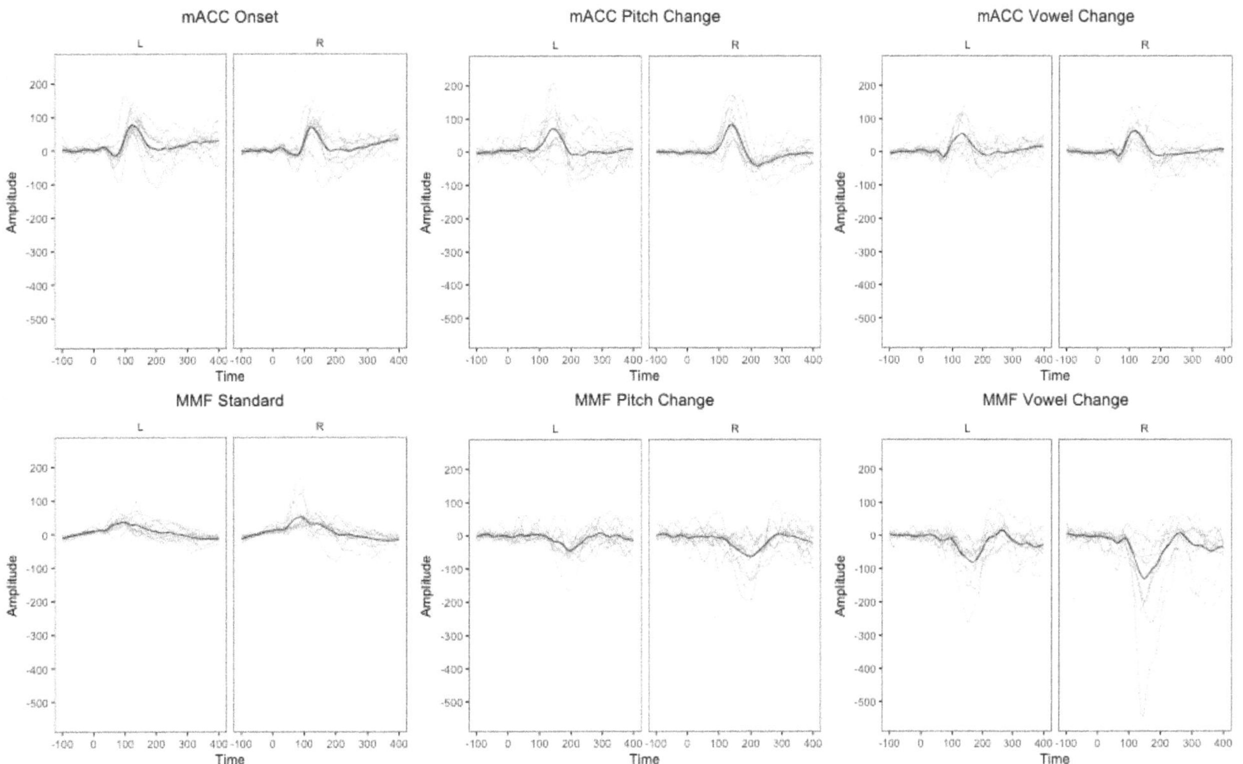

Figure 3. Left (L) and right (R) source waveforms for the mACC and MMF paradigms. Grey lines show the responses for individual subjects. Black lines show the mean of all subjects.

3. Results

Figure 4 shows the peak amplitude and SNR of the mACC and MMF responses. Consistent with the global field power and source waveforms (Figures 2 and 3), it suggests differential sensitivity of the two responses to the Pitch and Vowel stimuli—an impression confirmed by the analyses of variance.

ANOVA on the Peak Amplitude showed no overall effect of Paradigm (F[1,13] = 0.54, $p = 0.474$, $\eta_G^2 = 0.008$), but we did find a significant effect of Stimulus (F[1,13] = 6.10, $p = 0.028$, $\eta_G^2 = 0.017$), which was qualified by a Paradigm by Stimulus interaction (F[1,13] = 23.03, $p < 0.001$, $\eta_G^2 = 0.061$). ANOVAs conducted for each Paradigm separately both showed a main effect of Stimulus, but in opposite directions. For the MMF, the Vowel response was larger than the Pitch response (F[1,13] = 15.87, $p = 0.002$, $\eta_G^2 = 0.094$). For the mACC, the Pitch response was larger than the Vowel response (F[1,13] = 8.30, $p = 0.013$, $\eta_G^2 = 0.027$). No effects or interactions involving Hemisphere were significant.

For SNR, the results were similar. We again found no significant effect of Paradigm (F[1,13] = 2.64, $p = 0.128$, $\eta_G^2 = 0.048$], a significant effect of Stimulus (F[1,13] = 4.71, $p = 0.049$, $\eta_G^2 = 0.036$), and a significant Paradigm by Stimulus interaction (F[1,13] = 7.82, $p = 0.015$, $\eta_G^2 = 0.039$). Again, no effects of Hemisphere and no interactions involving Hemisphere were found to be significant. The Vowel MMF was larger than the Pitch MMF (F[1,13] = 9.39, $p = 0.009$, $\eta_G^2 = 0.192$). However, in contrast to the Peak Amplitude analysis, we found no difference between the Pitch and Vowel mACCs (F[1,13] = 0.01, p = 0.937, η_G^2 = 0.000). For Pitch stimuli, the SNR was higher for the mACC than for the MMF (F[1,13] = 9.45, p = 0.009, η_G^2 = 0.209), but there was no Paradigm effect for Vowel stimuli (F[1,13] = 0.02, p = 0.894, η_G^2 = 0.000).

Figure 4 shows one participant with a particularly large MMF response. We re-analyzed the Peak Amplitude and SNR data excluding this outlier. In both cases, the interaction between Paradigm and Stimulus remained significant, indicating that it could not be attributed to that outlying participant.

Finally, we determined whether each source waveform for each participant was reliably different to a null response (see Table 2). For the mACC, the Pitch and Vowel changes both elicited a significant response in at least one hemisphere for 12/14 and 13/14 of the participants respectively. The vowel-change MMF was present for 11/14 participants, but only 8/14 produced a reliable pitch-change MMF.

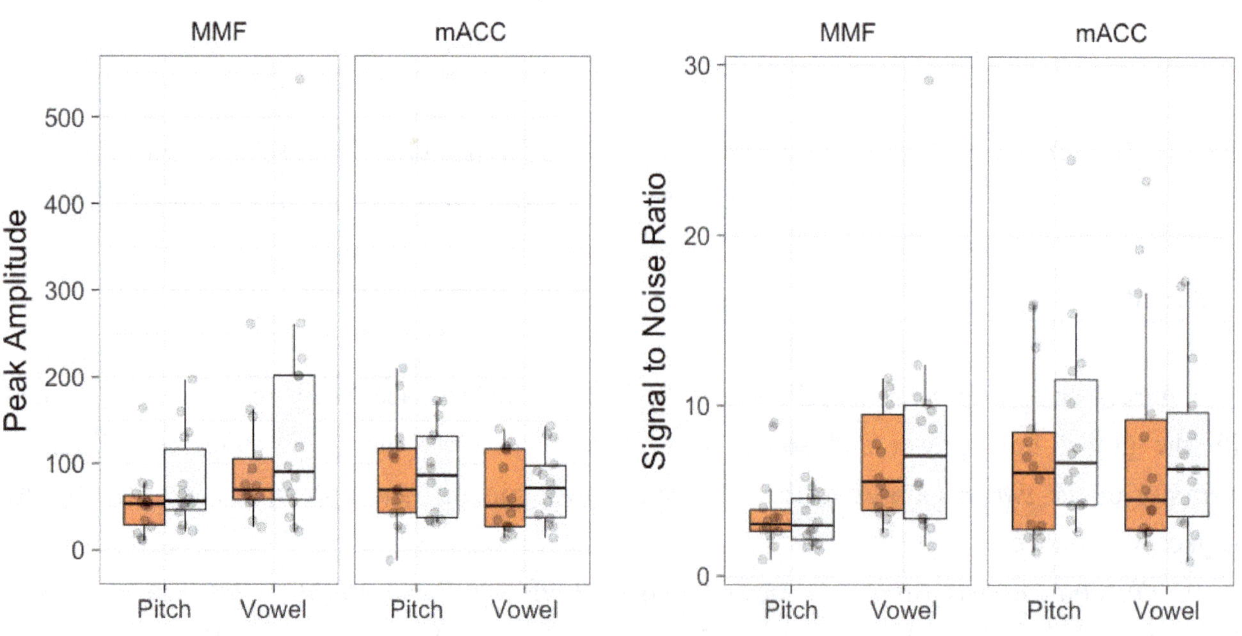

Figure 4. Boxplots showing peak amplitude (left panel) and signal-to-noise ratio (right panel) for mACC and MMF. Dots represent individual participants. Left and right hemisphere sources are in orange and white respectively.

Table 2. Presence of mACC and MMF for individual subjects in the left (L) and right (R) hemisphere. X indicates that the waveform contains at least one cluster of time points that was significantly different to zero (cluster-corrected).

	mACC				MMF			
	Pitch		Vowel		Pitch		Vowel	
Subject	L	R	L	R	L	R	L	R
1	X	X	X	X		X	X	X
2	X		X		X			
3	X	X	X	X	X	X	X	X
4		X		X		X	X	X
5	X	X						
6	X	X	X	X			X	
7	X	X	X	X	X	X	X	X
8	X	X	X	X				X
9		X		X			X	X
10		X		X		X		X
11				X			X	X
12		X	X	X		X	X	X
13	X	X	X	X	X	X	X	X
14				X				
Total	8	11	8	12	4	7	9	10

4. Discussion

The current study directly contrasted two complementary MEG paradigms for investigating auditory change detection, the MMF and the less commonly employed mACC. Although the MMN/MMF is much more widely used, the only previous study directly comparing the two responses found that the ACC is a larger and more robust response than the MMN elicited by the same auditory change [14]. The results of the current study indicate that the relative merits of the two paradigms may in fact be contingent on the stimuli used. For pitch changes, the mACC had a significantly higher SNR than the MMF and reliable responses were obtained more consistently. However, for vowel changes, the MMF had similar SNR to the mACC, and similar reliability at the individual subject level. Importantly, this interaction between Paradigm and Stimuli was also apparent in the global field power, which provides an assumption-free measure of brain responses across the sensors. As such, it would appear to reflect genuine differences in the relative sensitivity of the MMF and mACC to pitch and vowel changes, as opposed to differences in the quality of source model fit across conditions.

In seeking an explanation for this interaction, it is worth considering the putative mechanisms responsible for the mACC and MMF. The ACC/mACC is thought to arise due to the activation and deactivation of neural populations within the tonotopically organised auditory cortex [14,33,34]. The MMN/MMF on the other hand has sources in prefrontal areas [2,35–37] as well as auditory cortex [38–40] and, in addition to change detection, is thought to index processes of memory, attention switching, and the adjustment of internal models of the auditory environment [41–47]. The differential MMF response to vowel and pitch changes (in the presence of similar mACC responses) may, therefore, reflect the influence of one or more of these higher order functions, perhaps involving differences in frontal activation or fronto-temporal connectivity.

Whatever the precise explanation, the current results provide partial support for Martin and Boothroyd's contention that the ACC paradigm is the more efficient measure of auditory change detection. The mACC/ACC has now been found to have superior SNR for both pitch changes and complex tone to noise changes, with equivalent SNR for vowel changes. For the MMF procedure, there appears little scope to improve SNR without making the testing session considerably longer. In contrast, the efficiency of our mACC procedure could be further increased by eliminating the redundant e_{low} at the end of the stimulus, decreasing the duration preceding acoustic changes that are not of interest (e_{high} to e_{low} and u_{low} to e_{low}), and potentially, decreasing all durations and using deconvolution techniques to separate overlapping responses [48].

This is not to say, however, that MMN/MMF should be abandoned. The ACC paradigm is restricted to the study of discrete changes in steady state stimuli such as tones and vowel sounds. In contrast, the MMN can be used to index discrimination of consonant sounds (e.g., /ba/ vs /da/) and is also sensitive to more abstract representations of complex rules such as the conjunction of two different acoustic features [44,49–52]. Moreover, studies that use *both* paradigms may prove particularly informative. For example, in clinical populations, the profile of response across the mACC/ACC and the MMF/MMN may allow a distinction to be made between individuals with basic auditory discrimination deficits, and those with higher-order auditory processing difficulties. Ultimately, the choice of paradigm depends on the question at hand and, as the current results indicate, the precise nature of the acoustic change under investigation.

Acknowledgments

We thank Genevieve McArthur for comments on an earlier version of the manuscript.

Funding Disclosure

This work was supported in part by the HEARing CRC, established and supported under the Australian Cooperative Research Centres Program, an Australian Government Initiative and by support from the Australian Department of Health. Shu Hui Yau was supported by a Macquarie University Research Excellence Scholarship. Paul Sowman (DE130100868) and Jon Brock (DP098466) were supported by the Australian Research Council.

References

1. Ponton CW, Eggermont JJ, Kwong B, et al. (2000) Maturation of human central auditory system activity: evidence from multi-channel evoked potentials. *Clin Neurophysiol* 111: 220-236.
2. Alho K (1995) Cerebral generators of mismatch negativity (MMN) and its magnetic counterpart (MMNm) elicited by sound changes. *Ear Hear* 16: 38-51.
3. Hari R, Hamalainen M, Ilmoniemi R, et al. (1984) Responses of the primary auditory cortex to pitch changes in a sequence of tone pips: neuromagnetic recordings in man. *Neurosci Lett* 50: 127-132.
4. Amenedo E, Escera C (2000) The accuracy of sound duration representation in the human brain determines the accuracy of behavioural perception. *Eur J Neurosci* 12: 2570-2574.
5. Baldeweg T, Richardson A, Watkins S, et al. (1999) Impaired auditory frequency discrimination in dyslexia detected with mismatch evoked potentials. *Ann Neurol* 45: 495-503.
6. Lang AH, Eerola O, Korpilahti P, et al. (1995) Practical issues in the clinical application of mismatch negativity. *Ear Hear* 16: 118-130.
7. Kujala T, Kallio J, Tervaniemi M, et al. (2001) The mismatch negativity as an index of temporal processing in audition. *Clin Neurophysiol* 112: 1712-1719.
8. Dalebout SD, Fox LG (2001) Reliability of the mismatch negativity in the responses of individual listeners. *J Am Acad Audiol* 12: 245-253.
9. Kurtzberg D, Vaughan HG, Jr., Kreuzer JA, et al. (1995) Developmental studies and clinical application of mismatch negativity: problems and prospects. *Ear Hear* 16: 105-117.
10. Morr ML, Shafer VL, Kreuzer JA, et al. (2002) Maturation of mismatch negativity in typically developing infants and preschool children. *Ear Hear* 23: 118-136.
11. Uwer R, von Suchodoletz W (2000) Stability of mismatch negativities in children. *Clin Neurophysiol* 111: 45-52.
12. Wunderlich JL, Cone-Wesson BK (2001) Effects of stimulus frequency and complexity on the mismatch negativity and other components of the cortical auditory-evoked potential. *J Acoust Soc Am* 109: 1526-1537.
13. Martin BA, Boothroyd A (2000) Cortical, auditory, evoked potentials in response to changes of spectrum and amplitude. *J Acoust Soc Am* 107: 2155-2161.
14. Martin BA, Boothroyd A (1999) Cortical, auditory, event-related potentials in response to

periodic and aperiodic stimuli with the same spectral envelope. *Ear Hear* 20: 33-44.

15. Tremblay KL, Friesen L, Martin BA, et al. (2003) Test-retest reliability of cortical evoked potentials using naturally produced speech sounds. *Ear Hear* 24: 225-232.
16. He SM, Grose JH, Buchman CA (2012) Auditory discrimination: The relationship between psychophysical and electrophysiological measures. *Int J Audiol* 51: 771-782.
17. Martin BA (2007) Can the acoustic change complex be recorded in an individual with a cochlear implant? Separating neural responses from cochlear implant artifact. *J Am Acad Audiol.*
18. Hari R, Parkkonen L, Nangini C (2010) The brain in time: insights from neuromagnetic recordings. *Ann N Y Acad Sci* 1191: 89-109.
19. Roberts TP, Schmidt GL, Egeth M, et al. (2008) Electrophysiological signatures: magnetoencephalographic studies of the neural correlates of language impairment in autism spectrum disorders. *Int J Psychophysiol* 68: 149-160.
20. Johnson BW, McArthur G, Hautus M, et al. (2013) Lateralized auditory brain function in children with normal reading ability and in children with dyslexia. *Neuropsychologia* 51: 633-641.
21. Luck SJ (2005) An introduction to the event-related potential technique. Cambridge: MIT Press.
22. Oldfield RC (1971) The assessment and analysis of handedness: the Edinburgh inventory. *Neuropsychologia* 9: 97-113.
23. Wechsler D (2008) Wechsler adult intelligence scale - fourth edition. San Antonio, TX: Psychological Corporation.
24. Boersma P, Weenink D (2009) Praat: doing phonetics by computer (Version 5.1. 05).
25. Kado H, Higuchi M, Shimogawara M, et al. (1999) Magnetoencephalogram systems developed at KIT. *IEEE T Appl Supercon* 9: 4057-4062.
26. Uehara G, Adachi Y, Kawai J, et al. (2003) Multi-channel SQUID systems for biomagnetic measurement. *IEICE T Electron* E86c: 43-54.
27. Raicevich G, Burwood E, Dillon H, et al. (2010) Wide band pneumatic sound system for MEG. 20th International Congress on Acoustics: ICA. pp. 1-5.
28. Litvak V, Mattout J, Kiebel S, et al. (2011) EEG and MEG data analysis in SPM8. *Comput Intell Neurosci* 2011: 852961.
29. Bishop DV, Hardiman MJ (2010) Measurement of mismatch negativity in individuals: a study using single-trial analysis. *Psychophysiology* 47: 697-705.
30. Wager TD, Keller MC, Lacey SC, et al. (2005) Increased sensitivity in neuroimaging analyses using robust regression. *Neuroimage* 26: 99-113.
31. Lehmann D, Skrandies W (1980) Reference-free identification of components of checkerboard-evoked multichannel potential fields. *Electroencephalogr Clin Neurophysiol* 48: 609-621.
32. Delorme A, Makeig S (2004) EEGLAB: an open source toolbox for analysis of single-trial EEG dynamics including independent component analysis. *J Neurosci Methods* 134: 9-21.
33. Liegeois-Chauvel C, Giraud K, Badier JM, et al. (2001) Intracerebral evoked potentials in pitch perception reveal a functional asymmetry of the human auditory cortex. *Ann N Y Acad Sci* 930: 117-132.

34. Pratt H, Starr A, Michalewski HJ, et al. (2009) Auditory-evoked potentials to frequency increase and decrease of high- and low-frequency tones. *Clin Neurophysiol* 120: 360-373.
35. Alain C, Woods DL, Knight RT (1998) A distributed cortical network for auditory sensory memory in humans. *Brain Res* 812: 23-37.
36. Giard MH, Perrin F, Pernier J, et al. (1990) Brain generators implicated in the processing of auditory stimulus deviance: a topographic event-related potential study. *Psychophysiology* 27: 627-640.
37. Jemel B, Achenbach C, Muller BW, et al. (2002) Mismatch negativity results from bilateral asymmetric dipole sources in the frontal and temporal lobes. *Brain Topogr* 15: 13-27.
38. Jaaskelainen IP, Ahveninen J, Bonmassar G, et al. (2004) Human posterior auditory cortex gates novel sounds to consciousness. *P Natl Acad Sci USA* 101: 6809-6814.
39. May PJ, Tiitinen H (2010) Mismatch negativity (MMN), the deviance - elicited auditory deflection, explained. *Psychophysiology* 47: 66-122.
40. Scherg M, Vajsar J, Picton TW (1989) A source analysis of the late human auditory evoked potentials. *J Cogn Neurosci* 1: 336-355.
41. Escera C, Alho K, Schroger E, et al. (2000) Involuntary attention and distractibility as evaluated with event-related brain potentials. *Audiology and Neuro-Otology* 5: 151-166.
42. Garrido MI, Kilner JM, Stephan KE, et al. (2009) The mismatch negativity: a review of underlying mechanisms. *Clin Neurophysiol* 120: 453-463.
43. Naatanen R, Kujala T, Winkler I (2011) Auditory processing that leads to conscious perception: a unique window to central auditory processing opened by the mismatch negativity and related responses. *Psychophysiology* 48: 4-22.
44. Naatanen R, Tervaniemi M, Sussman E, et al. (2001) "Primitive intelligence" in the auditory cortex. *Trends Neurosci* 24: 283-288.
45. Rinne T, Alho K, Ilmoniemi RJ, et al. (2000) Separate time behaviors of the temporal and frontal mismatch negativity sources. *Neuroimage* 12: 14-19.
46. Todd J, Myers R, Pirillo R, et al. (2010) Neuropsychological correlates of auditory perceptual inference: a mismatch negativity (MMN) study. *Brain Res* 1310: 113-123.
47. Bendixen A, Schroger E, Winkler I (2009) I heard that coming: event-related potential evidence for stimulus-driven prediction in the auditory system. *J Neurosci* 29: 8447-8451.
48. Bardy F, McMahon CM, Yau SH, et al. (2014) Deconvolution of magnetic acoustic change complex (mACC). *Clin Neurophysiol* 125: 2220-2231.
49. Kujala T, Tervaniemi M, Schroger E (2007) The mismatch negativity in cognitive and clinical neuroscience: theoretical and methodological considerations. *Biol Psychol* 74: 1-19.
50. Naatanen R (2001) The perception of speech sounds by the human brain as reflected by the mismatch negativity (MMN) and its magnetic equivalent (MMNm). *Psychophysiology* 38: 1-21.
51. Pulvermuller F, Shtyrov Y (2006) Language outside the focus of attention: The mismatch negativity. as a tool for studying higher cognitive processes. *Prog Neurobiol* 79: 49-71.

2

Dominant and opponent relations in cortical function: An EEG study of exam performance and stress

Lucia P. Pavlova[1], **Dmitrii N. Berlov**[2,3] **and Andres Kurismaa**[4,*]

[1] Department of Higher Nervous Activity and Psychophysiology, Faculty of Biology, St. Petersburg State University, St.-Petersburg, Russia

[2] Department of Anatomy and Physiology of Humans and Animals, Herzen State Pedagogical University of Russia, St.-Petersburg, Russia

[3] International Research Center of the Functional Materials and Devices of Optoelectronics and Electronics, ITMO University, Saint Petersburg, Russia

[4] Department of History and Philosophy of Science, Faculty of Science, Charles University in Prague, Czech Republic

* **Correspondence:** Email: andres.kurismaa@gmail.com

Abstract: This paper analyzes the opponent dynamics of human motivational and affective processes, as conceptualized by RS Solomon, from the position of AA Ukhtomsky's neurophysiological principle of the dominant and its applications in the field of human electroencephalographic analysis. As an experimental model, we investigate the dynamics of cortical activity in students submitting university final course oral examinations in naturalistic settings, and show that successful performance in these settings depends on the presence of specific types of cortical activation patterns, involving high indices of left-hemispheric and frontal cortical dominance, whereas the lack thereof predicts poor performance on the task, and seems to be associated with difficulties in the executive regulation of cognitive (intellectual) and motivational processes in these highly demanding and stressful conditions. Based on such knowledge, improved educational and therapeutic interventions can be suggested which take into account individual variability in the neurocognitive mechanisms underlying adaptation to motivationally and intellectually challenging, stressful tasks, such as oral university exams. Some implications of this research for opponent-process theory and its closer integration into current neuroscience research on acquired motivations are discussed.

Keywords: cortical activity; dominant principle; electroencephalogram; functional asymmetry;

individual variability; opponent processes

1. Introduction

In the current paper, we focus on two basic, interrelated principles of systemic regulation of brain functions—the opponent process theory by R.S. Solomon [1–3], and A.A. Ukhtomsky's principle of the dominant [4,5], and apply them to electroencephalographic (EEG) analysis of human performance at university oral exams in naturalistic conditions [6]. By drawing on the experimental results of this pilot study, we demonstrate that successful adaptation of students to the requirements of an oral examination depends on the presence of individual types of cortical activation patterns (CAPs), involving high indices of left-hemispheric and frontal cortical dominance, whereas the lack thereof reliably predicts low achievement on the task, and seems to be associated with difficulties in the executive regulation of cognitive (intellectual) and acquired motivational processes in these highly challenging and stressful conditions. Findings from these studies seem to support several key tenets of Solomon's opponent process theory of motivation dynamics [3], and may help to analyze its so far relatively poorly understood neurophysiological mechanisms in the light of the dominant principle [4,5]. In particular, the widely prevalent, if not universal functional principle of coupled opposed dynamics (COD) of cortical activity, as revealed in the principle of the dominant, can be of fundamental importance for elucidating how functional cerebral systems with mutually exclusive and opposed effects interact in time, leading to both adaptive or maladaptive behavioral and cognitive responses. We introduce functional measures of COD, such as the coupled inversion of anterio-posterior (fronto-occipital) and bilateral (inter-hemispheric) activation gradients, to analyze these responses, and show how their dynamics change in different task conditions and cognitive states in a manner consistent with the opponent process theory.

Methodologically, analyzing the neurophysiological dynamics of motivational reactions in ecological settings may require specific approaches, and this has been rarely attempted in exam conditions. While numerous works are devoted to the role of emotions, stress and anxiety in the learning process [7–9], including the exam situation, virtually all such studies are limited to pre-examination and post-examination analysis [10–15], without affecting the exam itself, particularly with regard to measuring the brain's bioelectric activity in the course of the exam interaction and presumable peak stress experience. The current line of studies sought to validate the applicability of dynamic EEG analysis in these settings [6,16,17]. It may therefore represent particular interest for analysing not only the electrophysiological correlates of opponent processes, as understood by Solomon, but also for considering their so far little explored social and interpersonal aspects in relevant natural settings.

As will be shown, based on such knowledge, the individual variability of dominant and opponent processes can be analyzed, and improved pedagogical and therapeutic interventions suggested which take into account marked individual differences in the neural and cognitive mechanisms underlying adaptation to motivationally and intellectually challenging tasks, such as the oral exam. These aspects will be more extensively addressed in the discussion, after the concepts of the dominant and opponent processes have been introduced (section 2), and relevant empirical materials presented (section 3). Theoretically, the integrative approach developed here [6,16,17] corresponds to the widely recognized need for systemic frameworks and methodologies in the fields of behavioral and human neuroscience [18,19], and in the analysis of EEG [20,21], in particular.

2. Dominant and opponent processes

In the fields of neuroscience and psychophysiology, both the theory of opponent processes, as well as the principle of the dominant stand out by their systemic, heuristic predictions and specific applications in an unusually wide range of topics. Thus, Solomon and Corbit [1] proposed a general model of opponent processes to explain an apparently widespread mechanism securing the dynamic homeostasis of intense, contrastive emotional and motivational states [3]. The authors gathered evidence from physiology and psychology for a general model explaining how intense hedonic experiences can automatically induce in the nervous system a biphasic, compensatory motivational or affective process of opposite hedonic valence, before a return to stable affective baseline state occurs in the subject. However, the neurophysiological underpinnings of this dynamic homeostatic phenomenon have remained relatively elusive and little studied, in comparison to its behavioral and psychological effects.

Recently, some of the related methodical and methodological challenges have been discussed by Comer et al. [22]. In particular, the authors propose that the functional cerebral systems theory of A.R. Luria [23] may still provide "unsurpassed explanatory value and testability" in promoting the systemic-dynamic exploration of functional processes within the nervous system [22], including the relevant homeostatic and compensatory effects. Indeed, such aspects have remained largely underappreciated, and challenge current attempts to integrate opponent processes into mainstream neuroscience research, according to their view [22].

Here, we suggest that besides the works of A.R. Luria, valuable insights for the study of dynamic functional systems can be obtained from a historically and methodologically closely related tradition, namely A.A. Ukhtomsky's study on the dominant [4,5]. The fundamental basis informing this line of work concerns the unity of opposed functional processes in the brain—excitation and inhibition—as tonic neurophysiological states, and their reciprocal induction in cortical and neuronal excitability [24–26]. In particular, this approach may help to understand how intense work-load on any functional system—of immediate hedonic valence or not—can evoke its auto-inhibition and resultant "super-compensatory" effects, before a more stable baseline of excitability is restored or modified in the brain. In the present paper, we are limited to discussing this phenomenon in its cortical physiological aspects.[1]

[1]Currently, the concept of *hormesis* is widely discussed as a general biological model of state-dependent functional effects in physiological systems, particularly in relation to the varying and opposed effects which neurotransmitters and other substances may have at the cellular level, depending on their concentration (dose-response effects) or other conditions of exposure [77]. On the other hand, the conceptual and historical parallels of the hormetic research paradigm with the framework of parabiosis and paranecrosis, going back to Ukhtomsky's teacher N.E. Wedensky's and D.N. Nasonov's works [78,79], are also recognized [80,81]. These aspects lay beyond the scope of this paper, but are important to theoretically highlight, particularly given the recent interest in hormetic phenomena in the nervous system [82,83]. Without addressing such opposed phased functional effects, it may be difficult to develop a low-level neuronal interpretation of opponent processes in relation to particular transmitter systems, as currently sought [84,85], and thus firmly ground opponent process theory in biology. Interestingly, the school of Wedensky-Ukhtomsky appears to remain the only physiological tradition where principles characterizing homeostatic phenomena at the neuronal level, and the functional state parameters of general, brain-wide dynamics have been investigated from a common perspective [25,86].

The dominant approach allows to highlight how the opponent temporal dynamics of motivations and emotions may depend on the non-equilibrium properties of the cortical biopotential field as a whole. This field can be characterized by transitions in the *foci of maximal activation* (FMA), and by the localization of the accompanying coupled, collaterally inhibited areas in the surrounding cortical tissue. These two contrastive neurophysiological responses represent a pattern of *coupled opposed dynamics* (COD) in the cortex that seems to be of wide, perhaps universal relevance for interpreting neurophysiological coordination dynamics and mechanisms [6,17,27] (section 3).

In particular, this approach to opponent processes may allow to better understand the mechanisms governing dynamic changes in hemispheric dominance [22,28], as well as to demonstrate how shifts in inter-hemispheric and prefrontal dominance relate to changes in the motivational and higher cognitive processes of subjects as they adapt to diverse task conditions and cognitive work load [6,16,27]. Below, we show evidence for the hypothesis that opponent motivational processes may be directly related to changes in hemispheric and prefrontal dominance indices. While this hypothesis has been proposed and is supported by other experimental paradigms and evidence [22,28], the current approach allows to extend and generalize these findings by applying a novel experimental and methodological framework for their neurophysiologically rigorous and ecologically valid investigation—albeit in a small-scale pilot study.

It can be noted that respective materials raise also general theoretical problems, as they highlight that shifts in motivational states are most probably not limited to the sphere of "hedonic" processes or specific subcortical regions in the brain, but seem to involve widely distributed functional cerebral systems, including cortical ones associated with higher psychological processes and executive functions in humans. Although direct EEG evidence on opponent effects is so far limited, a recent study by Kline et al. [28] has obtained relevant results in this regard and should be shortly highlighted.

The authors revealed the role of prefrontal cortical regions in the opponent-type regulation of emotional experience, and showed how the organization of this experience depends on the dynamics of hemispheric functional asymmetry. In particular, it was shown that fear reactions evoked in a group of participants (in response to aversive pictures of human faces) are accompanied by increased relative right prefrontal activation, whereas the predominance of left prefrontal regions inhibits the same negative reaction and may, in well-coping subjects, respectively show enhanced and super-compensatory activity after the initial fear response. The authors interpret this increased leftward activation as a contrastive after-reaction necessary for suppressing, on an opponent process basis, the mainly right-hemispheric aversive response [28]. Although not obtained in an exam setting, these results seem to confirm the view that opponent affective processes, as conceived by Solomon, are closely associated with a corresponding contrastive dynamics in frontal lobe activity. A replication of this hypothesis in other experimental paradigms would be highly desirable, nevertheless, to demonstrate the pervasiveness of such opponent regulations and their possible functional contexts. This could also lead to a better understanding of the intra- and inter-individual variability which such opponent effects may have, their task-specificity, as well as association with other neural systems.

Close to the present focus, an early study by Craig and Siegel [29] has addressed the principle of opponent regulation in the exam situation. The authors investigated habituation to test-anxiety in college students and obtained evidence supporting Solomon's theory. In particular, by administering mood adjective checklists to students for self-rating just before and immediately after taking a final course exam, the authors quite expectably found a reliable decrease in dysphoria—but more significantly, also an increase in euphoria subsequent to the stressful test event, consistent with the opponent process model [29]. The important implication of the latter is the prediction of not simply attenuating apprehension, but also a surge in elation upon completing the exam. However, this study did not employ any physiological measures, and together with other related studies on exams [10–12,30], would clearly benefit from an integrated psychophysiological approach, allowing to analyze the neural substrates and mechanisms directly involved in the exam situation and interactions [16,17]. Likewise, most research on emotional and stress reactions has so far investigated EEG and peripheral signals separately [31], although their fusion and joint assessment may improve the robustness of both lines of findings [31], as our own data in the exam setting also suggests.

As shown below, our research on the higher cortical regulation of cognitive and motivational processes are in direct agreement with the above results [28,29], and may help to generalize and extend these findings on opponent-type regulation to more complex types of motivational and cognitive responses—such as involved in real-time exam situations. Before turning to the empirical findings obtained in this framework, we will briefly describe some methodological specifics of this line of studies based on A.A. Ukhtomsky's principle of the dominant. Further integration of this approach and findings with opponent-type processes is presented in the discussion.

3. Theoretical preliminaries: The dominant and human EEG

It's passing first to consider A.A. Ukhtomsky's pioneering insights on the functional role of EEG rhythms. Based on the concept of "operative rest" or calm (cf. [32,25]), his views were among the first to clarify the controversial issue of the quasi-periodic alpha-rhythm (8–10 Hz) and its significance in human brain activity. Ukhtomsky proceeded from the experimental fact that in humans, the resting state is dominated by coherent, low-frequency alpha-waves of high amplitude. Peripheral stimuli from sense organs are known to disturb this "resting-state oscillation" and to give rise to higher-frequency activation (beta rhythms > 12 Hz) in the cortical projections, further enhanced by the subject's endogenous attentional and emotional arousal. These facts led Ukhtomsky to conclude that it would be *incorrect to see coordination as being generally based on the synchronization of neuronal activity alone* [4]—more often than not, *it depends on a parallel increase in the desynchronization of neural networks* [4,6]. This constitutes a general principle of *coupled opposed dynamics* (COD) in brain function, as clarified below.

Elucidating the role and mechanisms of alpha-rhythm desynchronization continues to be an active area of research, where various general and more specific hypotheses have been offered to account for its functions. Jensen et al. [33] have framed an influential view on the gating and filtering properties of the cortical alpha, which through targeted suppression ("pulsed inhibition") of higher-frequency rhythms, particularly gamma oscillations (30–70 Hz), is assumed to have an active inhibitory role in shaping functional cortical architecture. Closely compatible interpretations have been recently proposed by Klimesch [34], who suggests an active inhibitory function for alpha activity in controlling attentional and conscious access to stored memory and knowledge; for this access to occur, information from competing sources must be temporarily excluded (suppressed). In more formal terms stemming from information theory, alpha desynchronization can be related to information richness in the brain, necessary for the encoding and retrieval of memory and other cognitive processes [35]; on the other hand, the degree of synchrony in neural firing patterns is inversely related to their information carrying capacity [35]. Indeed, hypersynchronized cortical activity in the alpha range has been associated with complete blockage of intracortical communication, leading to the breakdown in sensory processing and loss of consciousness [36]. Important studies, closely related to our own, have also been carried out in the framework of coupled event-related desynchornization/synchronization (ERD/ERS) by Pfurtscheller and colleagues, suggesting that cortical activation (reflected in ERD) may be more focused and concentrated when surrounded by fields of antagonistic inhibitory synchronization (ERS), particularly within the alpha band [37–39].

Thus, modern studies seem to offer numerous confirmations regarding the dominant concept and its application in the field of EEG study. At the same time, some methodological differences regarding the principles of EEG analysis should be noted. This concerns above all the problem of dynamic features of neural signals, specifically the non-stationary (discontinuous, segmentary) and stochastic properties they exhibit. While knowledge of such features has been available for a long time (and forms the basis of our work [40]), they have typically been ignored in current and classical frameworks of EEG interpretation due to methodical and theoretical premises [20,21]. On the other hand, while this may simplify signal analysis, neglecting such dynamic features has also lead to significant difficulties in constructing global models of the EEG phenomenon, and in relating it to problems of cognition and consciousness [20,21]. Thus, novel methodologies sensitive to the underlining quasi-stationary nature of the EEG signal are clearly necessary [21]. One of the earliest such frameworks has been developed in collaboration with one of the authors (L.P.) [17,40] on the basis of the dominant principle. Below, some of its key premises and methods are briefly outlined.

The principle of dominant introduces into cognitive science a factor rarely considered in other frameworks—the factor of non-equilibrium as an invariant principle in all neurocognitive phenomena. In its most general form, Ukhtomsky characterized dominant states as consisting of two coupled and inverse processes—a leading "focus" or excitatory link, and systemic propagation of inhibition over the remaining elements of the system. This divergent pattern constitutes a universal mechanism of coordination in his view, and the means by which superfluous degrees of freedom are eliminated in neural systems. In this context, dominance is not so much a theory or hypothesis, but an obvious feature of functional cerebral systems in his view. However, it can offer powerful heuristics for studying brain activity when constrained by specific models and analytic methods, and may prove to be its highly universal organizational feature.

It is thus instrumental to define an adequate model for dominant states and the associated non-equilibrium dynamics in brain networks. The dominance model outlined below presents methods for multi-parametric and multi-channel analysis of such functional dynamics according to coherence and synchrony parameters [6,40]. Accordingly, the activation gradients (AG) characterizing functional asymmetry indices along anterio-posterior (AP) and bilateral (LR) interhemispheric cortical zones define the structure of cortical activation patterns (CAPs), and their "non-equilibrium" (functional asymmetry). In our previous works, we elaborated optimal statistical quantitative measures for characterizing functional shifts in the brain's dominant CAP states, defined by the momentary activation gradients between α- and higher frequency rhythms [40,17] (Appendix 1).

In this model, a dominant CAP state is reflected in two coupled inverse shifts in regional biorhythm indices characterizing cortical areas: (1) a focus of maximal activation (FMA), with amplified β-rhythms in a given region and attenuated α-oscillations (down to their complete disappearance in that area); and (2) a state of coupled inhibition in the surrounding cortical regions, as reflected in the simultaneous appearance of amplified α- rhythm [6,17] (Appendix 1).

Additionally, an activation coefficient $K_{C/O}$ can be determined by the relation of latent reaction periods (LRP) after closing and opening the eyes—with LRP for closed eyes (LRP–CE) reflecting excitation inertia, and LRP for opened eyes (LRP–OE) reflecting inhibition inertia, or the inertial properties of inhibitory cortical states (Appendix 2).

4. Experimental studies on exam performance

Oral exams present one of the most intense forms of human mental activity, combining both intellectual, emotional, and stress-regulatory components in a highly dynamic social setting [6]. Examining their individual variability and neurocognitive structure may therefore present unique insights into the mechanisms of opponent processes in naturalistic conditions.

4.1. Methods and materials

Our studies were carried out in an experimental EEG recording facility in collaboration with Dr. N. Volkind from Krasnoyarsk Pedagogical Institute, with whom we conducted university term examinations on the subject “physiology of higher nervous activity” on volunteering student participants from St.-Petersburg State University’s Psychology Faculty. To ensure high performance criteria, students’ examination grades were recorded on exam sheets and reflected in their official study records.

Experimental conditions: In a group of 20 students (18 y.o., male, all right-handed), EEG was recorded continuously from 8 to 10 symmetrical anterior and posterior cortical sites (using the device “Biofizpribor”, 0.3–100 Hz bandwidth), simultaneously with electrocardiogram (ECG) data [6,17]. Electrode montage is specified in Appendix 3. On the eve of the exams, a test experiment was carried out on each participant to ensure habituation to exam settings and to the Eyes Closed/Eyes Open (EC/EO) test (Appendix 2). Each experimental session lasted for no less than 1.5 hours in a row, during daytime, under normal daylight conditions. EEG recordings were made as the subjects were seated in a comfortable chair, in a specially screened room (3×3 m^2) shielded from external noise. After installing the electrodes, the FAM test (Feeling, Activity, Mood) [41,42] was administered to students, who thereafter were left alone for 15 minutes to rest and prepare before starting the exam. After completing the exam, students were left to rest for 20 minutes, before being again administered a FAM test by the experimenter. Furthermore, prior to the experiment we tested subjects by the Hand [43], personal orientation inventory (POI), and Eysenck personality questionnaire (EPQ) psychological tests.

Students’ EEG and ECG were recorded continuously throughout 5 stages of the exam: I stage—students await for the examiner, corresponding to a state of operative rest (15 min); II stage—the examiner enters the room, students receive tickets (topics), read them in the examiner’s presence, the examiner leaves; III stage—students prepare independently an answer to the ticket (20 min); IV stage—students are orally examined on the ticket and on additional questions, are notified of their grade (20 min); V stage—period of post-exam rest, the examiner has left (20 min). Throughout the whole exam, short EC/EO tests were administered every 2–3 min.

It should be stressed that we did not assess FAM scores by averaging results across the participants, but distinguished between 2 experimental subgroups by their grades—a high-achieving group (A), who passed for "excellent", and a low-achieving group (B), who either failed the exam or passed it poorly. This strategy was used to reveal adequate correlations between CAP types and given sets of activity. While selecting students to be included in either group by their grade, we strove to maintain their homogeneity also by other indices, above all by high achievement motivation, which was present in all subjects. (In group A, all 5 students had "excellent" academic records exclusively in all subjects, and had all graduated with honors from highschool. In group B, students with high achievement motivation and generally good knowledge of the subject were chosen, but who failed to demonstrate this knowledge in the specific settings of an oral exam, both in the current study and during prior oral exams). These inclusion criteria were applied meticulously, particularly given the small sample size of the study.

Ethical conditions: The study was conducted on unpaid volunteers. Experimental procedures of study, including its ethical and medical aspects, were reviewed and approved by an expert committee at the A.A. Ukhtomsky Physiological Research Institute at St.-Petersburg State University. Participation in the study involved written consent from students and Deans of the Psychology and the Biology Faculties of the University.

4.2. Results

Most significant shifts in the level of cortical activation (by the coefficient $K_{C/O}$) (Appendix 2) and vegetative nervous activity (pulse rate) were observed in stages II and IV of the exam—while drawing the ticket and answering it, respectively. Signs of examination stress were particularly pronounced in highly anxious, poorly answering students (Figure 1).

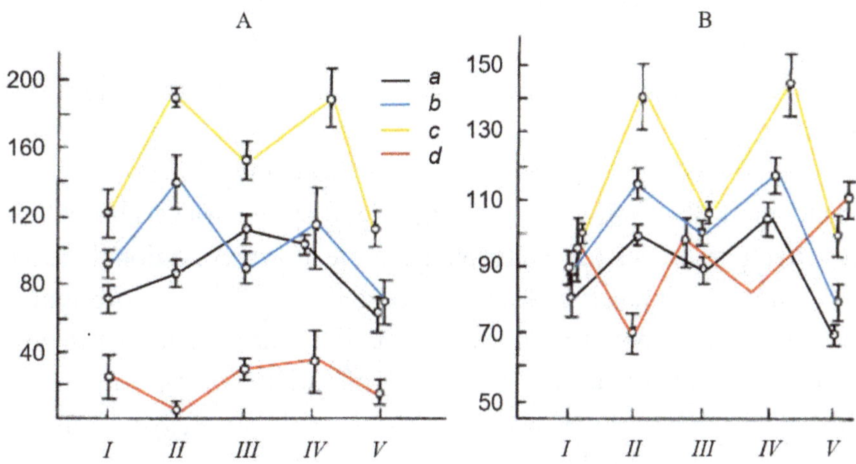

Figure 1. Shifts in general activation of cerebral cortex (A) and pulse rate (B) in consecutive stages (I–V) of oral examination in four variously graded groups (5 subjects in each group). *Ordinate*: A—average measures of general cortical activation ($\Sigma K_{C/O}$, in conditional units), B—pulse rate (bpm); *a, b, c, d*—grades received: excellent *(a)*, good *(b)*, average *(c)*, poor *(d)*, respectively. Abscissa—exam stages: *I*—waiting; *II*—drawing a ticket; *III*—preparing the answer; *VI*—exam response; *V*—after-effects.

Significant individual differences in the indices of general cortical activation by $K_{C/O}$ (Figure 1A) and pulse rate (Figure 1B) can be seen in relation to success rate at the exam. During all stages of the exam, students receiving excellent and good grades (groups a and b) showed intermediate values for these indices, in comparison to students receiving average and poor grades (groups c and d). Thus, less successful responders where characterized either by an excessive degree of cortical activation and pulse rate (group c), or an insufficient value of these functional indices (group d), in comparison to the high-achiving groups. The reliability of this data is increased by the identical conditions in which all examinees were tested, and the highly significant differences in functional brain states of high- and low-achieving participants (Figure 2).

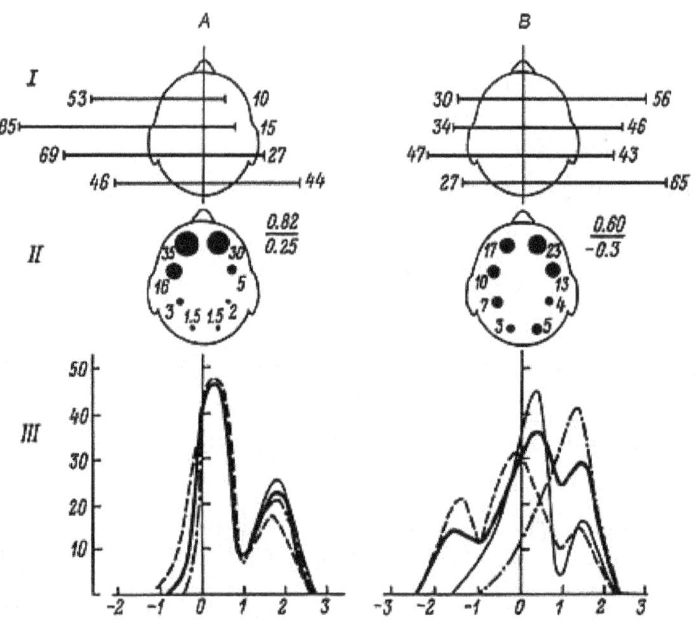

Figure 2. CAP types and mental work productivity at university exams (average data in 2 groups, 5 people in each). A—students with "excellent" results, generally high-achieving subjects; B—students with average or poor results, generally lower-achieving subjects. I—relative activation (by $K_{C/O}$) of left and right symmetrical cortical zones (%). II—regional activation indices (on hemispheric projections; conditional units); numbers on the right: numerator—anterio-posterior non-equilibrium ($K_{A/P}$), denominator—bilateral asymmetry index ($K_{L/R}$). III—variational distribution of $K_{C/O}$ values on logarithmic scale (on abscissa), number of variants (n = 400) for each value (on ordinate). One curve corresponds to one subject. Values within $K_{C/O} > 0$ reflect activation, values within $K_{C/O} < 0$ reflect marked inhibition, deactivation. For methods, cf Appendix 2.

Additionally, consideration of background EEG signals at the exam complements materials obtained by the EC/EO test, and allows to reveal symptoms of stress as well as mental fatigue in students. Most pronounced general cortical activation, determined by the coefficient of relative β- and α rhythm power ($K_{\beta/\alpha}$), was observed in stages II and IV of the exam, and was accompanied by most significant increases in pulse rate (by 1.5–2 times).

Below, we analyze the CAP types in two groups of students with most divergent results at the exam, respectively receiving "excellent" or "poor" (insufficient) grades. Both groups included five subjects, who were tested during the exam (by EC/EO test) no less than 60 times each. The high significance of obtained differences is reflected in the variational curves obtained from large sample sizes ($n = 400$) of the EC/EO test in the two student groups (Figure 2).

In the "excellent"—graded group of students (Figure 2A), stable FMA was observed in left frontal areas by the general activation level as well as by the percentage of prevalent left-sided activity on the background of high anterio-posterior (fronto-occipital) activation gradients (AGs). At the same time, the almost complete superposition of $K_{C/O}$ variational curve values, revealing the presence of a distinct FMA in left frontal areas, testifies to a largely identical functional brain state in all five high-achieving subjects. Double-peaking variational curves reveal a distinct FMA in left frontal areas on the background of significantly reduced activation range in the subdominant brain regions, with a non-significant transition rate in the deactivated areas (by $K_{C/O} < 0$; cf. Appendix 2). This allows to speak of a correspondence between the identified CAP type and requirements posed by the given class of verbal-logical tasks.

Among students receiving average and poor grades (group B), no distinct and stable FMA was found on the background of predominantly right-hemispheric activity (Figure 2B). In this group, diverse types of individual variational curves are seen, as well as a wider range of functional states (FSs). There is significant variation in regions with increased ($K_{C/O} > 0$), as well as decreased activation, the latter reflecting an inhibited cortical FS ($K_{C/O} < 0$) (Appendix 2). Reduced mental working capacity is accompanied by predominant activity in right prefrontal areas, on the background of significantly diminished anterio-posterior AG.

Comparing exam stages IV and V—the oral response and post-exam rest (after the examiner has left)—leads to the suggestion that opponent-type functional states, as described by R. Solomon [1–3], characterize also cognitive performance during exams. This is reflected in the shifting activation indices for the left and right hemispheres, and accompanying changes in mood and feeling by FAM test (discussed below). During exam stage V, an interesting paradoxical reaction can be seen in the brain activity of highly anxious subjects: a state of defensive cortical inhibition characterizing the response period typically changes, after the examiner has left, to a relatively normal state with FMA in frontal cortical regions; at the same time, speech functions recover that had been suppressed in the student during the response period in the examiner's presence.

Below, a detailed comparison of functional brain states during key stages of the exam, I, IV and V, are shown for two most highly contrastive students (Figures 3 and 4; Table 1). The students belong to different grade groups (Figure 2): Student R. was the best among high-achievers, while student G. the poorest performer in the weaker group. Data on intra-individual and comparative time-series variation can be particularly informative given the non-Gaussian distribution of obtained within- and between group measures (Figure 2), as well as considering the marked variabilty of individual EEG indices across various stages of the exam (Figures 3 and 4).

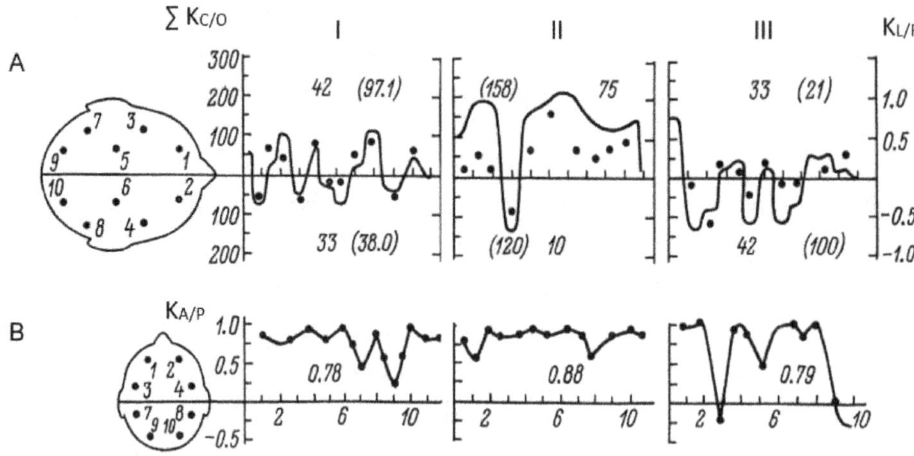

Figure 3. Examples of individual EEG dynamics during three examination stages in an excellently graded student (R.). A—diagram of the summed activation index of left and right cortical hemispheres (∑ $K_{C/O}$, left ordinate). Deviations above midline—functional predominance of left-hemispheric activity, below midline—right-hemispheric predominance; numbers above and below curves: in brackets—summed general cortical activation (∑ $K_{C/O}$), without brackets—relative activation predominance (%); isolated dots—values of inter-hemispheric asymmetry ($K_{L/R}$, right ordinate). B—magnitude of anterio-posterior non-equilibrium ($K_{A/P}$, ordinate); numbers below curves—averaged activation value; on abscissa—number of EC/EO trials (dots). I—before exam start; II—while answering the ticket; III—after exam termination (examiner has left). Differences in the scale for summed cortical activation in hemispheres (0–300) and their functional asymmetry (−1 to 1) are due to respective equations (measurement units are conditional) (Appendices 1 and 2).

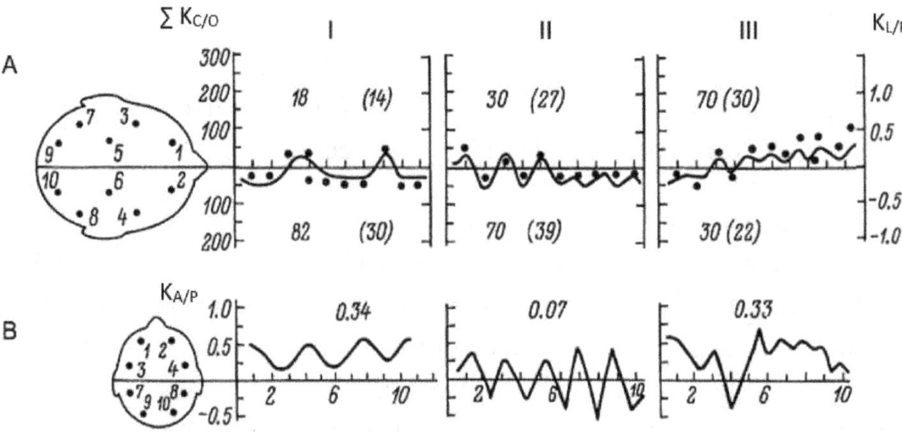

Figure 4. Examples of individual EEG dynamics during 3 examination stages in a poorly graded student (G.). Same designations as in Figure 3.

Table 1. Individual EEG, heart-rate and emotion indices of a highly-graded subject (R.) and a poorly graded subject (G.).

	Student R.			Student G.		
	I	IV	V	I	IV	V
Left hemisphere activation index	97	158	21	14	27	30
Left hemisphere dominance	42%	90%	33%	18%	30%	70%
Right hemisphere activation index	38	20	100	30	39	22
Right hemisphere dominance	33%	10%	42%	82%	70%	70%
$K_{L/R}$	0.4	0.7	−0.6	−0.3	−0.2	0.5
$K_{A/P}$	0.7	0.8	0.7	−0.3	−0.07	0.3
Heart-rate (bpm)	73	85	69	105	125	95
FAMai	6.0		4.5	2.2		5.3

Hemispheric activation indices are in conditional units (Appendix 2). I, IV, V—stage of experiment; $K_{L/R}$—bilateral asymmetry index; $K_{A/P}$—anterio-posterior asymmetry index; FAMai—FAM-test averaged scale index. Subject R. received an excellent evaluation, subject G.—poor evaluation.

Significant differences in the dynamics of cortical functional state can be seen in the representative highly-graded subject R. and poorly graded subject G. As seen on Figures 3–4, this difference is manifest already before exam onset, during the waiting stage (operative rest). This is reflected in the general level of cortical activation, which is significantly higher in student R. on the background of left-hemispheric dominance (shown as dots on Figures 3A, 4A), and the significantly higher (0.78) and more stable predominance of frontal cortical regions (Figures 3B, 4B). In student G., right-hemispheric dominance can be seen on the background of significantly reduced cortical activation and appearance on the EEG of slow hyper-synchronous delta-waves, reflecting cortical defensive inhibition already prior to exam onset. At the same time, anterio-posterior functional asymmetry is markedly diminished (0.34) due to deactivation of frontal brain regions.

These differences between students R. and G. increase during the response stage (II). In the high-achieving student R., left-hemispheric dominance is strongly amplified (with rising general activation), and the stability of frontal activity is increased. In student G., right-hemispheric dominance is retained on the background of reduced activation and instable dominance of frontal areas.

However, after exam completion, in both students rapid shifts occur in the opposite direction: in R., there is a transition to right-hemispheric dominance with a sharp drop in general cortical activation and reduced stability of frontal dominance, which can be interpreted as a reduction in neurocognitive work load. In student G., on the other hand, left-hemispheric dominance is quickly increased after the examiner has left, together with increases in inter-hemispheric functional asymmetry and frontal activation, *i.e.* cortical activation is increased.

On the example of these two students, strongly opposed intra-individual functional brain states can be seen by EEG and pulse measures when comparing stages 4 (response) and 5 (examiner's departure) (cf. Table 1 and Figure 5).

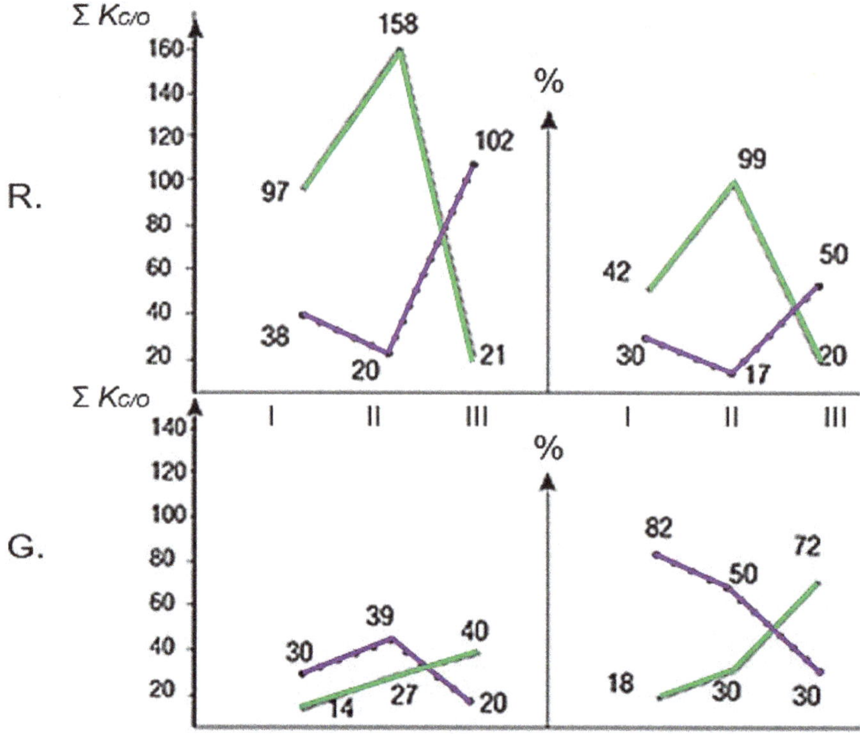

Figure 5. Prevalence of left- and right-hemispheric activation (by $K_{C/O}$) at three stages of the exam. Green—left hemisphere; purple—right hemisphere. Above—student R., excellent response. Below—student G., poor response. Abscissa: I—Initial state; II—response; III—after-effects. Left ordinate—activation sum by $K_{C/O}$ (curves in left columns); right ordinate—relative dominance of LH and RH, percentage (right columns).

Additionally, before and after the exam, we administered to all students the FAM test [41,42] on feeling, activity and mood changes (Table 1). The range of functional state (FS) shifts on this test lies on a scale from 1 to 6 points. Normal FS is considered to lie between 5.0–5.5 points; scores below 4 reflect poor FS and mood. In the high-performing group (Figure 2A), the average score prior to the exam was 5.5, and fell to 3.6 post-exam; in the unsuccessful group (Figure 2B) the average pre-exam score was 3.5, and rose to 4.9 after exam termination. In student R., the pre-exam score was 6.0 (highest in group A), but fell to 4.5 post-exam (by mood factor). In student G., the pre-exam score was 2.2 points; however, 20 minutes post-exam the score had risen to 5.3 (by mood factor) (Table 1).

Although these results are preliminary and need careful replication on larger samples, it should be noted that the corresponding changes in neural activity observed across task conditions in each group seem to confirm them. In particular, this concerns the widely reported associations of relative left frontal activation with positive emotions and approach motivation, versus the negative emotions and defensive motivation associated with right-hemispheric frontal functions [28,44–46]. This asymmetry has also been directly observed in the context of examination stress regulation [10]. In this light, let us consider the two students' indices more closely.

Student R., with low anxiety, prevalence of verbal intellect, and analytical cognitive style (by

Eysenck EPQ test), obtained an excellent grade. His initial functional state is characterized by left-hemispheric dominance, which increases during the exam response on the background of significant elevation of fronto-occipital AG and some increase in pulse rate. During this period, right-hemispheric activation decreases due to collateral inhibition from left-hemispheric dominants.

During the response, student R. shows positive emotions, apparently takes pleasure in answering the questions posed by the examiner. However, after responding, there is a clear drop in mood according to the FAM test (Table 1). At the same time, a significant reduction in left-hemispheric activation can be observed, together with increased activity and dominance of the right hemisphere, as well as diminished fronto-occipital AG, as shown in Table 1.

We can see from the above data how a clear transition takes place in student R., from a highly active physiological and cognitive state (and positive emotional experience) to an opposite functional state (accompanied by notably declined mood after the examiner has left). This is also reflected in the contrastive changes of EEG indices and pulse rate (Figure 5; Table 1).

Student G. shows high anxiety, has synthetic cognitive style, and prevalence of non-verbal intellect (by Eysenck's EPQ test). The subject knows the material, but has since school-years been afraid of exams. In the initial state, his cortical activity is reduced on the background of right-hemispheric dominance and markedly increased pulse rate (Figure 5; Table 1). Anterio-posterior AG and inter-hemispheric functional asymmetry are reduced. During the response, general cortical activation somewhat increases in the right hemisphere on the background of reduced activation and percentage of left-hemispheric activity, as well as deactivation of frontal regions (reflected in low fronto-occipital AG). However, as the examiner leaves, indices of functional brain state change contrastively—an increase is observed in left-hemispheric activation, together with increasing fronto-occipital AG on the background of collateral inhibition of the right hemisphere (Figure 5). In this case, a transition could be seen from negative emotional experience in the presence of the arousing stimuli (answering the ticket) to the appearance of a contrastive reaction—relief and satisfaction after the stressful situation has ended (as the examiner left).

A variety of methods were used to determine the emotional state of subjects. In addition to the oral response, the FAM test as well as certain behavioral characteristics and anamnesis were used. Student R., who received the excellent grade, had received during his two years of study at St.-Petersburg State University only the highest marks. Student G. did not manage to pass the exam and received a "poor"grade. During the response his speech was inhibited, and he did not seem to understand well the questions he was asked. Significant cortical deactivation was observed, and this coincided with markedly increased pulse rate (105 bpm) even before the exam, as well as during the response (125 bpm). This state can be defined as involving defensive inhibition ("functional pessimum") in the cerebral cortex on the background of simultaneous cardiac acceleration. It can be noted that this student, as well as others in the given group (Figure 2B), had frequent breakdowns during exams regardless of sufficiently good knowledge in the subjects. In all high-achieving students (Figure 2A), on the other hand, high mental productivity and composure were observed on the background of stable left frontal FMA while answering the ticket.

Apparently, the reason for CAP "dissolution" in stressful conditions is related to excessive stimulation of the cortex by the ascending activating systems. This gives rise to a flow of tonic impulses that are amplified in conditions of novelty and stress, and remain insufficiently regulated by the cortex. According to Luria's [23] and many later studies [47,48], key functions in the top-down regulation of ascending activating impulses are fulfilled by frontal cortical structures—a view supported also by Kline et al.'s [28], as well as our own findings.

Furthermore, prior to the exam we tested both subjects by the Hand [43] and POI psychological tests. In student R., we found high directiveness (13 points) and high self-actualization (40 points); in student G.—high frustration (88 points), high anxiety (44 points), and low self-actualization (6 points).

From a methodological perspective, it may be revealing to compare the above results with the findings by Dayan et al. [42], who used the FAM test and cardiac activity measures to study examination stress among high-school students enrolled in general educational classes versus differential classes (with more intensive coursework). FAM test scores demonstrated different dynamics of FS change depending on the type of class the students were enrolled in, as seen in Table 2.

Table 2. Average FAM-test scores in students of general and differential education programs.

Measurement time	Average FAM scores in general program	Average FAM scores in differential program
Regular day	5.24 ± 0.22	5.09 ± 0.19
Pre-exam	5.10 ± 0.25	4.85 ± 0.17
Post-exam	4.99 ± 0.25	4.95 ± 0.29.

FAM: Feeling, activity mood (test)

Thus, in the differential (intense coursework) class the scores were somewhat lower (4.85) than in the general class, possibly due to a sense of hightened responsibility for exam results. Higher examination stress was found in sympatotonics. However, in this study FAM scores were averaged across all students of a given class, without differentiating between highly and poorly performing subjects, as in our study. This may explain the less significant differences observed in the above summed FAM test results (Table 2). In other words, representative groups were not defined in either class by academic achievement motivation or actual progress, which may explain the differences from our findings.

Importantly, the above findings seem to indicate that processes with an opponent-type organization affect also higher cognitive functions dependent on strong motivational and emotional arousal. Of course, further similar studies including other groups of students and larger sample sizes are necessary to confirm and extend these findings. However, this should be done in representative groups (*e.g.*, highly motivated subjects), such as the reported groups of psychology students (all of whom were motivated to achieve high grades). Even then, regardless of possessing sufficient knowledge, some participants received low average or even poor grades since they were unable to concentrate, maintain composure, and cope with the stresses presented by the examination setting. In high-performing students, stable left-hemispheric dominance and strong fronto-occipital activation gradients helped to cope with the stressful situation. In low-performing students, on the other hand, no distinct left-hemispheric and frontal FMAs were observed, and this resulted in lower grades and stress-resistance in the same objective examination setting.

In sum, the above results reveal marked differences in the CAPs of successful and unsuccessful students at the exam, as reflected in the significantly higher activation of left frontal regions in high-achievers and of right frontal areas in those who failed the exam or passed it poorly. However, it should be stressed that in both groups, the characteristic CAP structure was regularly replaced by a symmetrically opposite one, with the predominant FMA periodically shifting to the right hemisphere in high-achievers, and conversely, to the left hemisphere in low-achievers, depending on particular stages of the exam. These inverse changes were combined with changes in pulse rate and the affective state of subjects, as registered by the FAM questionnaire and judged subjectively by the examiners at the exam interview. Together with available data on the contribution of prefrontal regions to the lateralization of emotions [10,22,44–46], these results suggest a key role of frontal brain regions' dominance shifts in the task-specific regulation of motivational and emotional states, including their opponent dynamics [28].

Further, the obtained results show not only the relevant role of activational asymmetries in bilateral hemispheric regions, but also in anterior and posterior brain regions, the relative dominance of which must likewise be regulated in accordance with task settings. Increases in left frontal activity in high-achievers were coupled to decreased, highly structured and stereotypical activation of posterior brain regions. On the other hand, the activation of right frontal regions in low-achievers was associated with higher, more generalized and individually varied activity in posterior cortical areas. Thus, the CAPs revealed in high-achievers were found to be relatively uniform in distribution (Figure 2) compared to low-achievers, in whom higher divergence between individual variational curves was observed, reflecting a wider range of distinct cortical functional states (Figure 2). Similar results on the higher variability of EEG indices during the exam period in low-achieving students have been reported by Wiet et al. [14].

5. Discussion

The present study has shown that in exam settings, individually specific reorganizations of CAPs can be observed in students, accompanied by corresponding shifts in their motivational-emotional and cognitive processes. In the light of the opponent process model of homeostasis, we find the indications of dynamic "super-compensatory" effects in inter-hemispheric and anterio-posterior interactions to be particularly interesting, as observed in students under high work-load and exam stress conditions (Figures 3, 4). Thus, after periods involving high activation and relative dominance of either hemisphere or prefrontal regions, these functional activation indices are typically not simply downregulated to the baseline, but show a steep decline below it, accompanied by increased activation in the opposite hemisphere, or posterior regions (Figures 3, 4), in comparison to the initial functional state. This type of super-compensatory regulation seems not to be addressed in the classical frameworks of homeostasis, although as revealed by current and earlier related studies [1,3,28,29], it may represent a phenomenon of potentially wide adaptive significance in the self-regulation of excitability in cerebral functional systems [22,28].[2] Theoretically, the opponent principle of regulation seems also consistent with current attempts to extend the classical frameworks of neural homeostasis by concepts such as anticipation and allostasis, to emphasize the inherent temporal variability and complexity of homeostatic processes in the brain [49–51].

Earlier, Craig et al. [29] investigated students' emotional dynamics during the high exam

---

[2]Interestinly, the problematic of super-compensation has a long history in Russian stress and sports physiology [87], as well as neurophysiology [25,88], although this has remained largely unknown in the West [5].

session, and found them to closely match Solomon's concept of opponent-type regulation. Our research has led to closely comparable findings. However, unlike in any prior studies, our study included integrated physiological and EEG measures, which were analyzed together with emotional and cognitive processes immediately in exam conditions, and while taking into account the various success rate of responders in high- and low-achiving groups. This is most important for distinguishing between the qualitatively different patterns of psychophysiological response expectable in subjects who not only achieve different grades, but who may experience the whole exam situation and challenge differently in terms of the motivational, stress-regulatory, and affective dynamics involved [9,52]. Indeed, in line with growing appreciation of the positive roles of stress in motivation and performance [53], Strack et al. [9] have recently shown how the stressful period immediately leading up to the exams can be experienced by some students as motivating rather than threatening or emotionally exhausting, indicating they interpret anxiety as facilitative to learning, and are less likely to appraise the exam stressor as a threat. While this ability is positively associated with academic performance, and prevents emotional exhaustion [9], it is also expectable that the opponent effects in such students would be manifestly different from those who experience the exam, or the days leading up to it, as primarily a negative and threatening stressor [9,52], with adverse health impacts [10,12].

Thus, although we have underscored the importance of differentiating between participants based on their performance to overcome such difficulties, there are further methodological and technical challenges to be addressed in this line of research. This includes, besides organizational difficulties, the relatively high diversity of motivational and emotional reactions involved in the exam situation, owing both to individual trait differences [30,54], as well as to individual expectations and experience in taking exams, the degree of preparation [55], and the subjective significance of the academic result [55,56]. For this reason, we enlisted only highly motivated and well prepared subjects in our study, and assigned them to different groups based on test scores before comparing the physiological data. Even then, besides group-averages, data on within-individual variability can be instrumental for understanding the neurocognitive structures and dynamics underlying successful and unsuccessful responses. In this way, the possible unique characteristics and strategies of responders can be characterized, together with their individual psychophysiological profile and state.

It should be noted here that most neurophysiological studies on opponent processes to date have looked at cases of pathological dysregulation, mainly addictive behavior and its underlying neurobiological circuitry, changes in which show obvious maladaptive dynamics—and probably involve pathological super-compensatory effects as described by the opponent-process model [57]. On the other hand, besides such obviously dysregulatory effects in neural substrates mediating motivational states [57], and other allostatic effects involved in pathology [49], the opponent type regulation seems to also reflect key principles underlying normal adaptation with a positive and adaptive temporal trend. For example, this has been revealed in sports and physical exercise, the accompanying motivational and affective dynamics of which seem to reveal similar biphasic fluctuations, at least under more strenuous and intense exercise leading to increased resilience and stress tolerance (*e.g.*, *via* stress-induced analgesia by endogenous opioids) [58]. Recently, this biphasic dynamics has been associated also with increased frontal asymmetry measures on a possible opponent process basis [59,60], similarly as we demonstrate here for the exam setting. Together, this may allow to hypothesize a close integration between higher cortical, emotional, and bodily stress-regulatory responses, on the basis of shared or similar opponent effects in the neural circuits mediating them.

Before turning to more general theoretical and methodological implications of our findings, it is therefore appropriate to comment on their potential applied significance. Indeed, the facts obtained in the current study reflect not only theoretical concerns, but also practical interest regarding the functional diagnostics of students' functional state in educational settings, and in particular, prior to stressful tasks such as (oral) exams. This offers the prospect of detecting "risk groups" most prone to the possible adverse health effects of such educational tasks. Given the increasing rates of anxiety and stress among college students found in recent research [61–63], and their close relation to depression and other mental health problems [63], these have become particularly urgent requirements today, and are now challenging universities to continually evaluate the mental health of students, as well as to tailor programs of prevention and treatment sensitive to their individual needs and work specifics [61,63]. Based on the dominant principle and relevant findings, we can suggest several non-invasive measures to increase the resilience of cortical functions and work dominants in easily stressed, highly anxious, and chronically tired students.

(1) In students practicing sports, symptoms of cortical over-excitation or defensive inhibition were generally not observed during exams. This allows to speak of optimal relations between intellectual, emotional, and stress-regulatory components of the exam response in physically trained subjects [6], and is in accord with numerous findings on the neurocognitive benefits of exercise [64,65], even if its relations to opponent neural dynamics require further study [58,59]. In particular, defining universal dose-response relations between excercise vigor, motivational and affective opponent effects, and health benefits has remained a difficult and largely elusive task [58]. From the present perspective, this further underscores the need to develop methods sensitive to the individual variability and specificity of such integrated physiological responses. Below, we discuss this question in more detail with respect to EEG analysis.

(2) Development of self-control through neurofeedback [66–68]. Our results have shown increased neurofeedback effectiveness if, in each individual, a most "controllable" cortical zone is selected, in which the alpha-rhythm can be most easily amplified by neurofeedback signals through visual, or other feedback channels [69]. Neurofeedback sessions are found to increase the efficiency of mental work and optimize cognitive performance on the background increased left-hemispheric dominance and fronto-occipital activation gradients [6,46], in accordance with the above reported results.

(3) The stress impact of an exam can be reduced by changing how students are engaged—*e.g.*, by allowing a written reply, additional time for preparing responses, encouraging attitudes by the examiners, etc. In anxious and neurotic subjects this creates conditions for forming a sufficiently stable frontal left FMA and is accompanied by improved quality of the exam response [6,16]. Furthermore, we have found evidence for possible personal compatibility effects in student-examiner interactions based on the similarity of their resting-state hemispheric dominance patterns [6,17]. The possible influence of such effects on a student's performance and grading should be taken into account, particularly in low-achieving students most prone to examination stress and anxiety.

Although traditionally, educational problems have been solved in the confines of humanities, the reported findings clearly indicate how a psychophysiological framework may support and enhance educational practices. This is particularly relevant for meeting special educational needs [16]. To best address these requirements, we propose that distinct types of integrative methods and concepts are needed to analyze not only inter-individual and quantitative, but also intra-individual and qualitative physiological measures of adaptation and human performance [70]. With regard to EEG analysis, this requires particular attention to the dynamic features of the EEG signal, such as its non-stationary stochastic properties [40]. While methods ignoring these complex properties have led to important discoveries, such as the functional specificity of individual EEG frequency bands, the initially rapid temporal resolution of the EEG signal is usually lost under such conditions [20,21], and makes its neurophysiological systemic interpretation more difficult. This limitation may particularly affect most dynamic experimental settings, such as those analyzed above, involving human psycho-social and socio-physiological functioning in exam conditions, or other conditions involving prolonged and conflicting motivational and stress responses.

In line with these requirements, we have presumed here that instead of individual frequency bands or correlational dependences between them, the neurophysiological units of cognitive processes should be sought in the rapidly shifting, discontinuous metastable states of the brain's biopotential field as a whole, characterized by anterio-posterior and inter-hemispheric activation gradients, as well as by global and regional changes in cortical states' inertial ("trace") properties (Appendices 1, 2). Such dynamic indices are highly variable both intra-and inter-individually, and this in close dependence on task conditions. Such methodological and methodical aspects may be fundamental if neuroscience research results are to be more directly applicable to educational settings and classroom scenarios, as currently called for [71]. Besides questions of methods and modeling, however, also ethical concerns should be further addressed in this line of research [72], including the possibilities of optimal educational and therapeutic interventions, preventive and rehabilitative measures at the individual level [16], as discussed above.

In our view, the framework of the dominant and the theory of opponent processes could provide valuable, mutually reinforcing concepts and models in this regard. These two frameworks are not only closely compatible, but both seem to possess the optimal levels of generality and complexity expected for integrative explanations and models in theoretical neuroscience [18]. Indeed, the necessity for such concepts—both sufficiently generalizable, yet well specifiable due to adequately chosen basic parameters—is becoming increasingly apparent in the field [18], together with some of the risks associated with prematurely formalizing its subject matter by methods drawn directly from other, non-biological disciplines (informatics, physics, etc.) [17,18,40,73]. These methodological considerations have played an important role in designing the current framework of EEG analysis on the basis of the dominant principle [6]. As such, it is hoped the presented materials encourage further research on the neural dynamics mediating opponent processes, and their integration into theoretical and applied human neuroscience.

Acknowledgments

The preparation of this work was supported by Charles University Grant Agency grant No. 926916. The authors wish to thank Dr. Aaro Toomela and an anonymous reviewer for comments and suggestions on an early version of this paper, and Mr. Sergey Tkachenko for his help with processing the image materials.

References

1. Solomon RL, Corbit J (1974) An opponent-process theory of motivation: I. Temporal dynamics of affect. *Psychol Rev* 81: 119–145.
2. Solomon RL (1980) The opponent-process theory of acquired motivation: The costs of pleasure and the benefits of pain. *Am Psychol* 35: 691–712.
3. Solomon RL (1991) Acquired motivation and affective opponent-processes. In: B M. J (ed.), *Neurobiology of Learning, Emotion, and Affect*. New York: Raven Press Ltd., 307–347.
4. Ukhtomsky AA (1966) *The Dominant*, Leningrad: Leningrad State University.
5. Nadin M (Ed.) (2015) *Anticipation: Learning from the Past.* Cham: Springer International Publishing, 13–150.
6. Pavlova LP (2017) *Dominants of the Working Brain: A Systemic Psychophysiological Approach to EEG Analysis*, St.-Petersburg: Inform-Navigator.
7. AlShorman O, Ali T, Irfan M (2017) EEG Analysis for Pre-learning Stress in the Brain. In: *Asian Simulation Conference*. Springer, Singapore, 447–455.
8. Robotham D, Julian C (2006) Stress and the higher education student: a critical review of the literature. *J Furth High Educ* 30: 107–117.
9. Strack J, Esteves F (2015) Exams? Why worry? Interpreting anxiety as facilitative and stress appraisals. *Anxiety Stress Coping* 28: 205–214.
10. Lewis RS, Weekes NY, Wang TH (2007) The effect of a naturalistic stressor on frontal EEG asymmetry, stress, and health. *Biol Psychol* 75: 239–247.
11. Jena SK (2015) Examination stress and its effect on EEG. *Int J Med Sci Pub Health* 11: 1493–1497.
12. Weekes N, Lewis R, Patel F, et al. (2006) Examination stress as an ecological inducer of cortisol and psychological responses to stress in undergraduate students. *Stress* 9: 199–206.
13. Hewig, J., Schlotz, W., Gerhards, F., et al. (2008) Associations of the cortisol awakening response (CAR) with cortical activation asymmetry during the course of an exam stress period. *Psychoneuroendocrinology* 33: 83–91.
14. Wiet SG, Goldstein L (1979) Successful and unsuccessful university students: Quantitative hemispheric EEG differences. *Biological Psychology* 8: 273–284.
15. Spangler, G., Pekrun, R., Kramer, K., et al. (2002) Students' emotions, physiological reactions, and coping in academic exams. *Anxiety Stress Coping* 15: 413–432.
16. Pavlova LP (2015) Individuality of brain dominants as a problem of special education and pedagogy. In: Nadin, M. (ed.) *Anticipation: Learning from the Past*, Cham: Springer International Publishing, 471–491.
17. Pavlova LP, Romanenko AF (1988) *A Systemic Approach to Psychophysiology of the Human Brain*, Leningrad: Nauka, 1988.
18. Kotchoubey B, Tretter F, Braun HA (2016) Methodological problems on the way to integrative human neuroscience. *Front Integr Neurosci* 10: 1–19.
19. Krakauer, JW, Ghazanfar AA, Gomez-Marin A., et al. (2017) Neuroscience needs behavior: correcting a reductionist Bias. *Neuron* 93: 480–490.
20. Fingelkurts AA, Fingelkurts AA (2010) Short-term EEG spectral pattern as a single event in EEG phenomenology. *Open Neuroimaging J* 4: 130–156.

21. Fingelkurts AA, Fingelkurts AA (2015) Operational architectonics methodology for EEG analysis: theory and results. In: Sakkalis V (ed.), *Modern Electroencephalographic Assessment Techniques: Theory and Applications,* New York: Humana Press, 1–59.
22. Comer CS, Harrison PK, Harrison DW (2015) The dynamic opponent relativity model: an integration and extension of capacity theory and existing theoretical perspectives on the neuropsychology of arousal and emotion. *SpringerPlus* 4: 345–366.
23. Luria AR (1980) *Higher Cortical Functions in Man,* New York: Basic Books.
24. Rusinov VS (1973) *The Dominant Focus: Electrophysiological Investigations*, New York: Springer Science & Business Media.
25. Kurismaa A (2015) Perspectives on Time and Anticipation in the Theory of Dominance, In: Nadin, M. (ed.), *Anticipation: Learning from the Past*, Cham: Springer International Publishing, 37–57.
26. Kositskiy GI, Smirnov VM (1972) *The Nervous System and Stress. The principle of Dominance in Pathology (Effect of Nonspecific Stimuli on Inhibition of Pathological Processes)*, Washington: National Aeronautics and Space Administration; Springfield, Va.
27. Kurismaa A, Pavlova LP (2016) The Dominant as a Model of Chronogenic Change: The Relevance of AA Ukhtomsky's and LS Vygotsky's Traditions for Systemic Cognitive Studies. In Krempe SR, Smith R (eds.), *Centrality of History for Theory Construction in Psychology,* Germany:Springer International Publishing, 125–149.
28. Kline JP, Blackhart GC, Williams WC (2007) Anterior EEG asymmetries and opponent process theory. *Int J Psychophysiol* 63: 302–307.
29. Craig RL, Siegel PS (1979) Does negative affect beget positive affect? A test of the opponent-process theory. *Bull Psycho Soc* 14: 404–406.
30. Spangler G (1997) Psychological and physiological responses during an exam and their relation to personality characteristics. *Psychoneuroendocrinology* 22: 423–441.
31. Chanel G (2009) Emotion Assessment for Affective Computing Based on Brain and Peripheral Signals. Doctoral dissertation, Geneva: University of Geneva., 2009.
32. Ilin YP (1975) "Operational calm" and the optimum regulation of human working capacity, In *Essays on the Psychology of Operator Labor*, Washington, D.C: National Aeronautics and Space Administration, 226–251.
33. Jensen O, Mazaheri A (2010) Shaping functional architecture by oscillatory alpha activity: gating by inhibition. *Fron Hum Neurosci* 4: 1–8.
34. Klimesch W (2012) Alpha-band oscillations, attention, and controlled access to stored information, *Trends Cognit Sci* 16: 606–617.
35. Hanslmayr S, Staudigl T, Fellner MC (2012) Oscillatory power decreases and long-term memory: the information via desynchronization hypothesis. *Front Hum Neurosci* 6: 1–12.
36. Supp GG, Siegel M, Hipp JF, et al. (2011) Cortical hypersynchrony predicts breakdown of sensory processing during loss of consciousness. *Curr Biol* 21: 1988–1993.
37. Pfurtscheller G, da Silva FHL (1999) Event-related EEG/MEG synchronization and desynchronization: basic principles. *Clin Neurophysiol* 110: 1842–1857.
38. Neuper C, Pfurtscheller G (2001) Event-related dynamics of cortical rhythms: frequency-specific features and functional correlates. *Int J Psychophysiol* 43: 41–58.
39. Neuper C, Wörtz M, Pfurtscheller G (2006) ERD/ERS patterns reflecting sensorimotor activation and deactivation. *Prog Brain Res* 159: 211–222.

40. Sergeev GA, Pavlova LP, Romanenko AF (1968) *Statistical Methods for Human Electroencephalogram Analysis*, Leningrad: Nauka.
41. Doskin VA, Lavrent'eva NA, Strongina OM, et al. (1975) “SAN” psychological test applicable to studies in the field of work physiology. *Gig Tr Prof Zabol* 28–32.
42. Dayan AV, Ogannisyan AO, Gevorkyan ES, et al. (2003) Reaction of cardiac activity of senior pupils of schools providing differentiated education upon examination stress. *Hum Physiol* 29: 160–165.
43. Wagner EE (1983) *The Hand Test: Manual*, Los Angeles: Western Psychological Services.
44. Demaree HA, Everhart DE, Youngstrom EA, et al. (2005) Brain lateralization of emotional processing: historical roots and a future incorporating “dominance”. *Behav Cognit Neurosci Rev* 4: 3–20.
45. Davidson RJ (2004) What does the prefrontal cortex “do” in affect: perspectives on frontal EEG asymmetry research. *Biol Psychol* 67: 219–234.
46. Kelley NJ, Hortensius R, Schutter DJ, et al. (2017) The relationship of approach/avoidance motivation and asymmetric frontal cortical activity: A review of studies manipulating frontal asymmetry. *Int J Psychophysiol* 119: 19–30.
47. Groenewegen HJ, Uylings HB (2000) The prefrontal cortex and the integration of sensory, limbic and autonomic information. *Prog Brain Res* 126: 3–28.
48. Sarter M, Givens B, Bruno JP (2001) The cognitive neuroscience of sustained attention: where top-down meets bottom-up. *Brain Res Rev* 35: 146–160.
49. Schulkin J (2004) *Allostasis, Homeostasis, and the Costs of Physiological Adaptation*, Cambridge: Cambridge University Press.
50. Sterling P (2012) Allostasis: a model of predictive regulation. *Physiol Behav* 106: 5–15.
51. Schulkin J (2003) Allostasis: a neural behavioral perspective. *Horm Behav* 43: 21–27.
52. Strack J, Lopes PN, Esteves F (2015) Will you thrive under pressure or burn out? Linking anxiety motivation and emotional exhaustion. *Cognition Emotion* 29: 578–591.
53. McGonigal K (2016) *The Upside of Stress: Why Stress is Good for You, and How to Get Good at it*. New York: Penguin.
54. Gilbert DG, Stunkard ME, Jensen RA, et al. (1996) Effects of exam stress on mood, cortisol, and immune functioning: Influences of neuroticism and smoker-non-smoker status. *Personal Individ Differences* 21: 235–246.
55. Mega C, Ronconi L, De Beni R (2014) What makes a good student? How emotions, self-regulated learning, and motivation contribute to academic achievement. *J Edu Psychol* 106: 121.
56. Pekrun R, Goetz T, Titz W, et al. (2002) Academic emotions in students' self-regulated learning and achievement: A program of qualitative and quantitative research. *Edu Psychol* 37: 91–105.
57. Koob GF, Le Moal M (2004) Drug addiction and allostasis. *Allostasis, Homeostasis, and the Costs Physiolog Adaptation*: 150–163.
58. Ekkekakis P, Hall EE, Petruzzello SJ (2005). Variation and homogeneity in affective responses to physical activity of varying intensities: an alternative perspective on dose–response based on evolutionary considerations. *J Sports Sci* 23: 477–500.
59. Woo M, Kim S, Kim J, et al. (2010) The influence of exercise intensity on frontal electroencephalographic asymmetry and self-reported affect. *Res Q Exerc Sport* 81: 349–359.
60. Woo M, Kim S, Kim J, et al. (2009) Examining the exercise-affect dose–response relationship:

Does duration influence frontal EEG asymmetry? *Int J Psychophysiol* 72: 166–172.

61. Regehr C, Glancy D, Pitts A (2013) Interventions to reduce stress in university students: A review and meta-analysis. *J Affec Disord* 148: 1–11.
62. Flatt AK (2013) A Suffering Generation: Six Factors Contributing to the Mental Health Crisis in North American Higher Education. *Coll Q* 16: 1–17.
63. Beiter R, Nash R, McCrady M, et al. (2015) The prevalence and correlates of depression, anxiety, and stress in a sample of college students. *J Affect Disord* 173: 90–96.
64. Loprinzi PD, Herod SM, Cardinal BJ (2013) Physical activity and the brain: a review of this dynamic, bi-directional relationship. *Brain Res* 1539: 95–104.
65. Heijnen S, Hommel B, Kibele A, et al. (2016) Neuromodulation of aerobic exercise—a review. *Front Psychol* 6: 1890-1896.
66. Hanslmayr S, Sauseng P, Doppelmayr M (2005) Increasing individual upper alpha power by neurofeedback improves cognitive performance in human subjects. *Appl Psychophysiol Biofeedback* 30: 1–10.
67. Gruzelier JH (2014) EEG-neurofeedback for optimising performance: A review of cognitive and affective outcome in healthy participants. *Neurosci Biobehav Revi* 44: 124–141.
68. Ratanasiripong P, Sverduk K, Prince J, et al. (2012) Biofeedback and counseling for stress and anxiety among college students. *J Coll Stud Dev* 53: 742–749.
69. Astafurov VI, Pavlova LP (1981) Some features of alpha-activity self-control through visual feedback. *All-Russian Inst Sci Tech Inf:* 4214–4281.
70. Molenaar PC (2007) Psychological methodology will change profoundly due to the necessity to focus on intra-individual variation. *Integrative Psychol Behav Sci* 41: 35–40.
71. de Jong T, Van Gog T, Jenks K, et al. (2009) *Explorations in Learning and the Brain: On the Potential of Cognitive Neuroscience for Educational Science*. New York: Springer Science & Business Media.
72. Stein Z, Fischer KW (2011) Directions for mind, brain, and education: Methods, models, and morality. *Edu Philos Theory* 43: 56–66.
73. de-Wit L, Alexander D, Ekroll V, et al. (2016) Is neuroimaging measuring information in the brain? *Psychon Bull Rev* 23: 1415–1429.
74. Barry RJ, Clarke AR, Johnstone SJ (2007) EEG differences between eyes-closed and eyes-open resting conditions. *Clin Neurophysiol* 118: 2765–2773.
75. Whitham EM, Pope KJ, Fitzgibbon SP (2007) Scalp electrical recording during paralysis: quantitative evidence that EEG frequencies above 20Hz are contaminated by EMG. *Clin Neurophysiol* 118: 1877–1888.
76. Corning HK (1946) *Lehrbuch der Topographischen Anatomie*. Berlin Heidelberg: Springer.
77. Mattson MP, Calabrese EJ (2014) *Hormesis. A Revolution in Biology, Toxicology and Medicine.* The United States: Humana Press.
78. Nasonov DN (1962) *Local Reaction of Protoplasm and Gradual Excitation.* Washington D.C: National Science Foundation.
79. Matveev VV (2005) Protoreaction of protoplasm. *Cell Mol Biol* 51: 715–723.
80. Agutter PS (2007) Cell mechanics and stress: from molecular details to the 'universal cell reaction' and hormesis. *BioEssays* 29: 324–333.
81. Agutter PS (2008) Elucidating the mechanism (s) of hormesis at the cellular level: the universal cell response. *Am J Pharmacol Toxicol* 3: 100–110.

82. Mattson MP (2008) Awareness of hormesis will enhance future research in basic and applied neuroscience. *Crit Rev Toxicol* 38: 633–639.
83. Calabrese EJ (2008) Neuroscience and hormesis: overview and general findings. *Crit Rev Toxicol* 38: 249–252.
84. Daw ND, Kakade S, Dayan P (2002) Opponent interactions between serotonin and dopamine. *Neural Networks* 15: 603–616.
85. Boureau YL, Dayan P (2011) Opponency revisited: competition and cooperation between dopamine and serotonin. *Neuropsychopharmacology* 36: 74–97.
86. Tsitolovsky LE (2015) Endogenous Generation of Goals and Homeostasis. In: *Anticipation: Learning from the Past* , Cham: Springer International Publishing, 175–191.
87. Viru A (2002) Early contributions of Russian stress and exercise physiologists. *J Appl Physiol* 92: 1378–1382.
88. Pavlova LP (2015) Work capacity and anticipation in AA Ukhtomsky's concept of dominance. *Int J General Syst* 44: 667–685.

3

Vascular biomarkers and ApoE4 expression in mild cognitive impairment and Alzheimer's disease

Diana C. Oviedo[1], Hector Lezcano[2], Ambar R. Perez[1,3], Alcibiades E. Villarreal[3], Maria B. Carreira[3], Baltasar Isaza[4], Lavinia Wesley[4], Shantal A. Grajales[3], Sara Fernandez[5], Ana Frank[6] and Gabrielle B. Britton[3,*]

[1] Universidad Católica Santa María La Antigua (USMA), Panamá
[2] Facultad de Medicina, Universidad de Panamá, Panamá
[3] Centro de Neurociencias y Unidad de Investigación Clínica, Instituto de Investigaciones Científicas y Servicios de Alta Tecnología (INDICASAT AIP), Panamá
[4] Servicio de Radiología, Complejo Hospitalario Arnulfo Arias Madrid, Caja del Seguro Social, Panamá
[5] Departmento de Psicología Básica II (Procesos Cognitivos), Facultad de Psicología, Universidad Complutense de Madrid, Madrid, España
[6] Servicio de Neurología, Hospital Universitario La Paz, Madrid, España

* **Correspondence:** Email: gbritton@indicasat.org.pa;

Abstract: Vascular pathology and genetic markers such as apolipoprotein E allele ε4 (ApoE ε4) are risk factors for the progression from mild cognitive impairment (MCI) to Alzheimer's disease (AD). In Panama, a high prevalence of vascular risk factors and an increase in the aging population, generate the need to investigate biomarkers using specific, sensitive, non-invasive and cost-efficient methods that could be used in primary care. The main objective of this study was to explore the association between vascular biomarkers such as intima-media thickness (IMT) and stenosis, ApoE ε4 and cognitive function in a sample of older adults, including healthy controls (n = 41), MCI (n = 33), and AD (n = 12). A descriptive and cross-sectional study was conducted. Participants were part of the Panama Aging Research Initiative (PARI), the first prospective study in aging in Panama. Assessments included a neuropsychological battery, ApoE ε4 genotyping and a Doppler ultrasound of the left carotid artery to examine the presence of vascular risk factors. Neuropsychological tests were combined to form six cognitive domains: Global cognition, language, visuospatial abilities, learning and memory, attention and executive functions. Multivariable analyses (using age, education, and ApoE ε4 expression as covariates) were conducted. Participants with increased IMT showed poorer performance in memory and those with carotid stenosis showed poorer performance in language, visuospatial abilities and attention, independent of age, education or ApoE ε4 expression. The results support the use of vascular markers in cognitive assessments of aged individuals.

Keywords: aging; cognition; atherosclerosis; intima-media thickness; stenosis; Latin America; Panama

---

Abbreviations: AD: Alzheimer's disease; ANCOVA: Analysis of Covariance; ANOVA: One-way Analysis of Variance; ApoE ε4: Apolipoprotein E ε4 allele; BMI: Body Mass Index; CSS: Social Security of Panama; EQ-5D-3L: Subjective Health Statuses; FAQ: Functional Activity Questionnaire; GDetS: Global Deterioration Scale; GDS-30: Geriatric Depression Scale; IMT: Intima-media thickness; LAC: Latin America and Caribbean; MANCOVA: Multivariable Analyses of Covariance; MCI: Mild Cognitive Impairment; MMSE: Mini Mental State Examination; NC: Normal Control; PARI: Panama Aging Research Initiative; PSV: Peak Systolic Velocity

1. Introduction

Multiple reports indicate that individuals over 60 years old are the fastest growing group on earth [1]. A reduced mortality rate and the advances in medicine in the last decades have resulted in an increase in life expectancy and in the elderly population [2]. As people age they are more likely to develop chronic diseases such as mild cognitive impairment (MCI) and Alzheimer's disease (AD) [3]. The Latin American and Caribbean (LAC) region is experiencing one of the fastest aging rates [4], and as a result the prevalence of dementia and MCI has increased causing economic, social and public health burdens. Therefore, one of the main objectives in AD research is to identify and study risk factors that could contribute to the discovery of specific, sensitive, non-invasive and cost-efficient methods that could be used in primary care for early detection of AD.

Numerous studies have shown that vascular pathologies such as cardiovascular disease are risk factors for AD and MCI [5,6]. Carotid atherosclerosis is a chronic inflammatory disorder characterized by the accumulation of plaques in the walls of large and medium arteries [7,8]. Atherosclerosis is a risk factor for cerebrovascular diseases such as stroke, silent brain micro infarcts and brain hemorrhages, causing white matter lesions, neural dysfunction and cognitive impairment [9,10].

During the process of aging, arteries undergo changes such as thickening of the intima-media and changes in the size and thickness of veins and arteries. The intima refers to the internal portion of the artery formed by an endothelium. The media or middle tunic is the middle layer of the artery. The distance between the intima and the media is known as the intima-media thickness (IMT) [11]. Several authors have reported associations between vascular risk factors such as IMT and stenosis and deficits in cognitive functions, although results have been inconsistent. An increased IMT can lead to a poor performance in memory and other cognitive functions such as language, attention, executive functions and psychomotor abilities [12–14]. However, other studies have not found such associations [15,16]. Therefore, the evaluation of these vascular markers can be a crucial step in identifying elderly individuals at risk of developing cognitive impairment.

Among genetic risk factors, apolipoprotein E ε4 (ApoE ε4) has been shown to be the strongest risk factor for AD [17,18]. ApoE ε4 expression increases the risk of developing dementia three to ten times [19]. ApoE ε4 and increased IMT have also been associated with cardiovascular disease [20]. Studies have shown that individuals with at least one copy of ApoE ε4 have a higher prevalence of cortical microinfarcts, atherosclerotic pathology, hemorrhages, thrombosis, cerebral amyloid angiopathy, cerebrovascular ischemia, pulsatility, hypertension, diabetes, among others [21]. In addition, ApoE ε4 is associated with an altered mechanism of cerebral circulation in older adults [22]. Evidence has stated that ApoE ε4 and vascular risk factors combined aggravate cognitive impairment [21] and their assessment can help in the understanding of the progression of MCI to AD [12].

To date, there are numerous studies focusing on the risk factors associated with cerebrovascular health and cognition in the elderly population, nevertheless most of this research has been carried out in developed countries. In the LAC region, the prevalence of vascular chronic diseases is increasing [23,24]. In Panamá, prevalence studies have shown that cardiovascular diseases are the leading cause of death [25]. To our knowledge, there are no studies that focus on the relationship between vascular pathologies, ApoE ε4 and cognitive impairment in LAC countries. In the present study, we examined the association between carotid IMT and stenosis, ApoE ε4 and cognitive function in a sample of elderly adults in Panama. Based on evidence from previous studies, we expected that vascular risk factors and ApoE ε4 would influence performance in specific cognitive domains.

2. Methods

2.1. Participants

Data were analyzed from 86 participants of the Panama Aging Research Initiative (PARI) cohort [26,27]. Volunteers were recruited from the outpatient geriatric services of the Social Security (CSS), the largest public hospital located in Panama City. Inclusion criteria encompassed being 65 years or older, having received the baseline cognitive assessment, willingness to participate in the follow-up visit and having signed the informed consent. Exclusion criteria consisted of any medical condition that interfered with the person's ability to attend the evaluation, illiteracy and participation in an ongoing clinical study at the time of enrollment. The protocol was approved by the Bioethics Committee of the CSS. Participants who were eligible for the study were explained the purpose of the study, the procedure, what was expected from them and then signed informed consent forms. Confidentiality was not breached in accordance with the principles of the Declaration of Helsinki (1964).

Participants underwent a standardized assessment protocol that included an interview to obtain information on sociodemographic characteristics, medical history, functional status and risk factors. A subsample of individuals (n = 70) underwent Doppler sonography to estimate the presence of vascular risk factors. A non-fasting blood sample was obtained to genotype for ApoE ε4. Interviews and evaluations were conducted in Spanish and reviewed by physicians, medical students and graduate students. Clinical data, medical records and imaging were examined by experienced clinicians. Approximately 17 months (M = 16.8 months, SD = 3.4) after baseline assessments participants underwent a follow-up interview, cognitive testing and assessment of functional status, subjective health status and presence of depressive symptoms. Interviews and neuropsychological evaluations were completed in a single visit (1.5–2 hours) and were conducted in Spanish by students and neuropsychologists.

2.2. *Variables and measurements*

2.2.1. Clinical and neuropsychological assessment

The neuropsychological test battery included measures of six cognitive domains: 1) global cognition (Mini-Mental State Examination, MMSE) [28]; 2) attention (Digit Span forward [29] and Trail Making Test part A [30]); 3) executive function (Trail Making Test part B [30] and Digit Span Backward [29]); 4) memory (10 word free recall immediate and delayed list [31]); 5) language (Boston Naming [32] and Semantic Verbal Fluency [33]); and 6) visuospatial abilities (Clock Drawing copy version [34] and Poppelreuter Test [35]). Basic and instrumental activities of daily living were assessed with the Lawton and Brody Instrumental Activities of Daily Living Scale [36] and Functional Activities Questionnaire (FAQ) [37]. Depression was assessed with the Spanish version of the 30-item Geriatric Depression Scale (GDS-30) [38], and health subjective status was evaluated using the European Quality of Life EuroQol Health Questionnaire (EGQ-5D-3L) [39]. Stages of cognitive function were rated according to the Global Deterioration Scale (GDetS) [40]. All information was reviewed by a consensus committee who diagnosed participants with AD, MCI or no cognitive impairment (normal controls; NC). Participants were included as controls if they performed within normal limits in the neuropsychological assessment and scored ≤ 10 in the GDS-30 (below the threshold for symptoms of depression). MCI diagnosis was based on core clinical criteria [41] and required deficits in at least one cognitive domain, independence in activities of daily living and a rating of GDetS ≤ 3. Diagnosis of AD was based on NINCDS-ADRDA [42] criteria and required evidence of impairments in memory and at least one other cognitive domain, impairments in everyday social and/or work-related activities, and a GDetS score of four or higher (range 1–7).

2.2.2. ApoE ε4 genotyping

For ApoE genotyping, DNA samples were obtained from whole blood leukocytes (EDTA plasma collection tubes) using QIAmp DNA Mini Kit (Qiagen) according to manufacturer recommendations. ApoE genotyping was conducted according to standardized PCR procedures [43].

2.2.3. Ultrasound assessment of carotid IMT and stenosis

High resolution B-mode ultrasonography (LOGIQ e GE Medical Systems, China) with 7.5 MHz high frequency linear transducer was used to measure the volume and speed of blood flow and IMT and stenosis in the left carotid artery. The exam was conducted while the participant was lying in a supine position with the head slightly rotated to 45° from the examiner, first from a cross-sectional view, starting from the base of the neck up to the bifurcation in the internal carotid and external carotid arteries. IMT was measured at the level of the distal portion of the left common carotid artery and was defined as the distance (in millimeters) between the leading edges of the lumen-intima and media-adventitia interfaces of the arterial wall. A cut-off value of 0.9 mm was considered abnormal thickening [44]. In addition, blood flow velocities and the presence of atheromatous plaques were evaluated. Carotid artery stenosis was determined using values of the peak systolic velocity (PSV) as follows: (1) normal when PSV < 125 cm/s without visible plaque or intimal thickening; (2) < 50% stenosis when PSV < 125 cm/s and visible plaque or intimal thickening; (3) 50–69% stenosis when

PSV 125–230 cm/s and visible plaque; (4) ≥ 70% stenosis to near occlusion when PSV > 230 cm/s and visible plaque and lumen narrowing are seen; (5) near occlusion when there was a markedly narrowed lumen; and (6) total occlusion when there was no detectable lumen [45]. Values were then dichotomized into absence (normal) or presence of stenosis (all other values).

2.3. Statistical analysis

Analyses were performed using SPSS 21.0 (Armonk, NY: IBM Corp). First, demographic and clinical characteristics were examined using descriptive statistics. Univariable one-way analysis of variance (ANOVA) and chi square (X^2) tests were applied to continuous and categorical variables, respectively, and post hoc comparisons were conducted with Bonferroni tests. Neuropsychological test scores were converted to z scores, then summed and averaged to calculate an average z score in six cognitive domains: Global cognition, language, visuospatial, memory, executive function and attention. Cognitive performance between groups was compared using analysis of covariance (ANCOVA) and using age, education and ApoE ε4 expression as covariates. Values of $p < 0.05$ were considered statistically significant.

Separate multivariable analyses of covariance (MANCOVA) were conducted in order to establish the influence of vascular risk factors and ApoE ε4 on cognitive performance across diagnostic groups. Covariates included age, education and ApoE ε4 expression.

3. Results

3.1. Sample characteristics

Diagnostic groups did not differ in sex, education, depressive symptoms, subjective health status, stenosis or ApoE ε4 expression (Table 1). The percentage of the AD group with IMT ≥ 0.9 mm was greater than the control and MCI groups, and the MCI group also differed from controls. As expected, groups differed in performance across all cognitive domains, independent of age, education and ApoE ε4 expression, although MANCOVA revealed greater deficits in global cognition in the AD group in the presence of ApoE ε4.

3.2. Association between IMT, stenosis, ApoE ε4, and cognitive performance

Tables 2 and 3 summarize the results of 2 × 3 MANCOVAs combining diagnostic groups and vascular markers. There was no significant interaction between diagnostic groups and IMT (Table 2) or stenosis (Table 3). Therefore, IMT groups were examined independent of diagnosis. This analysis showed that IMT values equal to or greater than 0.9 mm were associated with a lower performance in the learning and memory domain [$F(1,65) = 9.03$, $p = 0.004$] independent of age, education and ApoE ε4 expression (Table 4). Also, there was a tendency for poorer performance in the language and visuospatial domains ($ps < 0.07$). When participants were divided into those with and without stenosis (Table 5), stenosis was significantly associated with language [$F(1,65) = 12.81$, $p = 0.001$], visuospatial [$F(1,65) = 7.72$, $p = 0.007$], memory [$F(1,65) = 11.24$, $p = 0.001$], and attention [$F(1,65) = 5.08$, $p = 0.028$] deficits.

Table 1. Demographic characteristics

	Normal control ($n = 41$)	MCI ($n = 33$)	AD ($n = 12$)	*Test statistic*	p
Years of Study	10.7 (4.9)	9.5 (4.0)	7.9 (4.4)	$F(2,83) = 2.0$	0.141
Age	76.6 (5.6)	79.2 (7.8)	82.4 (7.9)[a]	$F(2,83) = 3.0$	0.030
% female sex	31 (75.6%)	21 (63.6%)	10 (83.3%)	$\chi^2 (2) = 2.2$	0.336
BMI	26.3 (4.9)	24.1 (4.4)	23.3 (6.1)	$F(2,83) = 2.6$	0.080
EQ-5D-3L	76.6 (18.6)	70.9 (22.7)	80.5 (17.1)	$F(2,82) = 1.2$	0.303
FAQ	1.2 (2.7)[b]	2.1 (2.7)	18.3 (6.6)[a]	$F(2,83) = 12.4$	0.000
Functionality Index	0.9 (0.2)[b]	0.9 (0.1)	0.4 (0.2)[a]	$F(2,83) = 78.7$	0.000
GDetS	1.5 (0.6)[b]	2.5 (0.5)[a]	4.9 (0.9)[a]	$F(2,83) = 9.5$	0.000
GDS-30	5.6 (4.9)	7.5 (5.2)	9.3 (5.9)	$F(2,83) = 2.7$	0.071
% IMT ≥ 0.9 mm	11/32 (34.4%)	15/27 (55.6%)	9/11 (81.8%)	$\chi (2) = 7.9$	0.019
% Stenosis	8/32 (25.0%)	11/27 (40.7%)	7/11 (63.6%)	$\chi (2) = 5.5$	0.065
ApoE ε4	9/40 (22.5%)	11/32 (34.4%)	6/12 (50.0%)	$\chi (2) = 3.6$	0.170
Global Cognition	0.5 (0.4)	0.2 (0.5)	−1.2 (1.3)[a b]	$F(2,77) = 25.7$	0.000
Language	0.4 (0.5)[b]	0.04 (0.7)	−1.0 (0.8)[a b]	$F(2,77) = 18.4$	0.000
Visuospatial	0.4 (0.3)	0.1 (0.5)	−1.1 (1.4)[a b]	$F(2,77) = 18.5$	0.000
Memory	0.6 (0.6)[b]	−0.3 (0.5)	−0.9 (0.7)[a b]	$F(2,77) = 32.0$	0.000
Attention	0.3 (0.5)[b]	−0.07 (0.6)	−0.7 (0.8)[a b]	$F(2,77) = 8.0$	0.001
Executive Function	0.4 (0.6)[b]	−0.2 (0.7)	−0.4 (0.4)[a]	$F(2,77) = 7.5$	0.001

Functionality Index: Number of activities on which the participant was independent divided by the total number of activities assessed; ApoE ε4: % ApoE with at least one copy of ε4 allele. Control, MCI and AD groups were compared using ANOVA for continuous variables and Pearson chi-square for categorical variables. ANOVA post hoc comparisons were conducted with Bonferroni tests. $p < 0.05$ was considered statistically significant. [a]Statistically different from control group. [b]Statistically different from MCI group. This table also describes the ANCOVA comparing z-scores for each cognitive domain between control, MCI and AD groups, controlling for age, education and ApoE4. The comparison was considered significant when $p < 0.05$.

Table 2. Association between IMT and diagnostic groups for each cognitive domain

Cognitive Domains	NC ($n = 32$)		MCI ($n = 27$)		AD ($n = 11$)		$F(2,61)$	p	η_p^2
	< 0.9 IMT	≥ 0.9 IMT	< 0.9 IMT	≥ 0.9 IMT	< 0.9 IMT	≥0.9 IMT			
Global Cognition	0.6 (0.2)	0.4 (0.4)	0.1 (0.4)	0.2 (0.6)	−1.1 (2.7)	−1.4 (1.2)	0.5	0.594	0.02
Language	0.5 (0.4)	0.5 (0.7)	0.1 (0.8)	−0.1 (0.6)	−0.6 (0.5)	−1.2 (0.8)	0.2	0.794	0.01
Visuospatial	0.4 (0.2)	0.4 (0.3)	0.2 (0.5)	0.04 (0.6)	−0.3 (1.2)	−1.5 (1.4)	1.9	0.148	0.06
Memory	0.9 (0.5)	0.2 (0.5)	−0.1 (0.6)	−0.3 (0.6)	−0.9 (0.1)	−0.9 (0.8)	1.3	0.273	0.04
Attention	0.4 (0.5)	0.3 (0.6)	−0.1 (0.5)	−0.2 (0.6)	−0.9 (0.2)	0.9 (0.8)	0.2	0.822	0.01
Executive Function	−0.4 (0.5)	−0.5 (0.6)	−0.5 (0.6)	−0.1 (0.6)	−0.8 (0.6)	−0.4 (0.3)	0.4	0.692	0.01

This table summarizes the average z scores for each cognitive domain. Statistics describe the MANCOVA comparing group IMT < 0.9 and IMT ≥ 0.9 within each diagnostic group for each cognitive domain, controlling for age, education and ApoE4. MANCOVA post hoc comparisons were conducted with Bonferroni tests. $p < 0.05$ was considered statistically significant.

Table 3. Association between stenosis and diagnostic groups for each cognitive domain

Cognitive Domains	NC ($n = 32$)		MCI ($n = 27$)		AD ($n = 11$)		$F(2,61)$	p	η_p^2
	No stenosis	Stenosis	No stenosis	Stenosis	No stenosis	Stenosis			
Global cognition	0.6 (0.3)	0.4 (0.4)	0.1 (0.5)	0.2 (0.5)	−1.4 (1.6)	−1.3 (1.3)	0.3	0.715	0.01
Language	0.6 (0.4)	0.4 (0.8)	0.1 (0.6)	−0.2 (0.7)	−0.9 (0.6)	−1.1 (0.9)	0.2	0.829	0.01
Visuospatial	0.4 (0.2)	0.4 (0.3)	0.2 (0.5)	0.02 (0.6)	−0.7 (0.9)	−1.6 (1.6)	2.5	0.094	0.08
Memory	0.8 (0.5)	0.2 (0.6)	−0.1 (0.6)	−0.5 (0.5)	−0.9 (0.1)	−0.9 (0.9)	0.9	0.400	0.03
Attention	0.3 (0.5)	0.5 (0.6)	−0.01 (0.6)	−0.4 (0.5)	−0.8 (0.1)	−0.9 (0.9)	1.0	0.371	0.03
Executive Function	0.4 (0.6)	0.6 (0.4)	0.3 (0.7)	−0.3 (0.6)	−0.6 (0.4)	−0.4 (0.3)	0.1	0.932	0.00

This table summarizes the average z scores for each cognitive domain. Statistics describe the MANCOVA comparing the group with no stenosis and with stenosis within each diagnostic group for each cognitive domain, controlling for age, education and ApoE4. MANCOVA post hoc comparisons were conducted with Bonferroni tests. $p < 0.05$ was considered statistically significant.

Table 4. Association between IMT and cognitive domains

Cognitive Domains	< 0.9 IMT (n = 35)	≥ 0.9 IMT (n = 35)	$F(1,65)$	p	η_p^2
Global Cognition	0.3 (0.7)	−0.2(1.0)	1.7	0.199	0.03
Language	0.3(0.6)	−0.2 (0.9)	3.5	0.065	0.05
Visuospatial	0.3 (0.4)	−0.2 (1.1)	4.0	0.051	0.06
Memory	0.5 (0.8)	−0.3 (0.7)	9.0	0.004	0.12
Attention	0.2 (0.6)	−0.2 (0.8)	2.7	0.107	0.04
Executive Function	0.02 (0.7)	0.0 (0.6)	0.8	0.367	0.01

This table summarizes the average z scores for each cognitive domain. Statistics describe the ANCOVA comparing group IMT < 0.9 and ≥ 0.9 for each cognitive domain, controlling for age, education and ApoE4. ANCOVA post hoc comparisons were conducted with Bonferroni tests. $p < 0.05$ was considered statistically significant.

Table 5. Association between stenosis and cognitive domains

Cognitive Domains	No stenosis (n = 44)	Stenosis (n = 26)	$F(1,65)$	p	η_p^2
Global Cognition	0.2 (0.8)	−0.1 (1.0)	2.2	0.148	0.03
Language	0.3 (0.7)	−0.3 (0.9)	12.8	0.001	0.17
Visuospatial	0.2 (0.5)	−0.3 (1.2)	7.7	0.007	0.11
Memory	0.3 (0.8)	−0.4 (0.7)	11.2	0.001	0.15
Attention	0.1 (0.6)	−0.3 (0.8)	5.1	0.028	0.07
Executive Function	0.03 (0.7)	−0.03 (0.6)	0.0	0.987	0.00

This table summarizes the average z scores for each cognitive domain. Statistics describe the ANCOVA comparing no stenosis versus stenosis groups for each cognitive domain, controlling for age, education and ApoE4. ANCOVA post hoc comparisons were conducted with Bonferroni tests. $p < 0.05$ was considered statistically significant.

4. Discussion

The main objective of this study was to explore the impact of vascular biomarkers such as IMT and stenosis on cognitive function in aged adults diagnosed with MCI or AD. Initially participants were assessed with a cognitive test battery, and as expected, groups performed differently across cognitive domains. The tests used in this study are common in AD research and diagnosis and have yielded similar results [46,47]. In addition, the combination of tests to form composite scores has generated comparable results in several studies [48,49] where the most frequently studied domains were attention, executive functions, global cognition, processing speed, episodic memory, verbal abilities and visuospatial abilities [50]. Our findings confirmed that participants with AD with at least one copy of ApoE ε4 had a significantly lower performance in global cognition [26].

Vascular markers were examined to identify their association with cognitive function. The results showed that there was no significant effect of IMT and stenosis when they are examined together with group diagnosis. However, when diagnosis was not considered, having an IMT ≥ 0.9 mm was associated with worse performance in memory; likewise the presence of carotid stenosis was related to worse performance in language, visuospatial abilities, memory and attention. These results were independent of age, education or ApoE ε4 expression.

Several studies have found a positive relationship between IMT and memory deficits [51]. Longitudinal studies that included older adults without a diagnosis of vascular pathologies or dementia, found that the higher the IMT, the lower the performance on memory tasks [51,52]. Memory alteration can be a preclinical manifestation of dementia, so the association between the vascular marker and the memory deficit can play a decisive role in establishing which subjects have a higher risk of progressing towards a more pronounced stage of cognitive deterioration. Consistent with our findings, others have found that vascular alterations were associated with lower cognitive performance in memory, attention, processing speed and executive function [53,54]. In contrast, other studies found no relationship between IMT and the memory domain, although greater IMT values were associated with deficits in executive functions and global cognition [48]. Likewise, as we observed, cognitive performance in multiple cognitive functions has been shown to be lower in subjects with stenosis [55,56]. In studies that compared cognitive performance of subjects with and without stenosis, subjects with stenosis had a worse performance in attention, psychomotor speed, memory, motor skills [57], visuospatial abilities and language [58,59].

There are different mechanisms that could explain the association between vascular alterations and cognitive impairment. First, changes in the arteries such as such as luminal narrowing or IMT thickening can reduce blood circulation and interrupt the flow of nutrients to the brain. As a result, different cognitive domains may be affected [5,60]. Also, it has been reported that an increase in IMT is a consequence of other vascular pathologies such as hypertension and atherosclerosis that may be related to brain changes, such as atrophy and white matter lesions, which also alter cognition [15,61]. Specifically, atrophy of temporal lobe structures is associated with difficulties learning and recovering information [62,63].

This study had several limitations, one of which was the small number of participants who were diagnosed with AD. A greater sample size would clarify further potential interactions among the variables examined. Also, the study was cross-sectional so we cannot draw causal inference about the variables measured and cognitive function. Another potential limitation involves the accuracy of AD and MCI diagnosis. Evidence has shown that the clinical diagnosis of AD has an accuracy of 70–90% [64] and the diagnosis of MCI is even more complex due do its mixed etiology that can be influenced by multiple factors. As such, our results should be interpreted with these limitations in mind. Each of these limitations is being addressed in ongoing studies. Study strengths include providing the first report of cognitive impairment associated with vascular markers and ApoE4 in the LAC region. The association between these measures reveals the possibility of incorporating markers (based on their association with neuropsychological tests) at the level of primary care in order to have additional information that could help establish the risk factors for cognitive impairment. Currently, no biological marker is used to detect individuals at risk of cognitive impairment in local public health facilities.

5. Conclusion

In Panama, research and policies focused on the health of older adults continue to be scarce. One of the main problems is that research on aging and associated conditions is insufficient making it difficult to develop biomarkers for diseases associated with cognitive impairment. On the other hand, there is a lack of adequate, consistent and timely diagnoses, especially in primary care. Thus our study contributes to the understanding of risk factors among Hispanics both within and outside

LAC. Our results indicate that including vascular markers in the assessment of older adults can provide a non-invasive tool that can facilitate early diagnosis of age-related impairments. These results support the notion that regardless of diagnosis, vascular pathologies are associated with worse performance in specific domains, which could serve to guide assessments in primary care.

Acknowledgments

Research reported in this publication was supported by the Melo Brain Project, Universidad Santa María la Antigua (DCO, ARP, and GBB), Sistema Nacional de Investigación of Panama (GBB, AEV, and MBC) and Secretaría Nacional de Ciencia, Tecnología e Innovación (SENACYT) of Panama (GBB, AEV, and MBC). We thank the support of administration and support staff of the Complejo Hospitalario Dr. Arnulfo Arias Madrid de la Caja de Seguro Social and the following collaborators from the Panama Aging Research Initiative for their assistance in conducting this study: Aquiles Aguilar, M.D.; Lissette Chang, M.D.; Frank Ferro, M.D.; Patricia González, M.D.; Vanessa González, M.D.; Luis Lee, M.D.; María Mendieta, M.D.; Ribana Molino, M.D.; Josué Morales, M.D.; Viterbo Osorio, M.D.; and Ramón Zarak, M.D.

Conflict of interest

The authors declare no conflict of interest.

Authors' contributions

D. Oviedo designed the study, conducted clinical data collection, interpreted data and wrote the manuscript. H. Lezcano assisted with laboratory data acquisition, interpretation of the data and drafting the manuscript. S. Grajales and A.Villarreal assisted with the design of the study, clinical and laboratory data collection and provided input to the manuscript. B. Isaza and L. Wesley assisted with laboratory data collection and drafting the manuscript. M. Carreira, A. Perez, S. Fernandez and A. Frank assisted with analyzing and interpreting the data and yielded input to the manuscript. G. Britton designed the study, conducted statistical analyses and wrote the manuscript. All authors read and approved the final version of the manuscript and agree to be responsible for all aspects of the study in ensuring questions regarding all aspects of the study are clarified and resolved.

References

1. Nations U (2017) World Population Aging.
2. Nations U (2015) Department of Economic and Social Affairs.
3. Hebert LE, Bienias JL, Aggarwal NT, et al. (2010) Change in risk of Alzheimer disease over time. *Neurology* 75: 786-791.
4. Palloni A, Pinto-Aguirre G, Pelaez M (2002) Demographic and health conditions of ageing in Latin America and the Caribbean. *Int J Epidemiol* 31: 762-771.
5. de la Torre JC (2012) Cerebral hemodynamics and vascular risk factors: setting the stage for Alzheimer's disease. *J Alzheimers Dis* 32: 553-567.

6. Viswanathan A, Rocca WA, Tzourio C (2009) Vascular risk factors and dementia: how to move forward? *Neurology* 72: 368-374.
7. Iadecola C (2003) Atherosclerosis and neurodegeneration: unexpected conspirators in Alzheimer's dementia. *Arterioscler Thromb Vasc Biol* 23: 1951-1953.
8. Roher AE, Esh C, Kokjohn TA, et al. (2003) Circle of willis atherosclerosis is a risk factor for sporadic Alzheimer's disease. *Arterioscler Thromb Vasc Biol* 23: 2055-2062.
9. Hofman A, Ott A, Breteler MM, et al. (1997) Atherosclerosis, apolipoprotein E, and prevalence of dementia and Alzheimer's disease in the Rotterdam Study. *Lancet* 349: 151-154.
10. Xiang J, Zhang T, Yang QW, et al. (2013) Carotid artery atherosclerosis is correlated with cognitive impairment in an elderly urban Chinese non-stroke population. *J Clin Neurosci* 20: 1571-1575.
11. Yamaura Y, Watanabe N, Obase K, et al. (2010) Relation between progression of aortic valve sclerosis and carotid intima-media thickening in asymptomatic subjects with cardiovascular risk factors. *J Echocardiogr* 8: 87-93.
12. Silvestrini M, Viticchi G, Falsetti L, et al. (2011) The role of carotid atherosclerosis in Alzheimer's disease progression. *J Alzheimers Dis* 25: 719-726.
13. Wendell CR, Waldstein SR, Evans MK, et al. (2016) Subclinical carotid atherosclerosis and neurocognitive function in an urban population. *Atherosclerosis* 249: 125-131.
14. Zeki Al Hazzouri A, Vittinghoff E, Sidney S, et al. (2015) Intima-Media Thickness and Cognitive Function in Stroke-Free Middle-Aged Adults: Findings From the Coronary Artery Risk Development in Young Adults Study. *Stroke* 46: 2190-2196.
15. Romero JR, Beiser A, Seshadri S, et al. (2009) Carotid artery atherosclerosis, MRI indices of brain ischemia, aging, and cognitive impairment: the Framingham study. *Stroke* 40: 1590-1596.
16. Arntzen KA, Schirmer H, Johnsen SH, et al. (2012) Carotid atherosclerosis predicts lower cognitive test results: a 7-year follow-up study of 4,371 stroke-free subjects—the Tromso study. *Cerebrovasc Dis* 33: 159-165.
17. Cervantes S, Samaranch L, Vidal-Taboada JM, et al. (2011) Genetic variation in APOE cluster region and Alzheimer's disease risk. *Neurobiol Aging* 32: e2107-2117.
18. Michaelson DM (2014) APOE epsilon4: the most prevalent yet understudied risk factor for Alzheimer's disease. *Alzheimers Dement* 10: 861-868.
19. Verghese PB, Castellano JM, Holtzman DM (2011) Apolipoprotein E in Alzheimer's disease and other neurological disorders. *Lancet Neurol* 10: 241-252.
20. Doliner B, Dong C, Blanton SH, et al. (2018) Apolipoprotein E Gene Polymorphism and Subclinical Carotid Atherosclerosis: The Northern Manhattan Study. *J Stroke Cerebrovasc Dis* 27: 645-652.
21. Bangen KJ, Beiser A, Delano-Wood L, et al. (2013) APOE genotype modifies the relationship between midlife vascular risk factors and later cognitive decline. *J Stroke Cerebrovasc Dis* 22: 1361-1369.
22. Filippini N, Ebmeier KP, MacIntosh BJ, et al. (2011) Differential effects of the APOE genotype on brain function across the lifespan. *Neuroimage* 54: 602-610.
23. Yusuf S, Hawken S, Ounpuu S, et al. (2004) Effect of potentially modifiable risk factors associated with myocardial infarction in 52 countries (the INTERHEART study): case-control study. *Lancet* 364: 937-952.

24. Gracia F, Benzadon A, Gonzalez-Castellon M, et al. (2014) The impact of cerebrovascular disease in Panama. *Int J Stroke* 9 Suppl A100: 28-30.
25. Carrion Donderis M, Moreno Velasquez I, Castro F, et al. (2016) Analysis of mortality trends due to cardiovascular diseases in Panama, 2001-2014. *Open Heart* 3: e000510.
26. Villarreal AE, Grajales S, O'Bryant SE, et al. (2016) Characterization of Alzheimer's Disease and Mild Cognitive Impairment in Older Adults in Panama. *J Alzheimers Dis* 54: 897-901.
27. Villarreal AE, O'Bryant SE, Edwards M, et al. (2016) Serum-based protein profiles of Alzheimer's disease and mild cognitive impairment in elderly Hispanics. *Neurodegener Dis Manag*.
28. Folstein MF, Folstein SE, McHugh PR (1975) "Mini-mental state". A practical method for grading the cognitive state of patients for the clinician. *J Psychiatr Res* 12: 189-198.
29. Wechsler D (1997) *WAIS-III administration and scoring manual*. San Antonio, TX: The Psychological Corporation.
30. Reitan RM (1958) Validity of the Trail Making Test as an Indicator or Organic Brain Damage. *Perceptual Motor Skills* 8: 271–276.
31. Connor DJ, Schafer K (1998) *Administration Manual for the Alzheimer's Disease Assessment Scale*. San Diego: Alzheimer's Disease Cooperative Study.
32. Kaplan EF, Goodglass H, Weintraub S (1983) The Boston Naming Test (2nd ed.). Philadelphia, PA: Lea & Febiger.
33. Spreen O, Benton AL (1977) *Neurosensory center comprehensive examination for aphasia: Manual of directions.* Vicotria, BC, Canada: Neuropsychology Laboratory, University of Victoria.
34. Sunderland T, Hill JL, Mellow AM, et al. (1989) Clock drawing in Alzheimer's disease. A novel measure of dementia severity. *J Am Geriatr Soc* 37: 725-729.
35. Poppelreuter W (1923) Zur Psychologie und Pathologie der optischen Wahrnehmung. *Zeitschrift für die Gesamte Neurologie und Psychiatrie* 83: 152.
36. Lawton MP, Brody EM (1969) Assessment of older people: self-maintaining and instrumental activities of daily living. *Gerontologist* 9: 179-186.
37. Pfeffer RI, Kurosaki TT, Harrah CH, Jr., et al. (1982) Measurement of functional activities in older adults in the community. *J Gerontol* 37: 323-329.
38. Yesavage JA, Brink TL, Rose TL, et al. (1982) Development and validation of a geriatric depression screening scale: a preliminary report. *J Psychiatr Res* 17: 37-49.
39. Badia X, Roset M, Montserrat S, et al. (1999) La versión española del EuroQol: Descripción y aplicaciones. *Medicina Clinica* 112 79–86.
40. Reisberg B, Ferris SH, de Leon MJ, et al. (1982) The Global Deterioration Scale for assessment of primary degenerative dementia. *Am J Psychiatry* 139: 1136-1139.
41. Albert MS, DeKosky ST, Dickson D, et al. (2011) The diagnosis of mild cognitive impairment due to Alzheimer's disease: recommendations from the National Institute on Aging-Alzheimer's Association workgroups on diagnostic guidelines for Alzheimer's disease. *Alzheimers Dement* 7: 270-279.
42. McKhann GM, Knopman DS, Chertkow H, et al. (2011) The diagnosis of dementia due to Alzheimer's disease: recommendations from the National Institute on Aging-Alzheimer's Association workgroups on diagnostic guidelines for Alzheimer's disease. *Alzheimers Dement* 7: 263-269.

43. Koch W, Ehrenhaft A, Griesser K, et al. (2002) TaqMan systems for genotyping of disease-related polymorphisms present in the gene encoding apolipoprotein E. *Clin Chem Lab Med* 40: 1123-1131.
44. Van Bortel LM (2005) What does intima-media thickness tell us? *J Hypertension.*
45. Grant EG, Benson CB, Moneta GL, et al. (2003) Carotid artery stenosis: gray-scale and Doppler US diagnosis--Society of Radiologists in Ultrasound Consensus Conference. *Radiology* 229: 340-346.
46. Cerami C, Dubois B, Boccardi M, et al. (2017) Clinical validity of delayed recall tests as a gateway biomarker for Alzheimer's disease in the context of a structured 5-phase development framework. *Neurobiol Aging* 52: 153-166.
47. Luna-Lario P, Azcarate-Jimenez L, Seijas-Gomez R, et al. (2015) Proposal for a neuropsychological cognitive evaluation battery for detecting and distinguishing between mild cognitive impairment and dementias. *Rev Neurol* 60: 553-561.
48. Lim SL, Gao Q, Nyunt MS, et al. (2016) Vascular Health Indices and Cognitive Domain Function: Singapore Longitudinal Ageing Studies. *J Alzheimers Dis* 50: 27-40.
49. Cloutier S, Chertkow H, Kergoat MJ, et al. (2015) Patterns of Cognitive Decline Prior to Dementia in Persons with Mild Cognitive Impairment. *J Alzheimers Dis* 47: 901-913.
50. Wisdom NM, Callahan JL, Hawkins KA (2011) The effects of apolipoprotein E on non-impaired cognitive functioning: a meta-analysis. *Neurobiol Aging* 32: 63-74.
51. Johnston SC, O'Meara ES, Manolio TA, et al. (2004) Cognitive impairment and decline are associated with carotid artery disease in patients without clinically evident cerebrovascular disease. *Ann Intern Med* 140: 237-247.
52. Vinkers DJ, Stek ML, van der Mast RC, et al. (2005) Generalized atherosclerosis, cognitive decline, and depressive symptoms in old age. *Neurology* 65: 107-112.
53. Mitchell GF, van Buchem MA, Sigurdsson S, et al. (2011) Arterial stiffness, pressure and flow pulsatility and brain structure and function: the Age, Gene/Environment Susceptibility—Reykjavik study. *Brain* 134: 3398-3407.
54. Zhong W, Cruickshanks KJ, Schubert CR, et al. (2014) Pulse wave velocity and cognitive function in older adults. *Alzheimer Dis Assoc Disord* 28: 44-49.
55. Li X, Ma X, Lin J, et al. (2017) Severe carotid artery stenosis evaluated by ultrasound is associated with post stroke vascular cognitive impairment. *Brain Behav* 7: e00606.
56. Wang T, Mei B, Zhang J (2016) Atherosclerotic carotid stenosis and cognitive function. *Clin Neurol Neurosurg* 146: 64-70.
57. Mathiesen EB, Waterloo K, Joakimsen O, et al. (2004) Reduced neuropsychological test performance in asymptomatic carotid stenosis: The Tromso Study. *Neurology* 62: 695-701.
58. Nemeth D, Sefcsik T, Nemeth K, et al. (2013) Impaired language production in asymptomatic carotid stenosis. *J Neurolinguistics* 6: 462–469.
59. Rocque BG, Jackson D, Varghese T, et al. (2012) Impaired cognitive function in patients with atherosclerotic carotid stenosis and correlation with ultrasound strain measurements. *J Neurol Sci* 322: 20-24.
60. Mataro M, Soriano-Raya JJ, Lopez-Oloriz J, et al. (2014) Cerebrovascular markers in lowered cognitive function. *J Alzheimers Dis* 42: S383-391.
61. Bots ML, van Swieten JC, Breteler MM, et al. (1993) Cerebral white matter lesions and atherosclerosis in the Rotterdam Study. *Lancet* 341: 1232-1237.

62. McDonald CR, Gharapetian L, McEvoy LK, et al. (2012) Relationship between regional atrophy rates and cognitive decline in mild cognitive impairment. *Neurobiol Aging* 33: 242-253.
63. Moretti DV (2015) Electroencephalography reveals lower regional blood perfusion and atrophy of the temporoparietal network associated with memory deficits and hippocampal volume reduction in mild cognitive impairment due to Alzheimer's disease. *Neuropsychiatr Dis Treat* 11: 461-470.
64. Korolev IO, Symonds LL, Bozoki AC, et al. (2016) Predicting Progression from Mild Cognitive Impairment to Alzheimer's Dementia Using Clinical, MRI, and Plasma Biomarkers via Probabilistic Pattern Classification. *PLoS One* 11: e0138866.

4

Nonlinear EEG parameters of emotional perception in patients with moderate traumatic brain injury, coma, stroke and schizophrenia

Galina V. Portnova[1,2,*] and Michael S. Atanov[1]

[1] Institute of Higher Nervous Activity and Neurophysiology of RAS, 5A Butlerova St., Moscow 117485, Russia
[2] The Pushkin State Russian Language Institute

* **Corresponding Author:** Email: caviter@list.ru;

Abstract: *Objective:* The aim of this study was to determine the EEG changes induced by emotional non-verbal sounds using nonlinear signals' features and also to examine the subjective emotional response in patients with different neurological and psychiatric disorders. *Methods:* 141 subjects participated in our study: patients after moderate TBI, patients in acute coma, patients after stroke, patients with schizophrenia and controls. 7 types of emotionally charged stimuli were presented. Non-comatose participants were asked to assess the levels of experienced emotions. We analyzed fractal dimension, signal's envelope parameters and Hjorth mobility and complexity. *Results:* The Hjorth parameters were negatively correlated with irritation. The fractal dimension was positively correlated with arousal and empathy levels. The only presentation of laughter to post-stroke patients induced the reaction similar to the control group. *Conclusions:* The results showed that the investigated nonlinear features of resting state EEG are quite group-specific and also specific to the emotional state. *Significance:* The investigated features could serve to diagnose emotional impairments.

Keywords: EEG; fractal dimension; EEG envelope; Hjorth; schizophrenia; stroke; coma; traumatic brain injury

---

1. Introduction

In this study we examined a set of time-domain and nonlinear features of EEG signal in patients with different neurological and psychiatric disorders. These features were shown to differ in patients with neurological disorders such as epilepsy, attention-deficit/hyperactivity disorder (ADHD) and Alzheimer's disease [1]. So, we expect that the complexity and chaotic nature of EEG data are useful to discriminate these disorders by their specific emotional traits. As reported by some researchers [2], quantitative measures of chaos and nonlinear features characterize electrophysiological abnormalities in neuropsychiatric disorders that are not evident in linear analysis. To show the effectiveness of these features to diagnose a concussion, in an approach similar to power analysis, the features can be calculated for both usual EEG frequency bands (rhythms) and individual EEG frequencies (2-Hz wide bands). This method came from a study on concussed athletes [2]. The investigated signal features: time domain Hjorth parameters, approximate entropy, and the Hurst exponent, didn't differ between the groups of the athletes and their healthy peers if calculated in the rhythm-band filtered case but they did differ in the narrow-band filtered case.

The observation of significantly different nonlinear features also revealed important notions about concussed athletes: they exhibited a decrease in Hjorth complexity and mobility. It has been reported by Pezard with colleagues [3] that depressive subjects tend to display lower complexity than controls. Moreover, it was reported that decreased complexity and mobility are associated with insomniac subjects [4]. Approximate entropy quantifies the amount of regularity in the data by calculating the upcoming amplitude values of the signal based on the knowledge of the preceding amplitude values [5]. Sohn with colleagues [6] reported about significantly lower approximate entropy for a group of ADHD subjects compared to matched controls and hypothesized that the patients might not have sufficient levels of cortical activation to reach the requirements for attention-demanding tasks. Following their hypothesis, the approximate entropy is discriminative in this case, we suppose it reflects the altered cortical information processing. Moreover, pathological disorder studies on schizophrenia, posttraumatic stress disorder, panic disorder, and epilepsy have reported lower Hjorth complexity in pathological states compared to healthy subjects [7]. We claim that lower EEG complexity is attributed to the abnormal neural integration in the above-mentioned mental disorders.

Nonlinear EEG parameters were previously shown to be related to emotional states and affective reactions. For example, fractal dimension of EEG signals provides comparative performance for both facial [8] and auditory [9] emotion recognition. Differential entropy of EEG signals proved to be more suitable for emotion recognition than traditional frequency domain EEG features [10]. Hjorth parameters can be used for happiness/sadness recognition of visual stimuli [11] and emotional components of music [12]. Thus, nonlinear parameters are a good choice in the paradigm of emotional processes investigation.

Nonlinear features are also a good tool for emotional processes research in neurological and psychiatric disorders of our interest. For example, fractal dimension decreases in the acute phase of a stroke and was also associated with worse clinical recovery [13]. Other researchers have reported that spectral entropy reflects the slowing of brain activity in patients with post-stroke vascular dementia and stroke-related cognitive impairment, whereas permutation entropy and Tsallis entropy reflect the complexity of the examined signals [14]. Using the support vector machine algorithm Chu and co-authors [15] even succeeded in classifying the type of induced emotion by EEG signal in groups of patients with moderate and severe schizophrenia and their healthy counterparts.

In our studies, we attempt to determine the specificity of emotional auditory nonverbal perception using nonlinear EEG parameters. In the present study we investigated four groups of patients with different diagnoses and therefore different types of emotional impairment, i.e., patients after: severe TBI (in coma), moderate TBI, stroke, and with schizophrenia. It is well known that mood depression is a typical post-stroke complication [16] and is associated with a disability [17] and with a worse rehabilitation outcome in stroke survivors [18]. Patients with moderate TBI demonstrate significant emotional and behavioral maladjustment, increased difficulties with anger management, antisocial behavior and abnormal self-monitoring [19]. Severe TBI is often accompanied by the lack of empathy, reduced behavioral regulation and impaired social function [20]. In our previous research on patients with TBI we found the EEG response on emotional stimulation to vary depending on the severity of trauma [21] Namely, patients with severe TBI showed decreased theta-rhythm power in the frontal areas during unpleasant sounds presentation, while the patients with moderate TBI exhibited increased alpha-rhythm power in the occipital areas during both pleasant and unpleasant stimulation. Patients with schizophrenia usually lack outward expression of emotion, diminished motivation and reduced experience of pleasure [22]. The described emotional changes in different groups of patients are polymorphic and have different origins and pathogeneses. We expect that nonlinear features of EEG signals could reveal the dynamics accompanying the emotional processes and discriminate these groups of patients.

2. Materials and methods

2.1. Participants

5 groups of adult subjects participated in our study (N = 141): healthy (control group), patients after moderate TBI (mTBI), patients in acute coma (caused by severe TBI), patients after stroke in the left middle cerebral artery and patients with schizophrenia. The exclusion criteria were: any history of epileptic seizures, tumors, and massive brain hematomas, additional medications or accompanying diseases. The resulting structure of the groups is depicted in Table 1. Glasgow Coma Scale was used for diagnostic purposes only.

Access to patients after TBI by the Central Clinical Hospital of Russian Academy of Science, access to patients with schizophrenia was provided by the 1st Psychiatric Clinical Hospital named by N.A. Alexeev.

No participants took any anticonvulsants, nootropics or antianxiolytics. All the comatose patients received identical acute care therapy according to local standards (the medication's doses were similar for each patient). All participants with schizophrenia received medical therapy of haloperidol (the same medication's doses). Patients after stroke received antihypertensive therapy (the medication's doses were similar for each patient). Patients after mTBI and healthy subjects were not under medication.

The outcome of comatose patients was as follows: 6 patients recovered within two weeks of the study, 8 patients remained in a vegetative state for the following three months, 5 patients were transferred to other hospital departments due to extracranial complications.

We analyzed hearing function in healthy subjects and patients after moderate TBI as we presented auditory stimulation. We used PDD-401 audiometer (Piston Ltd., Budapest, Hungary) to identify hearing threshold levels. None of the examined subjects had any symptoms of hearing loss.

Table 1. Descriptive statistics of subjects.

Groups	Number of subjects	Age	Sex (f/m)	Glasgow Coma Scale	Duration of the disease
Control group	37	31.6 ± 7.1	22/25	-	-
Patients with schizophrenia	26	25.9 ± 4.7	11/15	-	3 ± 0.6 years
Moderate TBI patients	31	31.2 ± 6.6	15/16	13.0 ± 1.9	10.5 ± 7.7 months
Patients after stroke	28	55.2 ± 5.1	13/15	-	7.9 ± 1.3 months
Patients in coma	19	27.1 ± 5.3	8/11	4.3 ± 1.7	5.9 ± 2.9 days

Note: Mean ± std.dev. where applicable.

All participants (or their authorized relatives) gave written informed consent prior to participating in the study. The protocol of the study was approved by the Ethics Committee of the Institute of Higher Nervous Activity and Neurophysiology of RAS.

2.2. Stimuli

We presented 30 second long sounds as stimuli. There was initially a large list (about 40) of such sounds, then a group of 198 healthy experts (mean age about 30 years) assessed all the stimuli on scales of pleasantness, arousal, fear, gladness, etc. We selected 7 stimuli for this study—most emotionally charged with most stable assessment: a dog barking, a crying infant, vomiting, coughing, scratching nails on a glass, a bird singing, and human laughter. Each stimulus was presented randomly 8 times, the interstimulus interval was 700–2000 msec long (randomly conducted): the obtained ~ 240 sec EEG fragments for each stimulus were further analyzed. Resting states with open and closed eyes were recorded for 2 minutes in the beginning and at the end of the study.

The subjects of the control, schizophrenia, stroke and mTBI groups assessed emotional valence and arousal level of the stimuli by the scales pleasantness (from −5 to 5), arousal (from 0 to 10), fear (from 0 to 10), empathy (from 0 to 10) and irritation (from 0 to 10). The stimuli were presented in a random order for 30 seconds (8–10 times each) with 0.7–2.0 second gaps between them (Table S1); the whole experiment lasted about 50 minutes.

2.3. EEG registration

The subjects sat in a comfortable position in an armchair in an acoustically and electrically shielded chamber, the comatose patients laid in a hospital bed in a resuscitation unit. The participants were instructed to remain calm and to listen to the presented sounds keeping their eyes closed (to avoid visual interference) and not to fall asleep. The stimuli were presented via earphones. EEG was recorded using the "Encephalan" (Medicom MTD, Taganrog, Russian Federation) device. Polygraphic channels were also recorded although these data are not presented. 19 AgCl electrodes (Fp1, Fp2, F7, F3, Fz, F4, F8, T3, C3, Cz, C4, T4, T5, P3, Pz, P4, T6, O1, O2) were placed according to the

International 10–20 system. The electrodes placed on the left and right mastoids served as joint references under unipolar montage. The vertical electrooculogram (EOG) was measured with AgCl cup electrodes placed 1 cm above and below the left eye, and the horizontal EOG was measured with electrodes placed 1 cm lateral from the outer canthi of both eyes. The sampling rate was 250 Hz, the filtering was set to bandpass 1.6–30 Hz. The electrode impedances were maintained at less than 10 kΩ. The small artifacts were deleted manually. EMG-related artifacts were deleted manually and using filtering 1.6–30 Hz. Eyes movement artifacts were cleaned out using EOG data by Encephalan device.

3. Data analysis

The artifact correction was conducted by the following way: the small artifacts were deleted manually, eyes movement artifacts were cleaned out using EOG data by "Encephalan" device.

3.1. Fractal dimension (FD)

We conducted the calculations of the examined signal bandpass-filtered in the range of interest (2–20 Hz), Butterworth filter of order 12 was used. FD was evaluated using the Higuchi algorithm [23].

3.2. Envelope mean frequency (EMF)

To express the (de-)synchronization dynamics of the rhythms we applied the following method. First, we calculated the envelope of the EEG signal for the whole frequency range (1.6–30 Hz) and for the alpha rhythm (8–13 Hz) using the Hilbert transform [24]. Second, we assessed the (in-)stability of the envelope's amplitude by calculating its average frequency using FFT (wideband—EMF, alpha—EMFA) and the ratio of its standard deviation to its mean (wideband only—RAT).

3.3. Hjorth parameters

Hjorth complexity [25] represents the change in frequency and indicates how the shape of a signal is similar to a pure sine wave. This parameter was calculated for wideband 1.6–30 Hz filtered signal in the following way:

$$complexity(y(t)) = \frac{mobility(y'(t))}{mobility(y(t))},$$

where

$$mobility(y(t)) = \sqrt{\frac{var(y'(t))}{var(y(t))}},$$

y(t)—a signal, y'(t)—its derivative, and var(...)—the variance.

The Hjorth complexity and mobility showed very similar results in our research, so we refer to them both as Hjorth parameters.

3.4. Power spectral density

Fast Fourier Transform (FFT) was used to evaluate the PSD, the resulting data were integrated over intervals of unit width in the range of interest (2–3 Hz, 3–4 Hz, …, 19–20 Hz). It was carried out for each EEG fragment and then used in correlation analysis with nonlinear EEG features.

3.5. Statistical analysis

A repeated-measures ANOVA with Bonferroni correction for multiple comparisons ($p < 0.05$) was used to determine group effects on EEG metrics (post-hoc Tukey). We analyzed separately group effect for non-linear features for the resting state and the group effect of differences between the features during stimulation was compared to the values during rest. The Pearson correlation coefficient between PSD and nonlinear features was calculated. Only significant ($p < 0.05$) correlation values were used for further analysis.

4. Results

4.1. Power spectral density

Comatose patients had higher 2–7 Hz PSD compared to other groups of subjects ($F(4, 141) = 8.928$, $p < 0.00001$) in all electrodes. Patients after stroke had higher 5–9 Hz PSD compared to TBI, schizophrenia and control groups ($F(4, 141) = 10.318$, $p < 0.00001$) (except T5, T6 electrodes). The alpha-rhythm PSD (10–13 Hz) was significantly higher in control group ($F(4, 141) = 7.0168$, $p < 0.0001$) in central, parietal and occipital areas: electrodes C3, Cz, C4, P3, Pz, P4, O1, O2 (depicted in Figure 1).

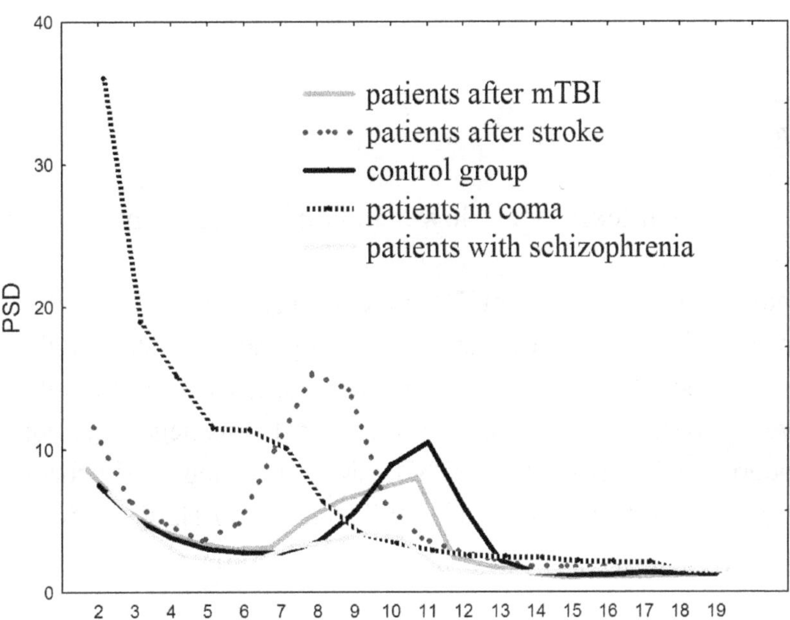

Figure 1. PSD values 2–20 Hz averaged over electrodes C3, Cz, C4: x—frequency in Hz, y—PSD in $\mu V^2/Hz$.

4.2. Group differences during rest

In this subsection the values during rest were compared between the groups.

4.2.1. FD

1. Lower in patients after stroke (except C3, T4, P3, Pz, P4), $F(4, 141) = 3.47050$, $p < 0.03$.
2. Higher in patients with schizophrenia (C3, T5, P3, Pz, P4, T6, O1, O2), $F(4, 141) = 4.7050$, $p < 0.005$.

4.2.2. EMF

1. Lower in patients after stroke (all except F7, C3, P3, Pz, P4, O1).
2. Lower in comatose patients (all except P4, T6).
3. Higher in patients with schizophrenia (all except C4, T4, T6), $F(4, 137) = 5.2412$, $p < 0.001$.

4.2.3. EMFA

Higher in patients with schizophrenia (Fp1, Fp2, F7, F3, Fz), $F(4, 137) = 5.9452$, $p < 0.0005$.

4.2.4. RAT

Higher in comatose patients (Fp1, F7, Fz, T3, C3, T5, P3, Pz, O1, O2), $F(4, 141) = 5.97050$, $p < 0.001$.

4.3. Hjorth parameters

Both mobility and complexity were lower in comatose patients (all except F3, F4, T5), $F(4, 141) = 6.1986$, $p < 0.001$.

Notably, no feature differed between mTBI and control groups.

The correlation analysis between linear and nonlinear parameters showed that FD was negatively correlated with 2–10 Hz and 13–14 Hz PSD, Hjorth parameters were negatively correlated with 2–8 Hz PSD and positively correlated with 15–20 Hz PSD. EMF was negatively correlated with 2–6 Hz PSD and positively correlated with 15–19 Hz PSD. EMFA was negatively correlated with 10–12 Hz PSD. RAD was positively correlated with 2–8 Hz PSD and 16–17 Hz PSD (depicted in Figure 2).

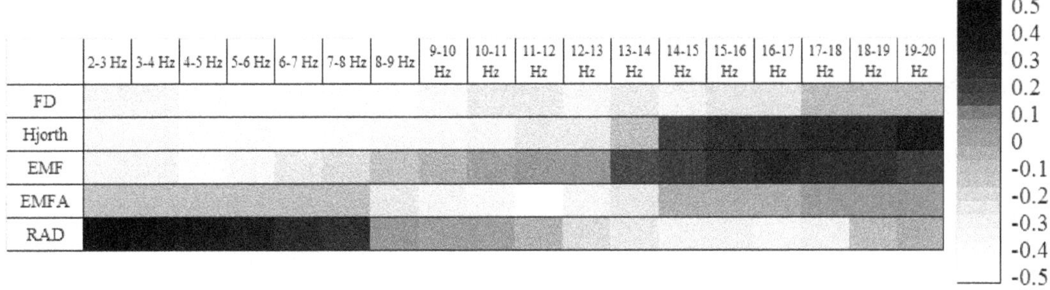

Figure 2. Significant (|r| > 0.35, $p < 0.05$) correlations between PSD and nonlinear EEG features.

4.4. Group differences during stimulation

The features during stimulation were compared to the values during rest.

4.4.1. FD

1. Higher in control group during presentation of crying (except F7, C3, Cz, C4, O2), $p < 0.03$.
2. Lower in patients with moderate TBI during presentation of coughing and vomiting (Fp1, Fp2, F7, Fz, F3, F4, C3, C4), $p < 0.009$.
3. Higher in comatose patients during these stimuli (Fp1, Fp2, F7, F3, Fz, F8, O1, T4), $p < 0.03$.
4. Higher in patients with schizophrenia during animal sounds presentation (barking and singing) (Fz, Fp2, F8, Cz, F4, C4, T4, P4, T6, O1), $p < 0.04$.
5. Lower in patients after stroke during animal sounds (barking and singing) presentation (F4, Fz, Pz, P4), $p < 0.01$, and higher during presentation of laughter (Fp1, Fz, F3, T3), $p < 0.02$.

4.4.2. *EMF*

1. Lower in control group during vomiting, coughing and scratching presentation (except T4, P4, T6), $p < 0.05$.
2. Lower in patients with moderate TBI during scratching (P4,T6, Cz, C4), $p < 0.007$.
3. Lower in comatose patients during vomiting, coughing and scratching presentation (Fp2, F4, F8, T4, T6, P4), $p < 0.03$ and higher during laughter and crying presentation (F4, F8, C4, T4, Pz, P4, T6, O1, O2).
4. Higher in patients with schizophrenia during bird song presentation (except Fp1, T3, T5, O2), $p < 0.009$.

4.4.3. EMFA

1. Lower in control group during presentation of vomiting, coughing, scratching, bird singing and barking (all channels).
2. Higher in patients with schizophrenia during presentation of bird singing, laughter, crying, coughing and vomiting (all except O2) and barking (Cz, C4, P4, T6).

4.4.4. RAT

1. Higher in patients after moderate TBI during presentation of crying (Cz, C4, T4,T6), $p < 0.04$ and laughter (C3, Cz, C4, T4), $p < 0.05$.
2. Higher in comatose patients during presentation of pleasant stimuli (laughter and bird singing) (F8, Cz, T6, Pz, O1, O2), $p < 0.02$.
3. Higher in patients with schizophrenia during presentation of coughing, laughter, scratching and bird singing (except T3, C3, T5, T6, O1, O2), $p < 0.03$, and lower during presentation of crying and barking (F3, T3, C3, Cz, C4, Pz, O1, O2), $p < 0.01$.

4.5. Hjorth parameters

1. Lower in patients after moderate TBI during all emotional stimuli (all channels), $p < 0.05$.
2. Lower in comatose patients during presentation of bird singing, barking and crying (F7, T3, C3, C4, P4, P3), $p < 0.01$.
3. Lower in patients with schizophrenia during presentation of laughter, barking and crying (Fp1, Fz, F3, F8, Cz, P3, Pz), $p < 0.03$, and higher during presentation of scratching (P3, Pz, O1), $p < 0.04$.
4. Lower in patients after stroke during presentation of barking (Fz, C3, Cz, Pz), $p < 0.05$.

The results of this subsection are summarized in Table 2.

Table 2. Significant differences of the features between stimuli presentation and rest ("+"—higher in rest, "–"—lower in rest).

	Bird song					Barking					Crying				
	FD	EMF	EMFA	RAD	Hjorth	FD	EMF	EMFA	RAD	Hjorth	FD	EMF	EMFA	RAD	Hjorth
Control group			–								+				
Schizophrenia	+	+	+	+		+			–	–			+	–	–
Moderate TBI					–					–				+	–
Stroke	–					–				–					
Coma				–	–					–		+		–	–

Continued on next page

	Coughing and Vomiting				Scratching				Laughter				
Control group	+	–	–		–	–							
Schizophrenia			+				+				+	+	–
Moderate TBI	–			–	–			–				+	–
Stroke									+				
Coma	+	–			–					+			

The assessment of emotional stimuli showed that participants of the control group reported significantly higher pleasantness of laughter ($F(4, 141) = 7.124, p < 0.0005$) and lower pleasantness of crying ($F(4, 141) = 3.945, p < 0.05$), compared to the groups of patients (depicted in Figure 3). Arousal was significantly higher in mTBI group during the presentation of unpleasant stimuli (coughing, vomiting) compared to other groups of subjects ($F(4, 141) = 8.61, p < 0.0001$).

4.6. The correlations between emotional assessment of stimuli and non-linear features

The empathy values (Table S1) were positively correlated with FD in the control group during the presentation of all stimuli ($r > 0.46, p < 0.05$). The arousal values were positively correlated with FD in patients with schizophrenia during the presentation of animal sounds (barking and bird singing) ($r > 0.37, p < 0.05$). The irritation values were negatively correlated with Hjorth parameters for all types of stimuli in all groups ($r < -0.39, p < 0.05$).

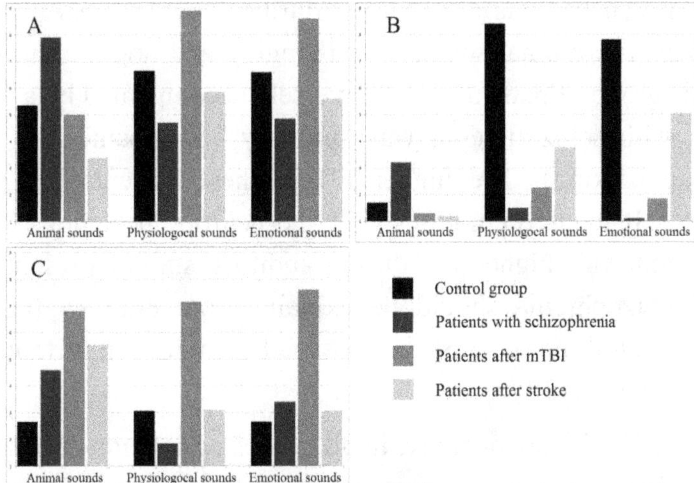

Figure 3. Emotional assessment of stimuli. A—arousal (0 10), B—empathy (0 10), C—irritation (0 10).

5. Discussion

In the present study, we found that the examined nonlinear features of resting state EEG are quite group-specific. Particularly, RAT was higher, Hjorth parameters and EMF were lower in comatose patients; EMF and FD were lower in patients after stroke. Having the correlation of these parameters with delta- and theta-rhythm PSD we suppose that the found specificity is related to the higher slow-wave activity [26,27] in these patients. These results match the previous data about reduced FD in patients with Alzheimer's disease [28] and studies reported that spectral entropy reflects the slowing of brain activity in post-stroke vascular dementia and stroke-related cognitive impairment patients [13].

EMFA and FD were oppositely higher in patients with schizophrenia. The negative correlations of these parameters with alpha-rhythm PSD may support the previous data of unusual alpha-rhythm activity of EEG in this group of patients [29]. This activity also proved to be related to clinical symptoms [30]. EMFA was shown to be sensitive to the emotional reaction of patients with schizophrenia: we observed the increase of EMFA during emotional stimulation only in this group, it even decreased in control group and demonstrated no significant changes in other groups. We supposed that the unusual emotional perception of patients with schizophrenia caused the abnormal changes in the EEG nonlinear parameters. Further, alpha activity during coma is not the same as physiological alpha rhythm [31] and patients after stroke and traumatic brain injury appeared to show a decreased frequency and magnitude of the alpha-rhythm [32], therefore EMFA didn't reflect their EEG changes.

We also found that some nonlinear EEG parameters can be associated with certain emotional states. For example, the control group showed an increase of FD during stimuli presentation (crying, coughing, and vomiting) which evoked arousal and empathy. These FD values also correlated with the subjective assessment of these emotions levels during the presentation. Some previous studies have reported that higher emotional response is associated with higher FD [33]; the "acute" or sudden emotions can also be determined using FD [34]; furthermore, FD was found to be useful to detect the level of arousal [35]. In our previous study [36] we also observed a significant positive correlation between FD of the EEG signal and fMRI BOLD-signal in some regions including the limbic system. Thus, FD in the control group could be used as a measure of arousal. We also observed this "normal" response in patients after stroke during laughter presentation, which was correlated with arousal feelings. The animal sounds (bird singing and dog barking), which evoked mostly irritation feelings in this group of patients, were inversely accompanied by a decrease in FD.

FD increase in patients with schizophrenia was similarly accompanied by higher reported arousal (bird singing and dog barking). The higher FD in these patients has previously been explained by other effects like self-focused emotions [37] and neurotic behavior [38], and the latter was also shown to be correlated with higher FD during auditory stimuli presentation. Thus, the higher FD in patients with schizophrenia should be explained not only by their more intense emotional reaction, i.e. higher arousal, but also by the loosened organization of thoughts and mental suggestions of certain superior abilities [39].

Hjorth parameters showed a significant decrease in all groups of patients during stimulation, but not in healthy subjects. This effect was most pronounced in comatose patients in response to animal sounds (bird singing, dog barking) and crying. Hjorth parameters were previously shown to be useful for recognition of emotional state: happy, sad, neutral and afraid [11], though using pictures as stimuli. We expected we could determine the pleasantness of our stimuli but the changes in the parameters didn't represent pleasantness in any way. Moreover, our results showed a negative correlation of Hjorth parameters during stimulation with the irritation level, which was most demonstrative considering barking sounds.

This study has some limitations which have to be pointed out. First of all, in spite of controlled medication's dozes, we are not sure that the emotional assessment and accompanying EEG changes in patients with schizophrenia were related only with their emotional disturbances. We also assume that the expanded amount of emotional sounds (we presented only seven types) and the presentation of emotional stimulation in other modalities could provide more detailed information about emotional impairment in patients.

6. Conclusions

We've shown that FD can be used to detect arousal in response to emotional stimulation.

EMFA reaction to the stimulation was observed only in patients with schizophrenia (increase) and controls (decrease).

The emotional stimuli (coughing and vomiting) that induced empathy in healthy subjects induced not empathy but irritation in patients with moderate TBI and led to opposite FD changes in this group. We've found that the presentation of laughter induced the same EEG changes in patients after stroke and comatose patients as in control group.

Hjorth parameters are useful to detect the abnormal increased irritation during stimulation.

In upcoming research we are planning to build a classification procedure to diagnose emotional impairments in different psychical and neurological diseases using these nonlinear parameters.

Acknowledgements

The research was supported by the grant #16-04-00092 of the Russian Foundation for Basic Research and by Russian Academy of Science.

References

1. Stam CJ (2005) Nonlinear dynamical analysis of EEG and MEG: review of an emerging field. *Clin Neurophysiol* 116: 2266–2301.
2. Mohammadi MR, Khaleghi A, Nasrabadi AM, et al. (2016) EEG classification of ADHD and normal children using non-linear features and neural network. *Biomed Eng Lett* 6: 66–73.
3. Pezard L, Nandrino J, Renault B, et al. (1996) Depression as a dynamical disease. *Biol Psychiatry* 39: 991–999.
4. Hamida ST, Ahmed B, Penzel T. A novel insomnia identification method based on Hjorth parameters. 2015 IEEE International Symposium on Signal Processing and Information Technology (ISSPIT); 2015 Dec 7–10; Abu Dhabi, UAE. New Jersey: IEEE; c2016. p. 548–552.
5. Bruhn J, Röpcke H, Hoeft A (2000) Approximate entropy as an electroencephalographic measure of anesthetic drug effect during desflurane anesthesia. *Anesthesiology* 92: 715–726.
6. Sohn H, Kim I, Lee W, et al. (2010) Linear and non-linear EEG analysis of adolescents with

attention-deficit/hyperactivity disorder during a cognitive task. *Clin Neurophysiol* 121: 1863–1870.

7. Takahashi T (2013) Complexity of spontaneous brain activity in mental disorders. *Prog Neuro-Psychopharmacol Biol Psychiatry* 45: 258–266.
8. Takehara T, Ochiai F, Watanabe H, et al. (2013) The relationship between fractal dimension and other-race and inversion effects in recognising facial emotions. *Cogn Emot* 27: 577–588.
9. Cheng M, Tsoi AC (2017) Fractal dimension pattern-based multiresolution analysis for rough estimator of speaker-dependent audio emotion recognition. *Int J Wavelets Multiresolut Inf Process* 15: 1750042.
10. Duan R, Zhu J, Lu B. Differential entropy feature for EEG-based emotion classification. 6th International IEEE/EMBS Conference on Neural Engineering (NER); 2013 Nov 6–8; San Diego, USA. New Jersey: IEEE; c2014. p. 81–84.
11. Mehmood RM, Lee HJ (2015) EEG based emotion recognition from human brain using hjorth parameters and SVM. *International Journal of Bio-Science and Bio-Technology* 7: 23–32.
12. Unterlöhner i Salvat N. Classifying music by their emotional content by using machine learning [master's thesis]. [Barcelona (Spain)]: Univ. Politecnica de Catalunya; 2013.
13. Zappasodi F, Olejarczyk E, Marzetti L, et al. (2014) Fractal dimension of EEG activity senses neuronal impairment in acute stroke. PLoS One 9: e100199.
14. Al-Qazzaz NK, Ali S, Ahmad SA, Islam MS, Escudero J. Entropy-based markers of EEG background activity of stroke-related mild cognitive impairment and vascular dementia patients. In: Yurish S, Malayeri A, editors. Sensors and electronic instrumentation advances: proceedings of the 2nd international conference on sensors and electronic instrumentation advances; 2016 Sep 22-23; Barcelona, Castelldefels, Spain. Barcelona: IFSA Publishing; c2016. p. 92–95.
15. Chu W, Huang M, Jian B, et al. (2017) Analysis of EEG entropy during visual evocation of emotion in schizophrenia. *Ann Gen Psychiatry* 16: 34–43.
16. Paolucci S (2008). Epidemiology and treatment of post-stroke depression. *Neuropsychiatr Dis Treat* 4: 145–154.
17. Pohjasvaara T, Vataja R, Leppävuori A, et al. (2001) Depression is an independent predictor of poor long-term functional outcome post-stroke. *European Journal of Neurology* 8: 315–319.
18. Gillen R, Tennen H, McKee TE, et al. (2001) Depressive symptoms and history of depression predict rehabilitation efficiency in stroke patients. *Arch Phys Med Rehabil* 82: 1645–1649.
19. Hanks RA, Temkin N, Machamer J, et al. (1999) Emotional and behavioral adjustment after traumatic brain injury. *Arch Phys Med Rehabil* 80: 991–997.
20. Williams C, Wood RL (2010) Alexithymia and emotional empathy following traumatic brain injury. *J Clin Exp Neuropsychol* 32: 259–267.
21. Galina P, Gladun K, Alexey I (2014) The EEG analysis of auditory emotional stimuli perception in TBI patients with different SCG score. *Open Journal of Modern Neurosurgery* 4: 81–96.
22. Kring AM, Caponigro JM (2010) Emotion in schizophrenia: where feeling meets thinking. *Curr Dir Psychol Sci* 19: 255–259.
23. Higuchi T (1988) Approach to an irregular time series on the basis of the fractal theory. *Physica D: Nonlinear Phenomena* 31: 277–283.
24. Ktonas PY, Papp N (1980) Instantaneous envelope and phase extraction from real signals: theory, implementation, and an application to EEG analysis. *Signal Processing* 2: 373–385.

25. Hjorth B (1970). EEG analysis based on time domain properties. *Electroencephalogr Clin Neurophysiol* 29: 306–310.
26. Sutter R, Kaplan PW (2012) Electroencephalographic patterns in coma: when things slow down. *Epileptologie* 29: 201–209.
27. Faught E (1993) Current role of electroencephalography in cerebral ischemia. *Stroke* 24: 609–613.
28. Gómez C, Mediavilla Á, Hornero R, et al. (2009) Abásolo D., Fernández A. Use of the Higuchi's fractal dimension for the analysis of MEG recordings from Alzheimer's disease patients. *Med Eng Phys* 31: 306–313.
29. Hinkley LB, Vinogradov S, Guggisberg AG, et al. (2011) Clinical symptoms and alpha band resting-state functional connectivity imaging in patients with schizophrenia: implications for novel approaches to treatment. *Biol Psychiatry* 70: 1134–1142.
30. Uhlhaas PJ, Haenschel C, Nikolić D, et al. (2008) The role of oscillations and synchrony in cortical networks and their putative relevance for the pathophysiology of schizophrenia. *Schizophr Bull* 34: 927–943.
31. Iragui VJ, McCutchen CB (1983) Physiologic and prognostic significance of" alpha coma". *J Neurol Neurosurg Psychiatry* 46: 632–638.
32. Angelakis E, Lubar JF, Stathopoulou S, et al. (2004) Peak alpha frequency: an electroencephalographic measure of cognitive preparedness. *Clin Neurophysiol* 115: 887–897.
33. Fuss FK (2016) A method for quantifying the emotional intensity and duration of a startle reaction with customized fractal dimensions of EEG signals. *Applied Mathematics* 7: 355–364.
34. Ekman P, Friesen WV, Simons RC (1985) Is the startle reaction an emotion?. *J Pers Soc Psychol* 49: 1416–1426.
35. Liu Y, Sourina O, Nguyen MK (2011) Real-time EEG-based emotion recognition and its applications, In: Gavrilova ML, Tan CJK Authors, *Transactions on computational science XII*, Berlin: Springer, 256–277.
36. Portnova G, Balaev V, Tetereva A, et al. (2018) Correlation of BOLD Signal with Linear and Nonlinear Patterns of EEG in Resting State EEG-Informed fMRI. *Front Hum Neurosci* 11: 654.
37. Bornas X, Tortella-Feliu M, Balle M, et al. (2013) Self-focused cognitive emotion regulation style as associated with widespread diminished EEG fractal dimension. *Int J Psychol* 48: 695–703.
38. Georgiev S, Minchev Z, Christova C, et al. (2009) EEG fractal dimension measurement before and after human auditory stimulation. *Bioautomation* 12: 70–81.
39. Koukkou M, Lehmann D, Wackermann J, et al. (1993) Dimensional complexity of EEG brain mechanisms in untreated schizophrenia. *Biol Psychiatry* 33: 397–407.

5

Effect of correlating adjacent neurons for identifying communications: Feasibility experiment in a cultured neuronal network

Yoshi Nishitani[1,*], Chie Hosokawa[2], Yuko Mizuno-Matsumoto[3], Tomomitsu Miyoshi[4] and Shinichi Tamura[5]

[1] Department of Radiology, Graduate School of Medicine, Osaka University, Suita 565-0871, Japan
[2] Biomedical Research Institute and Advanced Photonics and Biosensing Open Innovation Laboratory, AIST, Ikeda, Osaka 563-8577, Japan
[3] Graduate School of Applied Informatics, University of Hyogo, Kobe 650-0044, Japan
[4] Department of Integrative Physiology, Graduate School of Medicine, Osaka University, Suita 565-0871, Japan
[5] NBL Technovator Co., Ltd., Sennan 590-0522, Japan

* **Correspondence:** Email: ynishitani1027@gmail.com

Abstract: Neuronal networks have fluctuating characteristics, unlike the stable characteristics seen in computers. The underlying mechanisms that drive reliable communication among neuronal networks and their ability to perform intelligible tasks remain unknown. Recently, in an attempt to resolve this issue, we showed that stimulated neurons communicate *via* spikes that propagate temporally, in the form of spike trains. We named this phenomenon "*spike wave propagation*". In these previous studies, using neural networks cultured from rat hippocampal neurons, we found that multiple neurons, *e.g.*, 3 neurons, correlate to identify various spike wave propagations in a cultured neuronal network. Specifically, the number of *classifiable neurons* in the neuronal network increased through correlation of spike trains between current and adjacent neurons. Although we previously obtained similar findings through stimulation, here we report these observations on a physiological level. Considering that individual spike wave propagation corresponds to individual communication, a correlation between some adjacent neurons to improve the quality of communication classification in a neuronal network, similar to a diversity antenna, which is used to improve the quality of communication in artificial data communication systems, is suggested.

Keywords: cultured neuronal network; spike wave propagation; adjacent neurons; identifying communications; microelectrode array

1. Introduction

The brain is a well-known large neuronal network assembled through spike propagation (action potentials) through synapses [1–5]. How can neuronal networks comprising neurons with fluctuating characteristics reliably communicate (transmit information)? Many previous studies have attempted to answer this question, using spike-coding metrics [6], spatiotemporal coding models [7–13], and synchronous action models [14–18]. Since neuronal networks are considered spatiotemporal spike propagation fields and since the spatiotemporal form of spike activity is considered the fundamental generator of intelligence in the brain, these studies primarily aimed to investigate the principles of spike propagation in detail; however, these studies could not elucidate the basic means of communication between neurons. Therefore, the mechanisms underlying communication in the brain remain unknown.

In our previous studies attempting to resolve this issue, we reported that spikes propagating from stimulated neurons are received by afferent neurons as random-like sequences in simulated and natural asynchronous neuronal networks [19–24]. This phenomenon is similar to radio wave propagation in artificial data communication systems; hence, this phenomenon was referred to as "spike wave propagation." In these studies, we showed that stimulated neurons were able to identify various spatiotemporal patterns of spike wave propagation in specific areas (receiving area) of the neuronal network. From the viewpoint of communication, individual spike waves propagating from specific neurons are regarded as individual communication, thereby suggesting that distinct communications occur in multiple brain neuronal networks. In addition, certain adjacent neurons correlate to classify communications, in simulated neuronal networks [23].

On in-depth investigation, numerous neurons seem involved in communication, *e.g.*, 3 neurons in the receiving area, and result in smooth and stable spike propagation, whereas fewer neurons make communication more difficult. This suggests a correlation between some adjacent neurons to improve the classification quality of communication in neuronal networks, similar to diversity antennae, used to improve the quality of communication in artificial data communication systems [25].

Although this observation was exclusive to simulation studies, remarkable similarities in the manner of correlation in some adjacent neurons for intelligence activity have been observed [26]. If these similarities hold true, they could provide evidence to determine the mechanism underlying communication in the brain. To accomplish this, we need to investigate whether the same phenomenon is observed physiologically as with simulation. Thus, this study aimed to investigate this phenomenon in a cultured neuronal network and determine if its physiological correlates are in line with those demonstrated in previous simulation studies.

2. Materials and method

2.1. Coding spike trains from a cultured neuronal network

Hippocampal neurons were dissected from Wistar rats on embryonic day 18. The procedure conformed to the protocols approved by the Institutional Animal Care and Use Committee of the National Institute of Advanced Industrial Science and Technology. Cell culturing, stimulated spike recording, and coding spike trains were performed as described previously [24]. Figure 1 depicts the deposition of an electrode in microelectrode array (MEA) dishes with 64 (8 × 8) planar microelectrodes (channels). In this study, we cultured 5 samples of neuronal networks named cultures 01, 02, 03 planted on MED-P515A (spacing between electrodes, 150 μm) and cultures 04 and 05 planted on MED-P545A (spacing between electrodes, 450 μm). Two channels in each culture were selected as stimulation channels and 5–20 recordings were obtained from them. In this study, the stimulated channels are referred to as StimA and StimB. This experiment aimed to classify the StimA and B in accordance with time sequence data based on spike trains in specific neurons (current channels) and their adjacent neurons. The difference in stimulation channel was regarded as the difference of spike wave propagation [24].

2.2. Time sequence data with spike timing lag from adjacent channel

To estimate improvement in the classification quality of communication through correlation of adjacent neurons, as shown in Figure 2, we constructed time sequence data which linked the spike train interval of current channels (ch) with the time lag in spike train intervals between current and adjacent channels. Although Figure 2 shows only one adjacent channel for simplicity, several adjacent channels were actually referred. We compared the time sequence based on three types of adjacent channel locations, as shown in Figure 3. Moreover, time differences from the current channel are signs of delayed (+1) or preceding (−1) spike trains; however, this figure shows only delayed spike trains. Further, the encoded time sequence was generated from these time sequence data for the back propagation of neuronal networks (BPN) method described below in detail. These procedures were performed for all 64 channels in each culture.

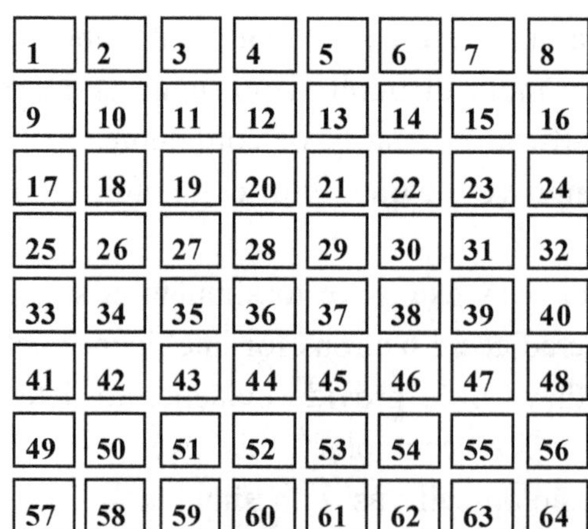

Figure 1. Deposition of electrodes in a microelectrode array. The size and spacing between electrodes were 50 × 50 μm^2 and 150 μm (MED-P515A) or 450 μm (MED-P545A), respectively. Each electrode corresponds to a channel of spike recording. The number indicates the electrode (channel) number.

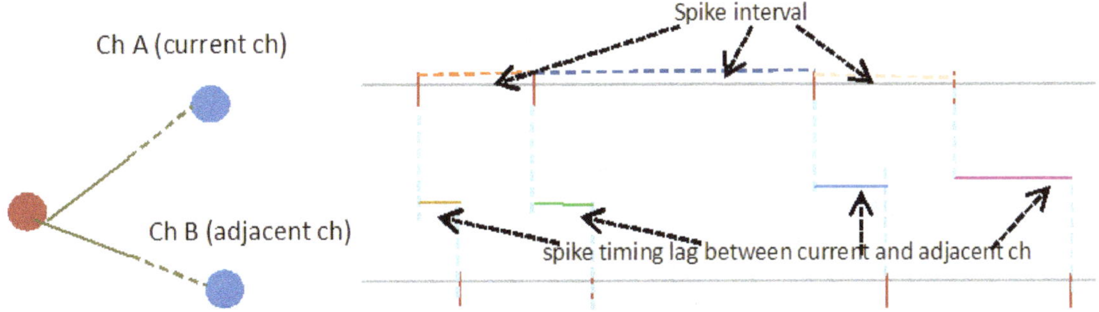

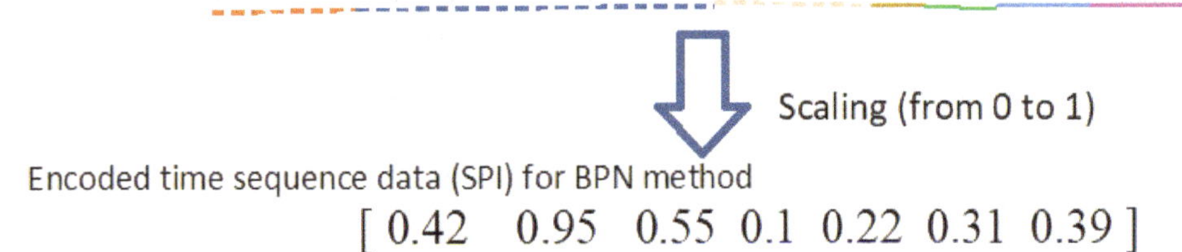

Figure 2. Procedure of generating time sequence data. The dashed color lines represent spike intervals in the current channel. Solid color lines are spike timing lags between the current and their adjacent neurons. The sequence data are spike train intervals in the current channel followed by the time lag in spike train intervals between current and adjacent channels. These time sequence data are encoded for the BPN method.

2.3. Classification by BPN method

On fluctuating conditions in neuronal networks, *e.g.*, synaptic weight, refractory period, and others, spatiotemporal patterns of spike wave propagations were not the same even if they were stimulated at the same channel in the same culture. Therefore, identifying the stimulated channels by only observing wave propagation is not easy. In our previous study, we used our original simple learning algorithm based on the arithmetic mean method for classification [24]. However, the resolution was not adequate to classify spike wave propagations completely. Thus, we believe that the BPN method has moderately strong pattern recognition ability [27] and could hence be applied to show the feasibility of classifying spatiotemporal patterns of spike wave propagation in neuronal networks, in this study.

Round–Robin learning and the test procedure for the BPN method are depicted in Figure 4. This figure depicts the example of the encoded data number and stimulation channel (stim ch) number in the case of culture 01 (stim ch 13 *vs* 54).

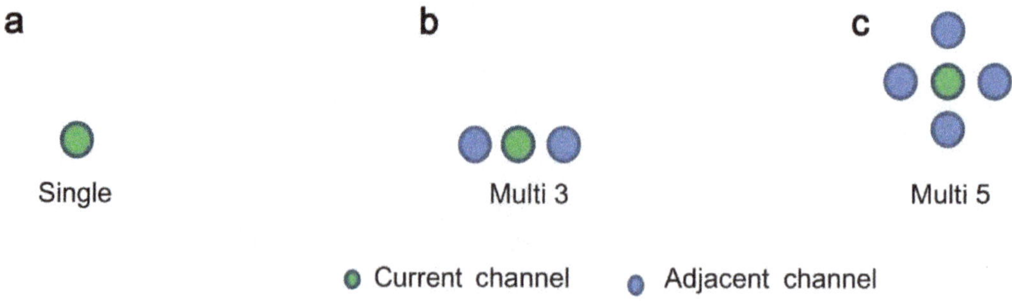

Figure 3. Location of adjacent channel. a: Without adjacent channels (only current channel) named *Single*; b: With right and left adjacent neurons named *Multi 3*; c: With right, left, upper, and lower adjacent neurons named *Multi 5*.

2.4. Estimation of the classification quality

To estimate the effect of correlation between current and adjacent channels and the classification quality, we calculated the rate of test data wherein the stimulation channel was detected correctly at the current channel in the BPN procedure; this was called "success rate ch" and the rate of test data wherein the stimulation channel was detected incorrectly (for example, in culture 01, the detection result was st54 when the real stimulating channel was channel 13) at current channel called fail rate ch. The equations for determining the success rate ch and fail rate ch are as follows:

$$\text{success rate}_{ch} = \frac{dtcablenum_{ch}}{test\ num} \times 100\ [\%] \tag{1}$$

$$\text{fail rate}_{ch} = \frac{eronum_{ch}}{test\ num} \times 100\ [\%] \tag{2}$$

In these equations, $dtcablenum_{ch}$ is the number of test data when the stimulation channel was detected correctly at the current channel, *test num* is the number of test data (5 to 10), $eronum_{ch}$ is the number of test data when the stimulation channel was detected incorrectly. In this study, we considered the $success\ rate_{ch} > 60\%$ as the *classifiable channel*. In other words, two different stimulations could correctly identify the *classifiable channel*. Furthermore, we regarded $fail\ rate_{ch} > 60\%$ as the *miss-classifiable channel*.

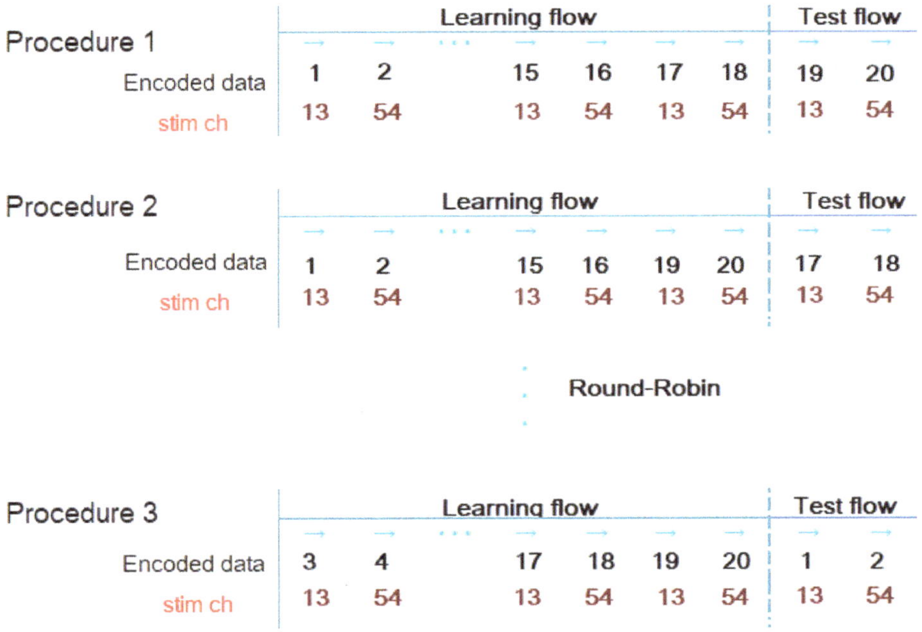

Procedure 1

	Learning flow						Test flow	
Encoded data	1	2	15	16	17	18	19	20
stim ch	13	54	13	54	13	54	13	54

Procedure 2

	Learning flow						Test flow	
Encoded data	1	2	15	16	19	20	17	18
stim ch	13	54	13	54	13	54	13	54

Round-Robin

Procedure 3

	Learning flow						Test flow	
Encoded data	3	4	17	18	19	20	1	2
stim ch	13	54	13	54	13	54	13	54

Figure 4. Round-Robin learning and test procedure for back propagation of neuronal networks (in culture 01). The example depicted here is of the encoded data number and stimulation channel (stim ch) number in the case of culture 01 (stim ch 13 *vs* 54). Twenty raster plot data (10 raster plot data stimulated from channel ch13 and 10 raster plot data stimulated from channel ch54) are encoded by the procedure shown in Figure 2; among them, two encoded data were selected for *Test Flow* and another 18 data were used for *Learning Flow*. Finally, all data were tested using the Round-Robin method.

3. Results and discussion

Figure 5 shows the number of *classifiable channels* and *miss-classifiable channels* in 64 channels in each culture in *Single*, *Multi3*, and *Multi5* (Figure 3). Though, in some cases, the number of *classifiable* channels is smaller in *Multi* than in *Single*, contrary to our assumption similar to that in Culture 03, we could confirm that the mean number of classifiable channels in all experiments in *Multi3* and *Multi5* was significantly larger than that in *Single* ($p < 0.05$). However, the difference between *Multi 5* and *Multi 3* was not significant; furthermore, *Multi 5* tended to be worse than *Multi 3*. Meanwhile, the number of *miss-classifiable channels* tended to be larger in *Multi* than in *Single*; however, in reality, they were fewer than the number of *classifiable channels*. These results show that the time lag in spike trains between adjacent neurons may effectively improve the quality of communication.

In these experiments, we could confirm the increase in the rate of classification through the schematic correlation of adjacent neurons. However, it remained unclear which neurons are classifiable by correlating adjacent neurons. Hence, we compared the distribution of classifiable channels in neuronal networks in *Single* and mul3 in Culture 1 and 3, as examples (Figure 6). We found that in culture 1, some unclassifiable channels in *Single* were classifiable in *Multi3* (indicated by yellow lattices in Figure 6). Moreover, these channels tended to concentrate in specific areas of the neuronal network. These tendencies were also observed in culture 3 despite the number of classifiable channels in *Multi3* being no more than that in *Single*, as shown in Figure 5(d). However, channels that classified only in *Single* (indicated by sky blue lattices in Figure 6) were also observed at similar numbers to that of the classifiable channels only in *Multi3* in culture 03. In contrast, in culture 01, the number of channels which classified only in *Single* was lower than those that became classifiable in *Multi3*. The difference between these results in Figure 5(a) and (d) corresponded to this. However, spacing between electrodes did not affect the experimental results (150 µm: culture 01, 02, and 03; 450 µm: culture 04 and 05).

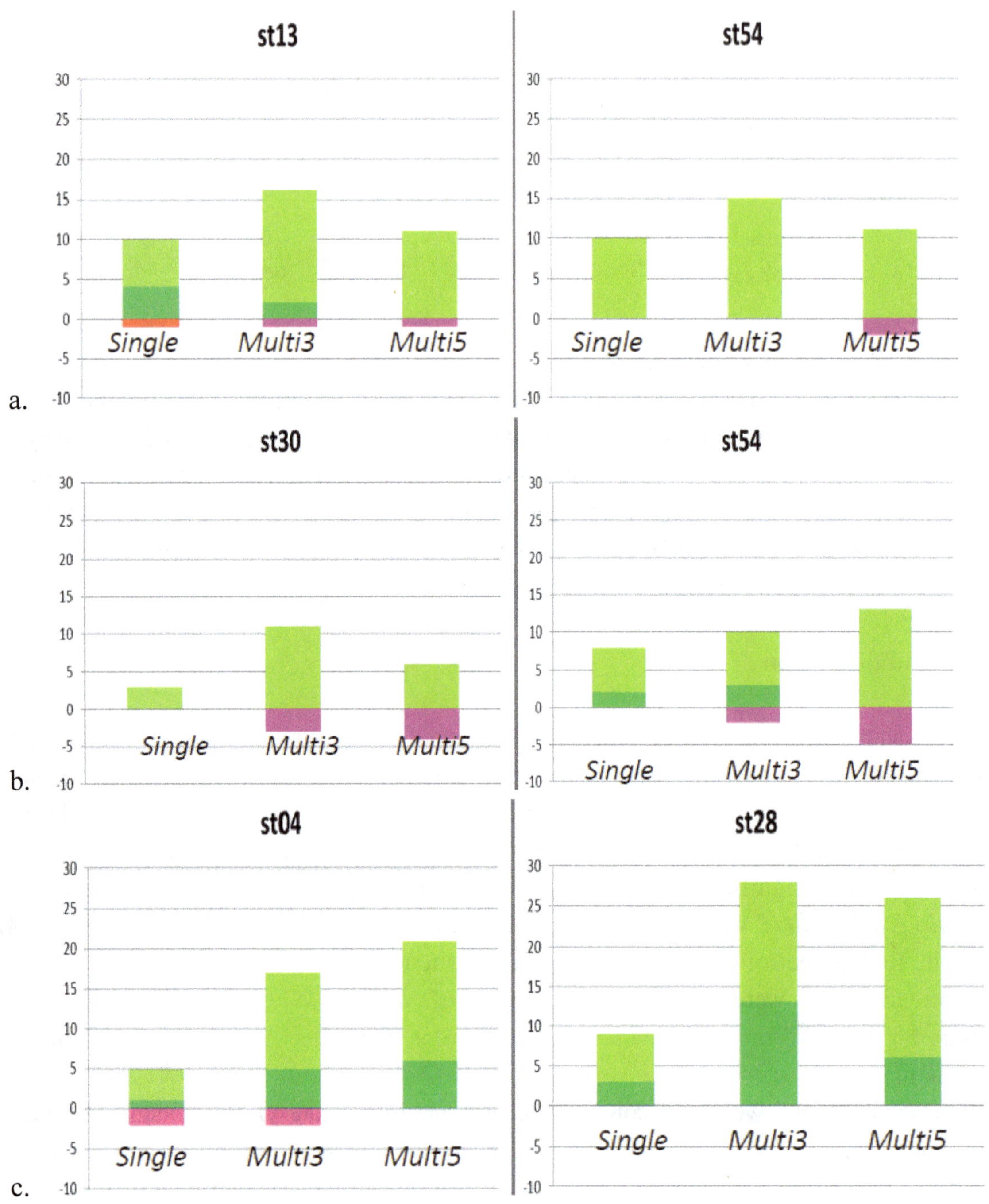

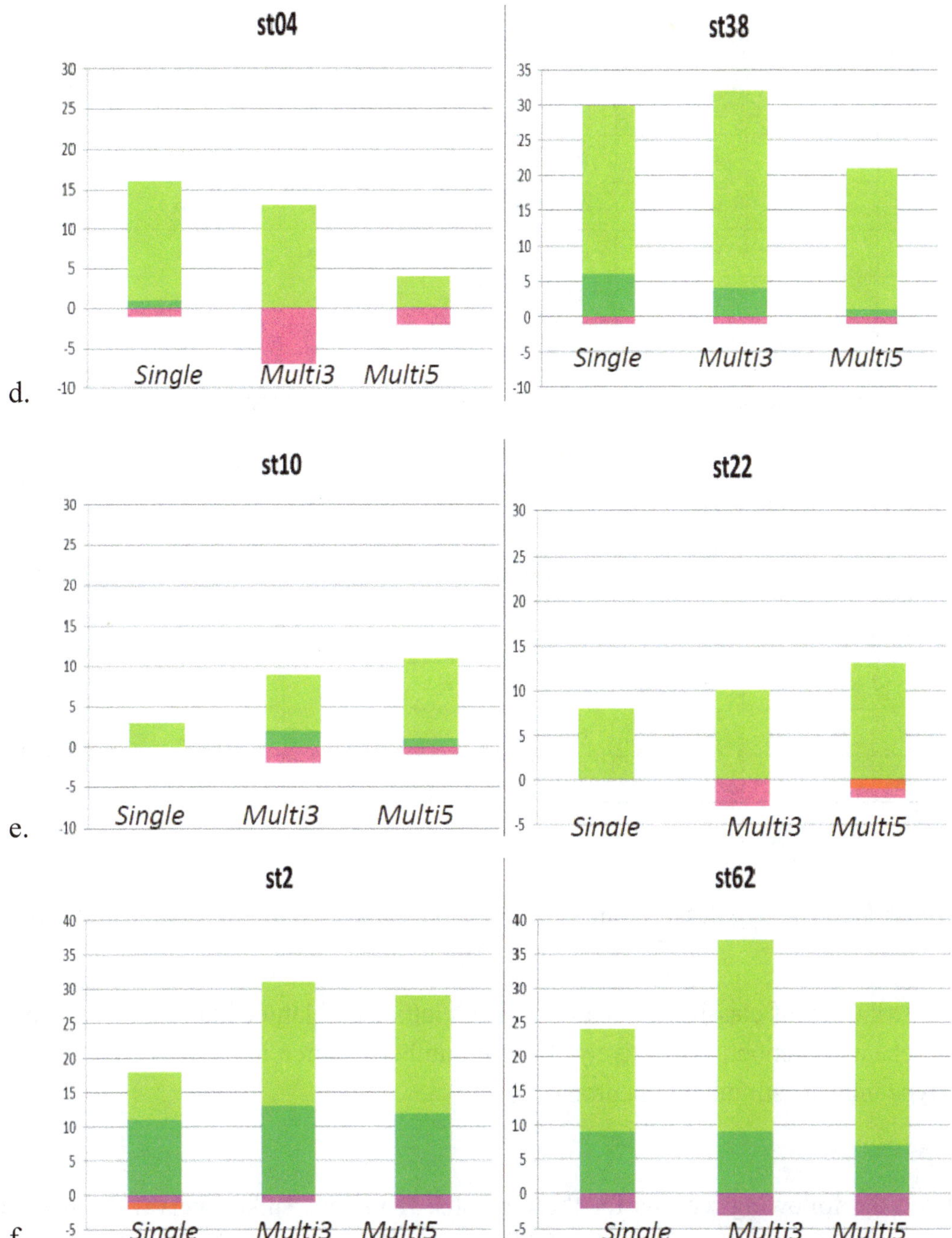

Figure 5. The number of classifiable channels in 64 channels in each culture.a: Culture 01 stimulation channel 13 *vs* 54; b: Culture 01 stimulation channel 30 *vs* 54; c: Culture 02 stimulation channel 04 *vs* 28; d: Culture 03 stimulation channel 04 *vs* 38; e: Culture 04 stimulation channel 10 *vs* 22; f: Culture 05 stimulation channel 2 *vs* 62. Vertical axis: Number of *classifiable channels* (positive) and *miss-classifiable channels* (negative); St: Stimulating channel.

1	2	3	4	5	6	7	8
9	10	11	12	***13***	14	15	16
17	18	19	20	21	22	23	24
25	26	27	28	29	30	31	32
33	34	35	36	37	38	39	40
41	42	43	44	45	46	47	48
49	50	51	52	53	***54***	55	56
57	58	59	60	61	62	63	64

st13 *vs* st54

1	2	3	4	5	6	7	8
9	10	11	12	***13***	14	15	16
17	18	19	20	21	22	23	24
25	26	27	28	29	30	31	32
33	34	35	36	37	38	39	40
41	42	43	44	45	46	47	48
49	50	51	52	53	***54***	55	56
57	58	59	60	61	62	63	64

st54 *vs* st13

1	2	3	***4***	5	6	7	8
9	10	11	12	13	14	15	16
17	18	19	20	21	22	23	24
25	26	27	28	29	30	31	32
33	34	35	36	37	***38***	39	40
41	42	43	44	45	46	47	48
49	50	51	52	53	54	55	56
57	58	59	60	61	62	63	64

st04 *vs* st38

1	2	3	***4***	5	6	7	8
9	10	11	12	13	14	15	16
17	18	19	20	21	22	23	24
25	26	27	28	29	30	31	32
33	34	35	36	37	***38***	39	40
41	42	43	44	45	46	47	48
49	50	51	52	53	54	55	56
57	58	59	60	61	62	63	64

st38 *vs* st04

Classified in *Multi3* only   Classified in *Single* only   Classified in both *Single* and *Multi3*

Figure 6. Distribution of classifiable channels. Each lattice and lattice number indicate a channel and channel number, respectively. Lattice numbers written in ***colored (red/blue) bold italic type*** indicate stimulating neurons.

We considered the following reasons for these results. If various spike interval trains of trials are large even in the same stimulation channel, it is difficult to detect the stimulation channel of only the spike interval train in the current channel. However, if the time lag in the spike trains between the current channel and the adjacent channel does not display variety, stimulated neurons could only be detected from the train of the time lag. The image so obtained is shown in Figure 7. In this case, the stimulation channel is detectable from the difference in spike timing between the current channel and the adjacent channel. When spike interval trains in all experiments in the current channel did not display variety, only the spike train intervals in the current channel were adequate to detect the stimulation channel. The image so obtained is shown in Figure 8. In this case, it is possible that the rate of classification is worse based on the variety of spike trains in the adjacent channel.

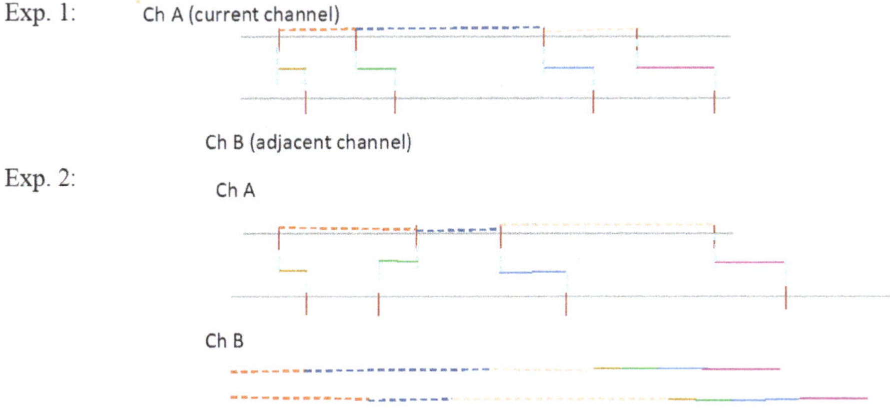

Figure 7. A case wherein correlating the adjacent neuron was effective. The meaning of the culler horizonal line and dashed culler horizonal line is the same as that in Figure 2.

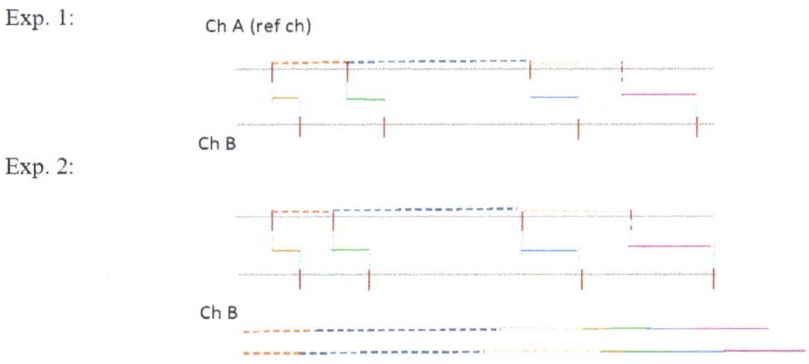

Figure 8. A case wherein correlating the adjacent neuron was not effective. The meaning of the culler horizonal line and dashed culler horizonal line is same as that in Figure 2.

To substantiate these assumptions, we decorrelated the current channel and adjacent channel by *channel shuffling* for all cultured samples; the procedure followed is shown in Figure 9. Thereafter, we performed the same experiments for the shuffled data, as for the original data.

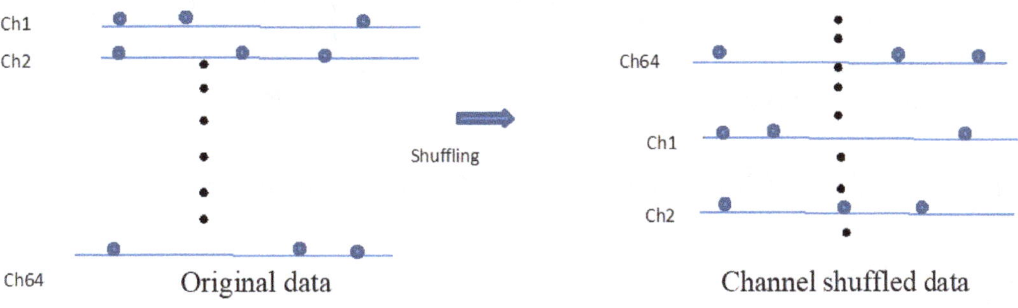

Figure 9. Channel shuffling. The row of channels was shuffled randomly, retaining the spike trains in each channel.

Figure 10 shows the number of *classifiable channels* and *miss-classifiable channels*, and Figure 11 depicts the example of the distribution of *classifiable channels* in neuronal networks in *Single* and *Multi3* for *channel shuffled data* of culture 01. Although data from other cultures are not shown owing to lack of space, results from these cultures were similar to those from culture 01, as described below. In this experiment, the detection of classifiable channels was performed only with *Multi3*, since it is adequate to determine the effect of neurons if this effect is observable in *Multi3* or *Multi5*; however, it is considered that the results after channel shuffling remain the same as before channel shuffling in *Single*.

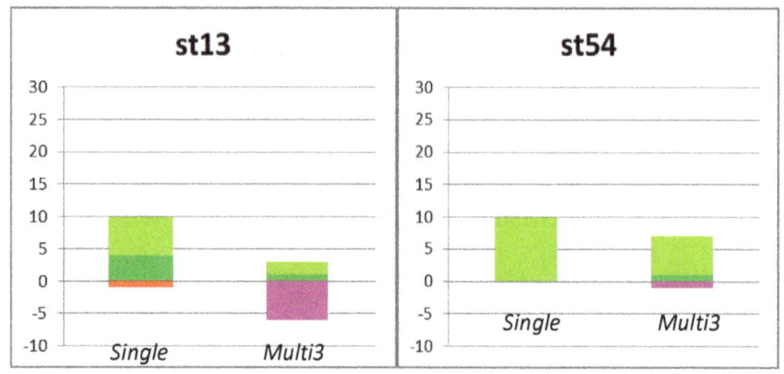

Figure 10. The number of detectable channels in 64 channels after ch shuffling in culture 01. Vertical axis: Number of *classifiable channels* (positive) and *miss-classifiable channels* (negative). st: Stimulating channel.

Multi3 mean values were remarkably lower than those of *Single*; however, there was no significant difference between their mean values in all cultures.

1	2	3	4	5	6	7	8
9	10	11	12	***13***	14	15	16
17	18	19	20	21	22	23	24
25	26	27	28	29	30	31	32
33	34	35	36	37	38	39	40
41	42	43	44	45	46	47	48
49	50	51	52	53	***54***	55	56
57	58	59	60	61	62	63	64

a. Classifiable st13 (*vs* st54)

1	2	3	4	5	6	7	8
9	10	11	12	***13***	14	15	16
17	18	19	20	21	22	23	24
25	26	27	28	29	30	31	32
33	34	35	36	37	38	39	40
41	42	43	44	45	46	47	48
49	50	51	52	53	***54***	55	56
57	58	59	60	61	62	63	64

b. Classifiable st54 (*vs* st13)

Classified in *Multi3* only Classified in *Single* only Classified in both *Single* and *Multi3*

Figure 11. Distribution of classifiable channels after ch shuffling in culture 01(st13 *vs* 54). Each lattice and lattice number indicates the channel and channel number, respectively. Lattice numbers written in colored (red/blue) bold italic type indicate stimulating neurons.

Based on the results from all cultures in this experiment, we could confirm that the number of *classifiable channels* in the shuffled data was significantly ($p < 0.05$) lower than that in the original data in *Multi3* (Cf. Figure 10 *vs* Figure 5(a), and Figure 11 *vs* Figure 6(a)). However, the difference between *Multi3* and *Single* was not significant in the shuffled data, although the values in *Multi3* were lower than those in *Single* in several cultures including culture 01 (Figure 10), against those in the original data.

In summary, we could confirm the effect of spike timing lag between the current and their adjacent neurons. The higher number of *classifiable channel*s in *Multi3,5* than in *Single* was not a chance event. Considering that individual stimulation channels correspond to individual communication, in this study, although the classification quality of communications was not always improved, various communications could be characterized by the correlating spike trains of adjacent neurons even when they could not be characterized by only the current neuron.

4. Conclusion

In our recent study, we showed that stimulated neurons could identify various spatiotemporal patterns of spike wave propagation in particular areas of neuronal networks. From the viewpoint of communication, this essentially suggests that distinct communications occur *via* multiple communicating links in the brain. Here, we showed that the quality of communication classification tends to improve *via* correlation of spike trains in current and their adjacent neurons. This shows that neighboring neurons work in harmony to identify communication. Assuming a communication path is a type of memory, it seems that the present results are concurrent with previous ones, indicating that some adjacent neurons work in harmony; however, this requires more detailed investigation.

Acknowledgments

The authors thank Y. Maezawa and M. Onishi (AIST) for the cell cultures. This study was partly supported by the Grants-in-Aid for Scientific Research of Exploratory Research JP21656100, JP25630176, JP16K12524, and Scientific Research (A) JP22246054 and JP16H06504 of the Japan Society for the Promotion of Science. We would like to thank Editage (www.editage.com) for English language editing.

References

1. Bonifazi P, Goldin M, Picardo MA, et al. (2009) GABAergic hub neurons orchestrate synchrony in developing hippocampal networks. *Science* 326: 1419–1424.
2. Lecerf C (1998) The double loop as a model of a learning neural system. Proceedings World Multiconference on Systemics. *Cybernetics Informatics* 1: 587–594.
3. Choe Y (2002) Analogical Cascade: A theory on the role of the thalamo-cortical loop in brain function. *Neurocomputing* 52: 713–719.

4. Tamura S, Mizuno-Matsumoto Y, Chen YW, et al. (2009) Association and abstraction on neural circuit loop and coding. *IIHMSP* 10-07: 546-549 (appears in IEEE Xplore)
5. Thorpre S, Fize D, Marlot C (1996) Speed of processing in the human visual system. *Nature* 381: 520.
6. Cessac B, Paugam-Moisy H, Viéville T (2010) Overview of facts and issues about neural coding by spike. *J Physiol-Paris* 104: 5–18.
7. Kliper O, Horn D, Quenet B, et al. (2004) Analysis of spatiotemporal patterns in a model of olfaction. *Neurocomputing* 58: 1027–1032.
8. Fujita K, Kashimori Y, Kambara T (2007) Spatiotemporal burst coding for extracting features of spatiotemporally varying stimuli. *Biol Cybern* 97: 293–305.
9. Tyukin I, Tyukina T, Van LC (2009) Invariant template matching in systems with spatiotemporal coding: A matter of instability. *Neural Networks* 22: 425–449.
10. Mohemmed A, Schliebs S, Matsuda S, et al. (2013) Training spiking neural networks to associate spatio-temporal input–output spike patterns. *Neurocomputing* 107: 3–10.
11. Olshausen BA, Field DJ (1996) Emergence of simple-cell receptive field properties by learning a sparse code for natural images. *Nature* 381: 607–609.
12. Bell AJ, Sejnowski TJ (1997) The "independent components" of natural scenes are edge filters. *Vision Res* 37: 3327–3338.
13. Aviel Y, Horn D, Abeles M (2004) Synfire waves in small balanced networks. *Neural Computation* 58-60: 123-127.
14. Abeles M (1982) Local Cortical Circuits: An Electrophysiological study, Springer, Berlin.
15. Abeles M (2009) Synfire chains. Scholarpedia 4: 1441. Available from: http://www.scholarpedia.org/article/Synfire_chains.
16. Izhikevich EM (2014) Polychronization: Computation with spikes. *Neural Comput* 18: 245–282.
17. Perc M (2007) Fluctuating excitability: A mechanism for self-sustained information flow in excite arrays. *Chaos Soliton Fract* 32: 1118–1124.
18. Zhang H, Wang Q, Perc M, et al. (2013) Synaptic plasticity induced transition of spike propagation in neuronal networks. *Commun Nonlinear Sci* 18: 601–615.
19. Mizuno-Matsumoto Y, Okazaki K, Kato A, et al. (1999) Visualization of epileptogenic phenomena using crosscorrelation analysis: Localization of epileptic foci and propagation of epileptiform discharges. *IEEE Trans Biomed Eng* 46: 271–279.
20. Mizuno-Matsumoto Y, Ishijima M, Shinosaki K, et al. (2001) Transient global amnesia (TGA) in an MEG study. *Brain Topogr* 13: 269–274.
21. Nishitani Y, Hosokawa C, Mizuno-Matsumoto Y, et al. (2012) Detection of M-sequences from spike sequence in neuronal networks. *Comput Intell Neurosci* 2012: 167–185.
22. Nishitani Y, Hosokawa C, Mizuno-Matsumoto Y, et al. (2014) Synchronized code sequences from spike trains in cultured neuronal networks. *Int J Eng Ind* 5: 13–24.
23. Tamura S, Nishitani Y, Hosokawa C, et al. (2016) Simulation of code spectrum and code flow of cultured neuronal networks. *Comput Intell Neurosci* 2016: 1–12.
24. Nishitani Y, Hosokawa C, Mizuno-Matsumoto Y, et al. (2016) Classification of spike wave propagations in a cultured neuronal network: Investigating a brain communication mechanism. *AIMS Neurosci* 4: 1–13.

25. Hourani H (2004) Overview of diversity techniques in wireless communication systems, postgraduate course in radio communications.
26. Buzsáki G (2010) Neural syntax: cell assemblies, synapsembles, and readers. *Neuron* 68: 362–385.
27. Rumelhart DE, Hinton GE, Williams RJ (1986) Learning representations by back-propagating errors. *Nature* 323: 533–536.

6

Reviving pragmatic theory of theory of mind

Chiyoko Kobayashi Frank[1,2,*]

[1] School of Psychology, Fielding Graduate University, Santa Barbara, CA, USA
[2] Center for Cognition and Communication, New York, NY, USA

* **Correspondence:** Email: ckobayashi@fielding.edu.

Abstract: Theory of Mind (ToM) refers to the ability to attribute mental states to self and others. It has been debated whether or not language capacity precedes ToM in development. Evidence from both neurological and developmental studies suggested that while linguistic capacity is important for ToM understanding, pragmatic component, which is a non-structural part of language, is more important for ToM. Moreover, given that pragmatic component of language is subserved by the right hemisphere of the brain, the evidence also indicates a significant overlap between the neural basis of ToM and that of pragmatic comprehension. The pragmatic theory of ToM, which I aim to revive in this review, firmly links pragmatics to ToM. It regards pragmatic aspects of language and ToM as extensively overlapping functions. I argue that research results from both developmental and neurological studies of ToM are beginning to converge to support this theory. Furthermore, I maintain that the pragmatic theory of ToM provides the best explanation for the seemingly incongruent results from recent child and infant studies on the developmental trajectory of ToM. Lastly, I will discuss whether this theory is in agreement with the domain-specific, the nativist framework, or neither.

Keywords: theory of mind; pragmatics; language; right-hemisphere damage; brain imaging; false-belief; domain-specificity

---

1. Introduction

Theory of Mind (ToM) refers to the ability to attribute mental states such as beliefs and intentions to self and/or others [1]. To date, ToM or *mentalizing* [2] has been tested with a variety of tasks in several psychiatric conditions. Many of these studies found aberrant patterns of performances in the clinical groups compared to the healthy control groups. Deficits in ToM or *under-mentalizing* has been found in several psychiatric conditions including autism spectrum conditions (ASC) [2–4] and schizophrenia [5–7], while *over-mentalizaing* has been found in a few conditions such as social anxiety disorder (SAD) [8] and borderline personality disorder (BPD) [9]. A core cognitive feature of individuals with ASC has been described as a difficulty in understanding others' mental states including their false-beliefs [3,4]. Likewise, a key feature of psychotic symptoms has been described as misrepresentation of one's own and others' intentions [5,6]. In contrast, it has been found that people with SAD and BPD show more excessive mentalizing than healthy adults [8,9].

The pragmatic component of language is difficult to define. But to state simply, it involves bringing in general world knowledge, integrating the individual utterances with the context, and making inferences based on one's prior knowledge [10]. Grice [11–13] proposed that our everyday conversations are based on a cooperative principle which has four maxims or rules; i.e., quantity, quality, relation or relevance, and manner. For instance, based on the relevance maxim, we generally do not tell someone about a book that we read in the middle of giving the person a direction to a hospital. Depending on the contexts, pragmatics can include understanding humors, ironies, metaphors, and indirect requests [14,15]. In a broader sense, pragmatics can be thought as *speech acts*, the main purpose of which is to change the attitudes or beliefs of the other conversant [12,16,17] and they may be present even in infants [16].

It has long been debated whether or not a person has to have sophisticated language skills in order to have ToM capacity. Some argue that ToM ability precedes language in development [18–20], while others maintain that language is a necessary precursor for ToM [21,22]. A seminal longitudinal study demonstrated that earlier language task competency predicts ToM performance later in development [21]. However, the reverse was not the case; i.e., earlier ToM task competency did not predict later language performance. A meta-analysis of more than a hundred studies that examined the relationship between language and ToM supported the latter, often dubbed "linguistic determinism" hypothesis of ToM [22,23]. The meta-analysis strengthened the seminal study's results by demonstrating that across different versions of the false-belief task, earlier language capacity independently contributes to later ToM and not the other way around [23]. However, the meta-analysis was limited in that it did not take into account the effects of pragmatics on ToM.

A more recent meta-analysis using a quantitative method found a significant overlap between the neural basis of ToM and that of pragmatic language comprehension [24]. The overlapping brain regions include typical ToM regions; i.e., the medial prefrontal cortex (mPFC) [25–29] and the bilateral temporo-parietal junction (TPJ) [27–30]. These results are in line with the observation that children with ASC have primary deficits in pragmatic aspects of language [31–33]. Children with ASC, for example, might understand a request, "Can you pass me the salt?" as a question about their ability to pass the salt because of the pragmatic deficit. Moreover, it has been shown that people with schizophrenia have impairments not only in ToM but also in understanding figurative, pragmatic aspects of language [6,34,35]. These findings point to a close relationship between pragmatics and ToM.

Over the past 10 years, the field of ToM research has changed dramatically. There are now numerous studies of infants aged 6–18 months using various non-verbal ToM tasks claiming that even the pre-verbal infants understand ToM [36–39]. These results presented challenge to the commonly accepted hypothesis that ToM develops only around 4 years of age [40]. In order to fill-in the seeming incongruence between results from child studies and those from infant studies of ToM, two main developmental hypotheses were presented. These are the two-system [41] and two-stage [42] hypotheses on the developmental trajectory of ToM (see below for more detailed explanations of these hypotheses). However, the seemingly large gap in the developmental trajectory of ToM can also be explained by the pragmatic hypothesis (as I will explain below).

There are two main aims for this review paper. One is to examine the pragmatic theory of ToM. The pragmatic theory of ToM is not new. Frith, for instance, described schizophrenia as a disorder of pragmatics and thereby, he equated pragmatics to ToM [6,34]. Likewise, Sperber and Wilson [43] described ToM as a specialized sub-module of pragmatics. Similarly, Malle [44] posited that ToM and pragmatics are co-evolved functions. Most recently, Westra and Carruthers [45] claimed that ToM development is largely dependent upon the pragmatic (i.e., perspective-taking) development. According to my version of the pragmatic theory of ToM, ToM and pragmatic aspects of language are so fused that they cannot be separable. In other words, mine is a stronger position than those mentioned above and is akin to Tom Givón's view [44]. While this theory is preliminary and subject to criticisms and challenges which I will explain in Section 7, results from recent developmental and neuroscientific studies all seem to point to this stronger position. I maintain that research evidence from both developmental and neurological studies including my (and my colleagues') own, has converged to support the long forgotten theory. The other main aim of this review is to delineate the seeming gap in the developmental trajectory of ToM. On this issue, I maintain that the pragmatic theory provides the best explanation for the seeming jump in the development of ToM. Thus my view is in agreement with Westra and Carruthers' [45]. Implications of this theory may or may not challenge the notion of domain-specificity and nativist framework of ToM.

There are several mainstream theories of ToM and pragmatics. The mainstream theories of ToM are modular [46,47], theory-theory [40,48], simulation [49,50], and the aforementioned linguistic determinism theory [22]. Current prominent theories of pragmatics are Grice's speech act (see above) and relevance theory [43]. Previously, these theories have received both validations and invalidations empirically by different researchers [40, 51–55]. However, none of these theories has fully delineated the relationship between pragmatics and ToM. In this short review, in order to provide focused arguments, I will discuss some of these theories only in relation to the pragmatic theory of ToM. Readers can refer to other reviews (including my own) [40, 51–56] that provide more extensive discussions or comparisons of these theories of ToM and/or pragmatics.

2. Evidence from developmental studies

If language is necessary for ToM, it follows that preverbal infants and toddlers do not understand ToM. Results from some studies of ToM in infants demonstrated otherwise. A series of infant studies that used looking-preference paradigm found that even 13–15 month-old infants have the capacity for ToM [36–39,57]. However, these results are seemingly inconsistent with the results from other studies that tested older preschool children using false-belief tasks [40]. In a typical false-belief test, a child is presented with a scenario, in which an object is moved by a protagonist while another protagonist is absent, so that the latter mistakenly believes the object is still in its last location. The child is then asked about the false-belief of the latter protagonist. The purpose of the false-belief test is to assess one's understanding of others' beliefs that may be different from his/her own [3,4]. The nearly universally observed results are that 4 and 5 year-olds are successful at the false-belief test, while 3 year-olds and older children with ASC are not [3,4,44]. Some posit that the seeming gap in the developmental trajectory of ToM can be explained by the two-stage or two-system hypothesis of ToM [41,42]. According to the former, the verbal, explicit ToM matures only after the non-verbal, implicit ToM [42]. According to the latter, the first subsystem that enables infants to discriminate multiple mental states emerges earlier than the second subsystem that capacitates 4 year-olds to discriminate reality incongruent informational states [41].

In contrary to the above hypotheses, Westra and Carruthers [45] posited that apparent incongruent results can better be accounted for by the development of pragmatics. According to this view, a child's success or failure in the false-belief task depends on whether the child can take the detached third person perspective. Because three year-old children can only take the second person perspective, they respond based on their interpretation of ostensive communicative intention [12,43]. The ostensive communicative intention (the main purpose of which is to produce a perceptual/cognitive/behavioral change in the recipient) can either be *cooperative* or *competitive* [58]. For instance, children fail the task because they try to help the main character in the story (cooperative bias) or to exhibit their knowledge and show the experimenter where the toy is now (competitive bias). Thus, according to the pragmatic hypothesis, children younger than three fail the false-belief task because of their immature pragmatic interpretation which can either be cooperative or competitive [45,58].

Ultimately, from the perspective of the full-fledged pragmatic theory of ToM, which I maintain in this review, the above seemingly incongruent results between studies on preschool children and those on preverbal infants are not inconsistent at all. This is because in a broader sense, pragmatic aspects of language include any communicative actions or speech acts such as turn-taking, pointing, cooing, or bubbling that typical infants display [59]. It has been shown that as early as 3 months, infants can coordinate their rhythms with caretakers' rhythms [59–61]. The turn-taking, the first prototypical pragmatic ability, appears as early as 3 to 6 months of age [62,63]. Pointing, another prototype of the speech act [64,65], emerges around 9 to 12 months of age [66].

Thus, according to the pragmatic theory of ToM, the seemingly incongruent research results from the infants and preschool children are not at all incogruent. This theory views that developmental trajectory of ToM is more continuous and gradual than the two-system or the two-stage hypothesis. At very early points in life, newborns already have the prototypical ToM/speech acts, which will later develop to the full-fledged speech acts. According to this scenario, children learn some prototypical pragmatic ability in early, preverbal stage of life and later these skills develop to an array of speech acts including making requests and conveying refusals, with appropriate inputs from adults [59]. Also, according to this scenario, as children acquire the expressive pragmatic skills along with other aspects of language; i.e., syntactic and semantic aspects, they develop higher levels of speech acts such as understanding of ironies, jokes, metaphors, and false-beliefs.

3. Evidence from brain lesion studies

It has been well-established that in human adults, syntactic and semantic aspects of language are specialized in the left hemisphere of the brain [67], while pragmatic aspects of language are specialized in the right hemisphere of the brain [68–70]. Several studies on patients with brain injuries showed that right-hemisphere-damaged (RHD) patients have difficulty with understanding non-literal verbal expressions while they have no problem in understanding literal expressions [69,70]. It has been shown that RHD patients have difficulty with understanding indirect speeches [71], non-literal and figurative expressions including idioms and proverbs [72,73], humors [74], lies and jokes [75], and sarcasms [76]. Likewise, it has been demonstrated that RHD patients have difficulty in recognizing prosodic cues such as tone of voices and facial expressions [77–79]. In a more recent study, the RHD patients with aphasia performed significantly worse in tasks involving formulaic or pragmatic language processing than the left-hemisphere-damaged (LHD) patients with aphasia [80]. On the contrary to the RHD group, the LHD group performed significantly better in tasks that involved literal language processing. Taken together, these results support a dual model of discourse processing which claims that *sentence grammar* and *discourse grammar* are processed in different hemispheres of the brain [81]. The discourse grammar involves non-literal, pragmatic aspects of language and is processed primarily in the right hemisphere of the brain, while the sentence grammar concerns constitutive aspects of language and is processed primarily in the left hemisphere of the brain [81,82].

Similar results were found in ToM studies on brain damaged patients. These studies consistently demonstrated that while RHD patients fail the false-belief task, LHD patients pass the task [83–85]. For instance, a study found a specific impairment in attributing mental states in the second-order format in a group of RHD patients [84]. Similar results were found in another study that used a non-verbal, cartoon-based task in which patients were asked to infer the intentions from geometric shapes. In this study, a group of RHD patients attributed intentions to geometric shapes more inappropriately compared to a group of people without brain damage [86]. Moreover, in a different study, RHD patients performed more poorly than the typical adults, both in a task that required understanding of pragmatic aspects of language and in another task that required ToM capacity [87]. Taken together, these results are in agreement with the pragmatic theory of ToM indicating that both ToM and pragmatics are subserved by the right hemisphere of the brain. However, the brain injury studies are relatively ambiguous about precisely which regions in the right hemisphere are involved in both ToM and pragmatics. In what follows, I will discuss brain imaging studies to address the issue of regional specificity of the neural basis of ToM/pragmatics.

4. Evidence from neuroimaging studies

As the results from the developmental studies and brain lesion studies, which I described above, results from brain imaging studies of ToM seem to be in agreement with the pragmatic theory of ToM. Among the ToM brain regions, the medial prefrontal cortex (mPFC) has been the most consistently implicated in ToM [25,88,89]. The dorsal mPFC (dmPFC), in particular, has been found to be activated during pragmatic language processing [90–92]. For instance, it has been demonstrated that understanding verbal ironies recruits the dmPFC [79,80]. This region has also been most frequently implicated in both verbal and nonverbal ToM [27,28,89,93,94]. Moreover, the dmPFC has been shown to be active during both a ToM task and another, different task that requires pragmatic language processing [90]. Results from my study are consistent with this line of results. Through a convergent analysis, I also found converged ToM-specific activity across 56 monolingual and bilingual adult and child participants in the right dmPFC, although the most robust convergence was found in a region more right-lateral than the dmPFC [52].

As I mentioned earlier, a large meta-analysis across more than a hundred of brain imaging studies found a significant functional and anatomical overlap between ToM and pragmatic language comprehension [24]. These results are consistent with a different, earlier meta-analysis that found an extended overlap between the neural correlates of ToM and those of pragmatics, even after excluding verbal ToM tasks [10]. Most recently, my colleagues and I examined whether pragmatic language or ToM has independent contribution to false-belief reasoning in adults [29]. In this study, we found no evidence for the independent contribution of ToM or pragmatics, in either men or women. Both men and women activated the TPJ during both the coherent story condition (that tapped pragmatic comprehension ability) and false-belief condition equally strongly (Figure 1). As I mentioned earlier, TPJ is another brain region most frequently implicated in ToM [26,28–30,89]. These results indicate that neural correlates of ToM and those of pragmatic comprehension are very similar if not the same.

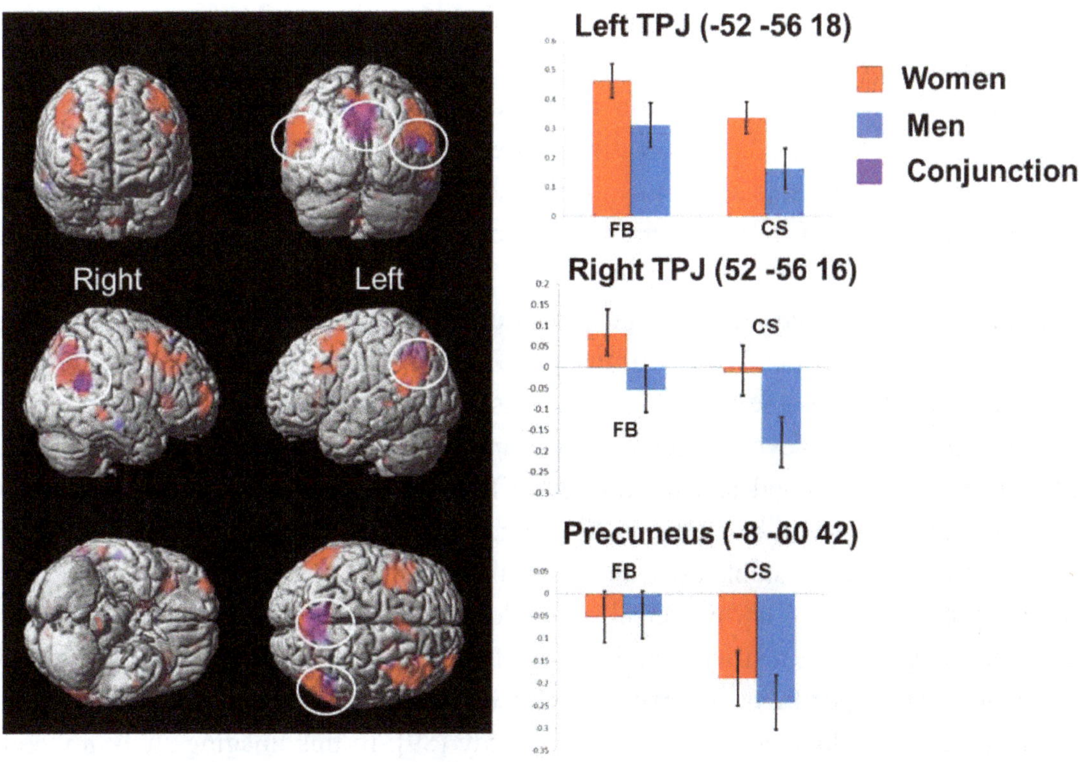

Figure 1. Convergent activity between sexes. The convergent brain activity between sexes was found in the TPJ bilaterally and the precuneus. However, we did not find any sex difference in the false-belief reasoning when we controlled for the coherence or pragmatic aspects in stories by the Coherent Story (CS) condition. Adapted, with permission [29].

Taken together, converged results from developmental, brain lesion and brain imaging studies of ToM and pragmatics are in agreement with the pragmatic theory of ToM. In contrast, as I maintained in my 2010 paper [52], these results are inconsistent with the constitutive language hypothesis or "linguistic determinism" hypothesis of ToM put forward by several others [21,22]. It is not an aim of this article to argue for that constitutive aspects of language are unimportant for ToM. However, the converged results indicate that these aspects are relatively less important than the pragmatic aspects for ToM.

5. Domain-specificity and pragmatic theory of ToM

It might be warranted to discuss whether or not the pragmatic theory of ToM is in agreement with the idea of domain-specificity. Some researchers argued for the modularity or domain-specificity of ToM [20,55,95–97] and others posited for the domain-generality of ToM [21,98,99]. The pragmatic theory of ToM is in line with neither of these extreme positions. Instead, it may be consistent with the *domain-relevance* hypothesis of ToM put forward by Karmiloff-Smith [100]. The domain-relevance hypothesis maintains that a domain-specificity develops from neither a tabula rasa start state nor a modular box state; but from a largely undifferentiated domain-general state to a more differentiated domain-specific state. Research evidence that I will describe below seems to support the domain-relevance hypothesis, but only in the reverse direction; i.e., from the domain-specificity to domain-general.

As I discussed earlier, the pragmatic theory of ToM views pragmatics as an equivalent function to ToM. Even though the pragmatics is a component of language, it is strongly tied to contexts unlike other components such as syntactic and semantic components. Pragmatic capacity or ability to understand communicative intentions cannot develop without appropriate environmental inputs or cultural influences. To support this point, while developmental, longitudinal studies of pragmatics are relatively scarce, there are numerous cross-cultural studies that showed evidence of cultural influences on pragmatics [101]. For instance, there are some significant cultural differences in how politeness [102], self-assertion [103], requests [104], and interrogative communicative acts [103] are recognized and conveyed. Likewise, there are equally numerous studies that demonstrated that mental states are understood and interpreted differently in different cultures [27,105,106]. In other words, research evidence has demonstrated that both ToM and pragmatics are significantly malleable and vulnerable to contextual or cultural influences. Thus, they are by no means "informationally encapsulated" or "universal" in Fodor's [96] sense. Therefore, I would argue that neither ToM nor pragmatics is a strictly modular function. However, ToM may become increasingly less modular or domain-specific as a person matures or develops as evidenced in the results of my (and my colleagues') developmental neuroimaging study [89]. In this imaging study my colleagues and I tested bilingual adults and children for their false-belief story understanding. The relevant results are that bilingual adults activated seemingly more dorsal mPFC area during the L1 (Japanese) ToM condition but more ventral mPFC area during the L2 (English) condition. However, bilingual children activated more converged or overlapping mPFC regions of the brain for both conditions. I would argue that it is bilingual adults' ToM that had experienced more contextual or cultural impacts cumulatively over the years. Similar results were found in research on pragmatics. A systematic meta-analysis of brain injury studies on adults indicated that pragmatic capacity is associated with an array of cognitive domains [107]. In this meta-analysis, the authors computed correlations between pragmatics and five key cognitive constructs (i.e., declarative memory, working memory, attention, executive functions, and social cognition). They found significant moderate-to-strong correlations between pragmatics and all of these constructs. These results demonstrate progressively less functional specialization and more generalization in adults' ToM/pragmatics than in children's ToM/pragmatics; therefore, they seem to support the progressively less domain-specificity or the domain-relevance hypothesis of ToM in the reverse direction.

6. Nativism and pragmatic hypothesis of ToM

Along with the domain-specificity, Fodor [96] included innateness as one of the criteria for modularity. It may not be an exaggeration to state that many of the aforementioned developmental studies were conducted in order to support the innateness of ToM because one can claim that if a cognitive function appears at a very early point in life, it is more likely that the function is innate. On this issue, my position is similar to the above on the domain-specificity. ToM/pragmatics may be considered as an innate capacity in the sense that some genetic components might be involved in ToM/pragmatics as evidenced in the case of ASC; but ToM/pragmatics may not be innate in the sense that it is considerably malleable or vulnerable to contextual inputs. In fact, as I maintained above, a defining feature of pragmatics is that it has a strong tie to social cognition and hence it is susceptible to contextual and cultural influences. But this does not necessarily rule out the involvement of genetic or biological basis of ToM/pragmatics. As I discussed above, it has been shown that even 13–15 month olds have been shown to have ToM capacity [36–39]. Likewise, a prototypical pragmatic capacity (i.e., turn-taking) is even demonstrated by 3 to 6 months-old infants [62,63].

However, it has been shown that children with ASC will develop ToM with appropriate environmental inputs or trainings that predominantly focus on various speech acts [108–110]. For example, a study showed that through an in-home verbal imitation training, toddlers with ASC can increase the usage of single words [109]. Likewise, a recent training/learning study demonstrated that ToM capacity improves in children who showed below average performance in ToM tasks initially [111]. Similar results were found in brain damaged patients. A group of brain damaged patients who initially showed below average performances in ToM tasks improved their performances through an adequate training [112]. Interestingly, however, the results from neither of these studies supported a strong tabula rasa hypothesis. In the former study, only those children who demonstrated some competency in the knowledge access, which is a precursor ability of ToM [113], improved their performances in the ToM task in a microgenetic [114–116] way [112]. In the latter study, only those brain damaged patients who were trained with a ToM (not executive functions) training protocol showed improvements [112]. Similarly, it has been demonstrated that augmentative and alternative communication (AAC) intervention, which utilizes a sign-based imitation technique, is not very effective for individuals with ASC who showed severe impairments in vocal skills [117]. Thus, similar to the above debate on the domain-specificity, these results are more in line with the reverse domain-relevance theory which supports neither the strong nativist nor the tabula rasa hypothesis of ToM/pragmatics.

7. Challenges and future directions

As other researchers [33,51,56] aptly addressed there are several challenges to confirming the present pragmatic theory of ToM. One of the challenges is associated with definitions of both pragmatics and ToM. Currently, neither ToM nor pragmatics is operationally and conceptually defined either clearly or consistently by different researchers. As Cummings [51] aptly expressed, ToM is currently very poorly defined construct. This difficulty seems to stem from the fact that ToM can encompass different functional components including volition, intentions, motivation, and beliefs. To make matters even more complicated, ToM can also include both affective and cognitive components such as empathizing and reasoning [29]. Any of these facets of ToM may overlap with some facets of pragmatics which also embraces both linguistic and intentional/volitional components. For instance, one broad definition of pragmatics is that by Levinson, "relations between language and context that are basic to an account of language understanding" [118]. This definition can encompass mental as well as non-mental aspects. Also, one of ToM's definitions, "ability to perceive intentions of others" [119,120] is practically identical to a hallmark definition of pragmatics; i.e., "understanding contexts and intentions of speakers" [121]. Moreover, the problem of conflation or semantic mish-mash may extend to developmental studies of ToM. For instance, turn-taking and joint-attention are considered to be precursors for both ToM and pragmatics [59,123]. These definitional challenges of ToM and pragmatics have generated confusions and lengthy debates among researchers.

To make matters even more challenging, many developmental and neurological studies of ToM have not distinguished between tasks that tap into pragmatics and those that test ToM. For instance, irony and metaphors are often used to test either ToM [123,124] or pragmatic language comprehension [125,126]. In these studies, the boundary between ToM and pragmatics is blurred and subject to individual interpretations. Likewise, several researchers pointed out problems associated with the use of false-belief task to test ToM [127,128]. One of these problems is that current false-belief tasks employ not only ToM but also other related but non-specific cognitive skills such as verbal memory and executive functions [51,129]. Therefore, it may be necessary for future studies, first, to clearly distinguish ToM from pragmatics by defining each of them operationally and, second, to devise tasks that specifically test the clearly and operationally defined ToM and/or pragmatics.

8. Concluding thoughts

In sum, in this article, I argued for the pragmatic theory of ToM. In order to reconcile apparent incongruent results between studies on infants and those on preschool children, two hypotheses were proposed; i.e., the two-system, and the two-stage hypothesis of ToM. As an alternative to these two hypotheses, I proposed the yet third hypothesis; i.e., the pragmatic theory of ToM. I discussed some results from developmental and neurological studies that clearly support the theory. The pragmatic theory of ToM equates ToM with pragmatic capacity which is present from very early, preverbal periods of life in the form of turn-taking. Thus, this theory explains the incongruent results between studies on infants and those on preschool children well by eliminating the requirement of verbal capacity for ToM.

As I delineated above, the pragmatic theory of ToM seems to be consistent with the domain-relevance theory of ToM in the reverse direction. This theory is also in agreement with the microgenetic theory [114,115] which, I would argue, is a mid-way between the nativist and tabula rasa theories of cognition. ToM/pragmatics may involve some genetic underpinnings; however, this capacity is too malleable and vulnerable to contextual and cultural influences to be considered as a domain-specific or innate capacity. In this review, I also discussed some definitional challenges of both ToM and pragmatics and problems in current task batteries to test either capacity. Until the definitional problem is solved, the pragmatic theory of ToM may remain as preliminary and subject to further refinement. Therefore, more research is definitely needed to confirm the theory. Lastly, once this theory is confirmed, an interesting clinical application drawn from it is that ToM or pragmatic deficits in individuals with brain damages or other psychiatric conditions can be attenuated through adequate trainings that will target either ToM and/or pragmatics.

Acknowledgements

The writing of this article was partially funded by a Faculty Research Fund from Fielding Graduate University to the author. A portion of the discussion in this article was presented as a poster at a scientific meeting, titled: "Of mice and mental health: Facilitating dialogue between basic and clinical neuroscientists" by the Royal Society in London, UK, in April, 2017. I would like to thank Randall Frank for assistance.

References

1. Dennet DC (1980) The milk of human intentionality (commentary on Searle). *Behav Brain Sci* 3: 428–430.
2. Frith U, Frith CD (2003) Development and neurophysiology of mentalizing. *Philos Trans R Soc London* 358: 459–473.
3. Baron-Cohen S, Leslie AM, Frith U (1985) Does the autistic child have a "theory of mind"? *Cognition* 21: 37–46.
4. Baron-Cohen S, Leslie AM, Frith U (1986) Mechanical, behavioural and Intentional understanding of picture stories in autistic children. *Br J Dev Psychol* 4: 113–125.
5. Brüne M (2005) "Theory of mind" in schizophrenia: A review of the literature. *Schizophrenia Bull* 31: 21–42.
6. Frith CD (1992) The cognitive neuropsychology of schizophrenia. Hove, England: Psychology Press.
7. Sprong M, Schothorst P, Vos E, et al. (2007) Theory of mind in schizophrenia: Meta-analysis. *Br J Psychiatry* 191: 5–13.
8. Washburn D, Wilson G, Rose M, et al. (2016) Theory of mind in social anxiety disorder, depression, and comorbid conditions. *J Anxiety Disord* 37: 71–77.
9. Vaskinn A, Antonsen BT, Fretland RA, et al. (2015) Theory of mind in women with borderline personality disorder or schizophrenia: Differences in overall ability and error patterns. *Front Psychol* 6: 1239.

10. Ferstl EC, Neumann J, Bogler C, et al. (2008) The extended language network: A meta-analysis of neuroimaging studies on text comprehension. *Hum Brain Mapp* 29: 581–593.
11. Grice HP (1969) Utterer's Meaning and Intentions. *Philos Rev* 78: 147–177.
12. Grice HP (1975) Logic and conversation, In: Cole P, Morgan JL, eds., *Speech Acts,* New York, NY: Academic Press, 41–58.
13. Grice HP (1989) Studies in the Way of Words. Cambridge, MA: Harvard University Press.
14. Ruiz-Gurillo L, Alvarado-Ortega MB (2013) The pragmatics of irony and humor, In: Ruiz-Gurillo L, Alvarado-Ortega MB, eds., *Irony and humor: From pragmatics to discourse,* Amsterdam, The Netherlands: John Benjamins, 1–14.
15. Van Ackeren MJ, Casasanto D, Bekkering H, et al. (2012) Pragmatics in action: Indirect requests engage theory of mind areas and the cortical motor network. *Cognit Neurosci J* 24: 2237–2247.
16. Austin JA (1962) How to do things with words. *Analysis* 23: 58–64.
17. Searle JR (1969) Seech acts. Cambridge, England: Cambridge University Press.
18. Baron-Cohen S (1995) Mindreading: An essay on autism and theory of mind. London, England: MIT Press.
19. Fodor JA (1975) The language of thought. New York, NY: Crowell. 22: 69–71.
20. Leslie AM, Friedman O, German TP (2004) Core mechanism in "theory of mind". *Trends Cognit Sci* 8: 528–533.
21. Astington JW, Jenkins JM (1999) A longitudinal study of the relation between language and theory of mind development. *Dev Psychol* 35: 1311–1320.
22. De Villiers JG, De Villiers PA (2000) Linguistic determinism and the understanding of false beliefs, In: Mitchell P, Riggs KJ, eds., *Children's reasoning and the mind,* East Sussex, England: Psychology Press, 191–228.
23. Milligan K, Astington JW, Dack LA (2007) Language and theory of mind: Meta-analysis of the relation between language ability and false-belief understanding. *Child Dev* 78: 622–648.
24. Mar RA (2011) The neural basis of social cognition and story comprehension. *Ann Rev Psychol* 62: 103–134.
25. Amodio DM, Frith CD (2006) Meeting of minds: The medial frontal cortex and social cognition. *Nat Rev Neurosci* 7: 268–277.
26. Krall SC, Rottschy C, Overwelland E, et al. (2015) The role of the right temporoprietal junction in attention and social interaction as revealed by ALE meta-analysis. *Brain Struct Funct* 220: 587–604.
27. Kobayashi C, Glover GH, Temple E (2006) Cultural and linguistic influence on neural bases of "Theory of Mind": An fMRI study with Japanese bilinguals. *Brain Lang* 98: 210–220.
28. Kobayashi C, Glover GH, Temple E (2007) Children's and adults' neural bases of verbal and nonverbal "Theory of Mind". *Neuropsychologia* 45: 1522–1532.
29. Frank CK, Baron-Cohen S, Ganzel BL (2015) Sex differences in the neural basis of false-belief and pragmatic language comprehension. *NeuroImage* 105: 300–311.
30. Saxe R, Wexler A (2005) Making sense of another mind: The role of the right tempro-parietal junction. *Neuropsychologia* 43: 1391–1399.
31. Frith U (2003) Autism: Explaining the enigma. Malden, MA: Blackwell.
32. Happé FG (1993) Communicative competence and theory of mind in autism: A test of relevance theory. *Cognition* 48: 101–119.

33. Tager-Flusberg H (2000) Language and Understanding Minds: Connections in autism, In: Baron-Cohen S, Tager-Flusberg H, Cohen DJ, eds., *Understanding other minds: Perspectives from autism and developmental cognitive neuroscience,* 2nd Edition., Oxford, England: Oxford University Press, 124–149.
34. Corcoran R, Frith CD (2003) Autobiographical memory and theory of mind: Evidence of a relationship in schizophrenia. *Psychol Med* 33: 897–905.
35. Gavilan IJM, Garcia-Albea RJE (2013) Theory of mind and language comprehension in schizophrenia. *Psiothema* 25: 440–445.
36. Buttelmann D, Carpenter M, Tomasello M (2009) Eighteen-month-old infants show false belief understanding in an active helping paradigm. *Cognition* 112: 337–342.
37. Buttleman D, Over H, Carpenter M, et al. (2014) Eighteen-month olds understand false beliefs in an unexpected contents task. *J Exp Child Psychol* 119: 120–126.
38. He Z, Bolz M, Baillargeon R (2012) 2.5-year-olds succeed at a verbal anticipatory-looking false-belief task. *Br J Dev Psychol* 30: 14–29.
39. Onishi KH, Baillargeon R (2005) Do 15-month-old infants understand false belief? *Science* 308: 255–258.
40. Wellman HM, Cross D, Watson J (2001) Meta-analysis of theory-of-mind development: The truth about false-belief. *Child Dev* 72: 655–684.
41. Baillargeon R, Scott RM, He Z (2010) False-belief understanding in infants. *Trends Cognit Sci* 14: 110–118.
42. Low J, Perner J (2012) Implicit and explicit theory of mind: State of the art. *Br J Dev Psychol* 30: 1–13.
43. Sperber D, Wilson D (2002) Pragmatics, modularity, and mindreading. *Mind Lang* 17: 3–23.
44. Malle BF (2002) The relation between language and theory of mind in development and evolution, In: Givón T, Malle BF, eds., *The evolution of language out of pre-language,* Amsterdam, The Netherlands: Benjamins, 265–284.
45. Westra E, Carruthers P (2017) Pragmatic development explains the theory-of-mind scale. *Cognition* 158: 165–176.
46. Leslie AM (1992) Autism and the "theory of mind" module. *Cur Dir Psych Sci* 1: 18–21.
47. Roth D, Leslie AM (1998) Solving belief problems: Towards a task analysis. *Cognition* 66: 1–31.
48. Gopnik A, Wellman HM (1992) Why the child's theory of mind really is a theory. *Mind Lang* 7: 145–171.
49. Goldman AI (1989) Interpretation psychologized. *Mind Lang* 4: 161–185
50. Harris PL (1992) From simulation to folk psychology: The case for development. *Mind Lang* 7: 120–144.
51. Cummings L (2013) Clinical pragmatics and theory of mind. *Springer Int Publishing* 2: 23–56.
52. Frank CK (2010) Linguistic effects on the neural basis of theory of mind. *Open Neuroimaging J* 4: 37–45.
53. Frank CK (2012) Cultural and linguistic influence on developmental neural basis of theory of mind: Whorfian hypothesis revisited. Hauppauge, NY: Nova Science Publishers.
54. Saxe R (2005) Against simulation: The argument from error. *Trends Cogit Sci* 9: 174–179.
55. Scholl BJ, Leslie AM (1999) Modularity, development and "Theory of Mind". *Mind Lang* 14: 131–153.

56. Zufferey S (2010) Lexical pragmatics and theory of mind. Amsterdam, The Netherlands: John Benjamins.
57. Surian L, Caldi S, Sperber D (2007) Attribution of beliefs by 13-month-old infants. *Psychol Sci* 18: 580–586.
58. Helming KA, Strickland B, Jacob P (2016) Solving the puzzle about early belief ascription. *Mind Lang* 31: 438–469.
59. Airenti G (2017) Pragmatic Development, In: Cummings L, ed., *Research in Pragmatics,* Cham, Switzerland: Springer, 3–28.
60. Malloch SN, Sharp DB, Campbell AM, et al. (1997) Measuring the human voice: Analyzing pitch, timing, loudness and voice quality in mother/infant communication. *Proc Inst Acoustics* 19: 495–500.
61. Trevarthen C, Kokkinaki T, Fiamenghi GA (1999) What infants' imitations communicate: With mothers with fathers and with peers, In: Nadel J, Butterworth G, eds., *Imitation in infancy,* Cambridge, England: Cambridge University Press, 127–185.
62. Butterworth GE, Cochran E (1980) Toward a mechanism of joint visual attention in human infancy. *Int J Behav Dev* 3: 253–272.
63. Stern HH (1975) What can we learn from the good language learner? *Can Mod Lang Rev* 34: 304–318.
64. Bates E, Camaion L, Volterra V (1975) The acquisition of performatives prior to speech. *Merrill-Palmer Quarterly* 21: 205–226.
65. Bruner JS (1975) The ontogenesis of speech acts. *J Child Lang* 2: 1–19.
66. Liszkowsku U, Brown P, Callaghan T, et al. (2012) A prelinguistic gestural universal of human communication. *Cognit Sci* 36: 698–713.
67. Friederici AD, Rüschemeyer SA, Hahne A, et al. (2003) The role of left inferior frontal and superior temporal cortex in sentence comprehension: Localizing syntactic and semantic processes. *Cereb Cortex* 13: 117–177.
68. Martin I, McDonalds S (2005) Exploring the cause of pragmatic deficits following traumatic brain injury. *Aphasiology* 19: 712–730.
69. Surian L, Siegal M (2001) Sources of performance on theory of mind tasks in the right hemisphere-damaged patients. *Brain Lang* 78: 224–232.
70. Weed E, Mcgregor W, Nielsen JF, et al. (2010) Theory of Mind in adults with right hemisphere data: What's the story? *Brain Lang* 113: 65–72.
71. Weylman ST, Brownell HH, Roman M, et al. (1989) Appreciation of indirect requests by left- and right-brain damaged patients: The effect of verbal context and conventionality of wording. *Brain Lang* 36: 580–591.
72. Brundage S (1996) Comparison of proverb interpretations provided by right-hemisphere damaged adults and adults with probable dementia of the Alzheimer type. *Clin Aphasiol* 24: 215–231.
73. Cutica I, Bucciarelli M, Bara BG (2006) Neuropragmatics: Extralinguistic pragmatic ability is better preserved in left-hemisphere-damaged patients than in right-hemisphere-damaged patients. *Brain Lang* 98: 12–25.
74. Cheang H, Pell M (2006) A study of humour and communicative intention following right hemisphere stroke. *Clin Linguist Phonetics* 20: 447–462.

75. Winner E, Brownell H, Happe F, et al. (1998) Distinguishing lies from jokes: Theory of mind deficits and discourse interpretation in right hemisphere brain damaged patients. *Brain Lang* 62: 89–106.
76. Mcdonald S (2000) Exploring the cognitive basis of right-hemisphere pragmatic language disorders. *Brain Lang* 75: 82–107.
77. Kucharskapietura K, Phillips ML, Germand W, et al. (2003) Perceptions of emotion from faces and voices following unilateral brain damage. *Neuropsychologia* 41: 1082–1090.
78. Parola A, Gabbatore I, Bosco FM, et al. (2016) Assessment of pragmatic impairment in right hemisphere damage. *J Neurolinguistics* 39: 10–25.
79. Shamaytsoory SG, Tomer R, Berger BD, et al. (2005) Impaired "affective theory of mind" is associated with right ventromedial prefrontal damage. *Cognit Behav Neurol* 18: 55–62.
80. Sidtis DVL, Yang S (2016) Formulaic language performance in left- and right-hemisphere damaged patients: Structured testing. *Aphasiology* 31: 82–99.
81. Heine B, Kuteva T, Kaltenöck G (2014) Discourse, grammar, the dual process model, and brain lateralization: Some correlations. *Lang Cognit* 6: 146–180.
82. Heine B, Kuteva T, Kaltenöck G, et al. (2015) On some correlations between grammar and brain lateralization, In: Oxford Handbooks Online, Oxford, England: OUP.
83. Brownell H, Griffin R, Winner E, et al. (2000) Cerebral lateralization and theory of mind, In: Baron-Cohen S, Tager-Flusberg H, Cohen D, eds., *Understanding other minds: Perspectives from developmental cognitive neuroscience,* 2, Oxford, UK: Oxford University Press, 306–333.
84. Griffin R, Friedman O, Ween J, et al. (2006) Theory of mind and the right cerebral hemisphere: Refining the scope of impairment. *Laterality* 11: 195–225.
85. Siegal M, Carrington J, Radel M (1996) Theory of mind understanding following right hemisphere damage. *Brain Lang* 53: 40–50.
86. Weed E (2011) What's left to learn about right hemisphere damage and pragmatic impairment? *Aphasiology* 25: 872–889.
87. Champagne-Lavau M, Joanette Y (2009) Pragmatics, theory of mind and executive functions after a right-hemisphere lesion: Different patterns of deficits. *J Neurolinguistics* 22: 413–426.
88. Frith CD, Frith U (2006) The neural basis of mentalizing. *Neuron* 50: 531–534.
89. Kobayashi C, Glover GH, Temple E (2008) Switching language switches mind: Linguistic effects on developmental neural bases of "Theory of Mind". *Soc Cogn Affect Neurosci* 3: 62–70.
90. Ferstl EC, Cramon DYV (2002) What does the frontomedian cortex contribute to language processing: Coherence or theory of mind? *Neuroimage* 17: 1599–1612.
91. Bašnáková J, Weber K, Petersson KM, et al. (2014) Beyond the language given: The neural correlates of inferring speaker meaning. *Cereb Cortex* 24: 2572–2578.
92. Spotorno N, Koun E, Prado J, et al. (2012) Neural evidence that utterance-processing entails mentalizing: The case of irony. *NeuroImage* 63: 25–39.
93. Castelli F, Frith C, Happé F, et al. (2002) Autism, Asperger syndrome and brain mechanisms for the attribution of mental states of animated shapes. *Brain* 125: 1839–1849.
94. Gallagher HL, Frith CD (2003) Functional imaging of "theory of mind". *Trends Cognit Sci* 7: 77–83.
95. Barrett HC, Kurzban R (2006) Modularity in cognition: Framing the debate. *Psychol Rev* 113: 628–647.
96. Fodor JA (1983) The modularity of mind. Cambridge, MA: MIT Press.

97. Scholl BJ, Leslie AM (2001) Minds, modules, and meta-analysis. *Child Dev* 72: 696–701.
98. Carlson SM, Moses LJ, Claxton LJ (2004) Individual differences in executive functioning and theory of mind: An investigation of inhibitory control and planning ability. *J Exp Child Psychol* 87: 299–319.
99. Perner J (1991) Understanding the representational mind. Cambridge, MA: MIT Press.
100. Karmiloffsmith A (2015) An alternative to domain-general or domain-specific frameworks for theorizing about human evolution and ontogenesis. *AIMS Neurosci* 2: 91–104.
101. Trosborg A (2010) Pragmatics across language and culture. Berlin, Germany: Walter de Gruyter.
102. Zhu J, Bao Y (2010) The pragmatic comparison of Chinese and Western "Politeness" in cross-cultural communication. *J Lang Teach Res* 1: 848–851.
103. Wierzbicka A (2003) Cross-cultural pragmatics: The semantics of human interaction. Berlin, Germany: Walter de Gruyter.
104. Wierzbicka A (2010) Cultural scripts and intercultural communication, In: Trosborg A, ed., *Pragmatics across language and culture,* Berlin, Germany: Walter de Gruyter, 43–78.
105. Liu D, Wellman HM, Tardif T, et al. (2008) Theory of mind development in Chinese children: A meta-analysis of false-belief understanding across cultures and languages. *Dev Psychol* 44: 523–531.
106. Kobayashi FC, Temple E (2009) Cultural effects on the neural basis of theory of mind. *Prog Brain Res* 178: 213–223.
107. Rowley DA, Rogish M, Alexander T, et al. (2017) Cognitive correlates of pragmatic language comprehension in adult traumatic brain injury: A systematic review and meta-analysis. *Brain Inj* 31: 1564–1574.
108. Landa R (2007) Early communication development and intervention for children with autism. *Dev Disabil Res Rev* 13: 16–25.
109. Seung HK, Siddiqi S, Elder JH (2006) Intervention outcomes of a bilingual child with autism. *J Med Speech Lang Pathol* 14: 53–63.
110. Thunberg G, Johansson M, Wikholm J (2015) Meeting the communicative rights of people with autism—using pictorial supports during assessment, intervention and hospital care, Chapter 15, Open Access, In: Fizgerald M, ed., *Autism spectrum disorder—Recent advances,* London, England: In Tech.
111. Rhodes M, Wellman H (2013) Constructing a new theory from old ideas and new evidence. *Cognit Sci* 37: 592–604.
112. Ludgren K, Brownell H (2015) Selective training of theory of mind in traumatic brain injury: A series of single subject training studies. *Open Behav Sci J* 9: 1–11.
113. Wellman H, Liu D (2004) Scaling of theory-of-mind tasks. *Child Dev* 75: 523–541.
114. Brown JW (1977) Mind, brain and consciousness. New York, NY: Academic Press.
115. Brown JW (2015) Microgenetic theory and process thought. New York, NY: Academic Press.
116. Siegler R, Stern E (1998) Conscious and unconscious strategy discoveries: A micrognetic analysis. *J Exp Psychol Gen* 127: 377–397.
117. Howlin P (2006) Augmentative and alternative communication systems for children with autism, In: Charman T, Stone W, eds., *Social and communication development in autism spectrum disorders,* New York, NY: Guilford Press, 236–266.
118. Levinson SC (1984) Pragmatics (Cambridge textbooks in linguistics). Cambridge, England: Cambridge University Press.

119. Blakemore SJ, Decety J (2001) From the perception of action to the understanding of intention. *Nat Rev Neurosci* 2: 561–567.
120. Iacoboni M, Dapretto M (2006) The mirror neuron system and the consequence of its dysfunction. *Nat Rev Neurosci* 7: 942–951.
121. Haugh M (2008) The place of intention in the interactional achievement of implicature, In: Kecskes I, Mey J, eds., *Intention, common ground and the egocentric speaker-hearer,* Berlin, Germany: Mouton de Gruyter, 45–86.
122. Charman T, Baroncohen S, Swetternham J, et al. (2000) Testing joint attention, imitation, and play as infancy precursors to language and theory of mind. *Cognit Dev* 15: 481–498.
123. Rapp AM, Felsenheimer AK, Langohr K, et al. (2018) The comprehension of familiar and novel metaphoric meanings in schizophrenia: A pilot study. *Front Psychol* 8: 2251.
124. Varga E, Simon M, Tényi T, et al. (2013) Irony comprehension and context processing in schizophrenia in remission—a functional MRI study. *Brain Lang* 126: 231–242.
125. Mo S, Su Y, Chan RC, et al. (2008) Comprehension of metaphor and irony in schizophrenia during remission: The role of theory of mind and IQ. *Psychiatry Res* 157: 21–29.
126. Wang AT, Lee SS, Sigman M, et al. (2006) Neural basis of irony comprehension in children with autism: The role of prosody and context. *Brain* 129: 932–943.
127. Apperly IA, Butterfill SA (2009) Do humans have two systems to track beliefs and belief like states? *Psychol Rev* 116: 953–970.
128. Bloom P, German TP (2000) Two reasons to abandon the false belief task as a test of theory of mind. *Cognition* 77: B25–B31.
129. Sabbagh MA, Xu F, Carison SM, et al. (2006) The development of executive functioning and theory of mind: A comparison of Chinese and U.S. preschoolers. *Psychol Sci* 17: 74–81.

7

Evolving robot empathy towards humans with motor disabilities through artificial pain generation

Muh Anshar[1] **and Mary-Anne Williams**[2,*]

[1] Social, Cognitive Robotics and Advanced Artificial Intelligent Research Centre, Department of Electrical Engineering, Universitas Hasanuddin UNHAS Makassar Indonesia
[2] Innovation and Enterprise Research Lab, Centre for Artificial Intelligence, University of Technology Sydney UTS Australia

* **Correspondence:** Email: muh.anshar@gmail.com/anshar@unhas.ac.id;

Abstract: In contact assistive robots, a prolonged physical engagement between robots and humans with motor disabilities due to shoulder injuries, for instance, may at times lead humans to experience pain. In this situation, robots will require sophisticated capabilities, such as the ability to recognize human pain in advance and generate counter-responses as follow up emphatic action. Hence, it is important for robots to acquire an appropriate pain concept that allows them to develop these capabilities. This paper conceptualizes empathy generation through the realization of synthetic pain classes integrated into a robot's self-awareness framework, and the implementation of fault detection on the robot body serves as a primary source of pain activation. Projection of human shoulder motion into the robot arm motion acts as a fusion process, which is used as a medium to gather information for analyses then to generate corresponding synthetic pain and emphatic responses. An experiment is designed to mirror a human peer's shoulder motion into an observer robot. The results demonstrate that the fusion takes place accurately whenever unified internal states are achieved, allowing accurate classification of synthetic pain categories and generation of empathy responses in a timely fashion. Future works will consider a pain activation mechanism development.

Keywords: cognitive; empathic reaction; assistive robots; synthetic pain; joint position; shoulder motion

1. Introduction

Social assistive robotics has been one of growing fields of study in human-robot interaction (HRI) that covers the utilization of robot technology to assist people through social interaction. A prolonged physical engagement between assistive robots and humans, particularly those with motor disabilities due to a shoulder injury for instance, may at times lead humans to experience pain. In this situation, robots are required to develop a more sophisticated HRI capability, namely the ability to recognize and predict human pain during an interaction, and at the same time, to adopt counter responses as empathic action when human pain experiences are predicted. Hence, it is critical for assistive robots to acquire an appropriate and relevant concept of pain that allows them to develop and generate effective empathic behaviors. This paper conceptualizes and implements the generation of empathy into two stages: (1) The realization of the concept of artificial pain through synthetic pain classes integrated into a robot self-awareness framework, and the utilization of robot body awareness to implement the fault detection as the primary source of synthetic pain activation; (2) the projection of the human shoulder motion into the robot arm motion using a fusion process that allows the gathered information to be used to generate a corresponding synthetic pain in the robot that allows it to adopt counter empathic responses.

A practical approach is designed to mirror the internal state of a human shoulder motion projected on a observer robot's shoulder. A special remark on the studies in human empathy suggests that an empathic state is obtained through perceptions towards another person's narrative. In other words, an empathic person does not directly experience what the other person is experiencing. By utilizing this concept, our approach is to have an observer robot which mirrors the internal state of the human peer by capturing the human shoulder motion through the robot's visual perception.

Our findings demonstrate that the projection of the human and the observer robot takes place accurately when they both share unified internal states. An accurate projection further allows better prediction results of the robot body behavior, accurate classification of synthetic pain categories/levels, and at the same time, appropriate generation of empathy responses in a timely fashion.

The reminder of the paper proceeds as follows: Section 2 presents an overview of related work in assistive robots highlighting self-awareness, human pain and empathy concepts. Section 3 gives a brief description of the proposed synthetic pain and empathy concepts within a self-awareness framework for robots, followed by section 4 which explains experiment stages and environmental set up. Section 5 provides evaluation and discussion. Finally, section 6 concludes the overall achievement and possible future developments.

2. Robot design

In this section we briefly present relevant background studies in the area of assistive robotics, self-awareness, pain and empathy concepts.

2.1. Assistive robotics

Assistive robotics is a growing field of study in HRI that focuses on assisting people with physical disabilities and the robots typically utilize a physical medium or physical contact when delivering assistance. As the physical contact interaction occurs, the element of embodiment plays a crucial role as the basis for a structural coupling that creates potential perturbation between robots and the environments. The design approaches commonly consider a biologically inspired approach or functionality designs which focus on the constrained operational and performance objectives [6]. Studies in assistive robotics cover a wide range of applications, such as rehabilitation robots, wheelchair robots, educational robots and manipulator arms for disable people [7]. People with physical disabilities, particularly with a motor disability, are people who suffer from conditions that restrict their abilities in moving and manipulating object tasks. This condition introduces a significant limitation in moving, controlling and coordinating the movement of body parts, such as wrist, hands, fingers or arms [2]. People with shoulder motor injury experience pain as the shoulder moves to specific positions which will evoke the sensation of pain.

2.2. *Cognitive designs*

In the theory of mind (ToM) literature, it is reported that humans have the ability to correctly attribute beliefs, goals, and perceptions towards themselves and other people [3]. A robot, with the ability to recognize human emotional, attentional, and cognitive states, can learn to develop counter reactions and modify its own behavior accordingly. This concept is central and plays a crucial role in human interactions, including in the field of assistive robotics. The mind is considered as the consciousness embodiment, where consciousness is defined as a function of consistent cognition and behavior performance [4,5]. Proposes that embodiment is one of the features of consciousness, and our self-concept utilizes this embodiment aspect in developing our empathic robot responses.

2.2.1. Self-awareness

According to [10] robots with self-awareness have the ability to behave more effectively in novel situations compared to those without it. Studies on the notion of robots being self-aware early appeared in [3,8], where [8] develops a capability for a robot to recognize itself in the mirror. Since then, self-aware robot studies continue to grow as reported in [9,11–15]. Propose a framework with a self-awareness based on the ability to focus attention on the internal state's representation. Much of literatures, however, identifies the lack of concept of "self" [1]. Propose a concept of self by deriving its definition postulated by [16] which divides the concept into two levels, subjective and objective awareness. Subjective awareness concerns the machinery level of the body and objective awareness concerns the focus of attention towards one's body, thought, actions and feelings. The authors further introduce a new framework which is capable of switching the robot awareness from subjective to objective, and vice versa.

2.2.2. Empathy for the pain of others

Studies of empathy have been growing in the last decade, particularly human empathy towards pain, as reported in [17–23]. A common understanding is emerging that suggests a complex structure in the human brain and the nerve cells assembly play a major role in the arousal of empathy and pain. With such complexity, generating empathy and pain should be developed by considering the current state-of-the-art of robot technology. The implementation of our robot empathy for pain is inspired by the work in [24], which proposes a shared-representation model of pain empathy. This model mentions that witnessing another person in pain activates pain representations in the observer, which reflects a relative capacity to understand pain experiences in others. Hence, our empathy for pain is generated by projecting humans' body, e.g. shoulder motions which suffer from a motor injury into a robot observer's shoulder. The observer robot visually captures the shoulder motions and projects them on its own arm, while analyzing the kinds of synthetic pain to be generated.

3. Self-awareness framework and synthetic pain

This paper utilizes a self-awareness framework proposed by [1], Adaptive Self-Awareness Framework for Robot (ASAF) and the kinds of synthetic pain definitions in developing our empathic reactions. The overall design of the ASAF is shown in Figure 1 below. In this new framework, the subjective awareness refers to the element of physical parts of robots or robot embodiment, such as motors and joints; while the objective awareness specifies the metaphysical aspects, such as robot's representation of its position towards an external reference. A brief overview of the ASAF is discussed in the following subsection.

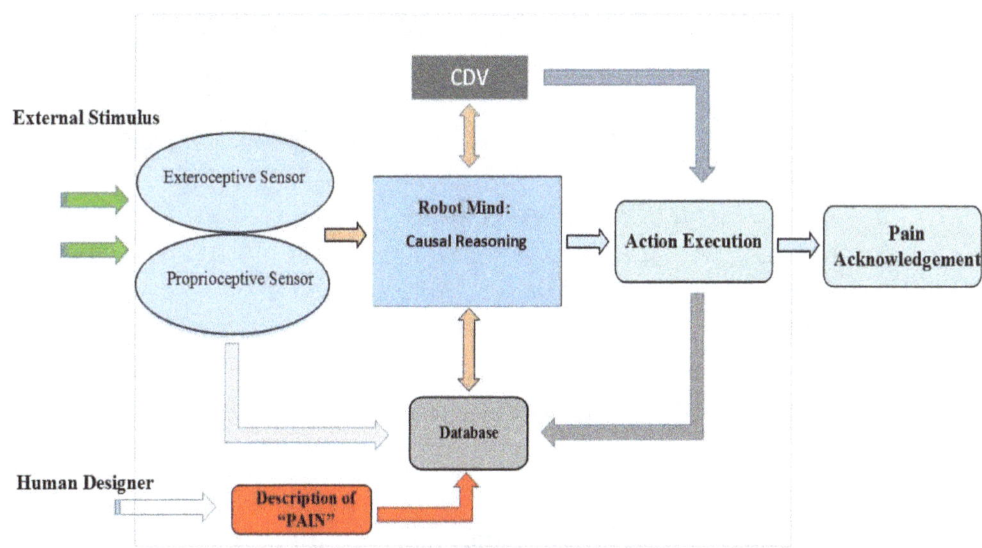

Figure 1. Adaptive self-awareness framework for the robot (ASAF).

3.1. Adaptive Self-awareness framework for robot (ASAF)

There are three elements that play pivotal roles in the performance of the framework, which we are going to further elaborate in the following subsections.

3.1.1. Consciousness direction

The term of consciousness in the ASAF is to signify the cognitive focus, which is the focus of attention and it should not be understood to mean human consciousness. Hence, consciousness direction is changeable between the two levels of awareness, subjective and objective awareness (see Figure 2). There are two predominant factors in directing robot consciousness: (i) The ability to focus attention on a specified physical aspect of self. (ii) The ability to foresee, and at the same time, to be aware of the consequences of predicted actions. Our approach formulates how to address these two aspects so that they can be developed and built into a robot self-awareness framework. Thus, the detection of synthetic pain can be acknowledged and responded to in an appropriate way. Robot awareness is mapped to a discrete range 1–3 for subjective and 4–6 for objective elements. Changing the value of Consciousness Direction (CDV) allows the exploration of these regions, and at the same time, changes the focus of robot attention. The robot mind governs the CDV modification and determines the conditions of exploration of robot awareness regions, either constrained or unconstrained conditions. The structure of robot awareness regions and CDV are illustrated in Figure 2 and for simplicity, we will use the abbreviations for each awareness region throughout the paper.

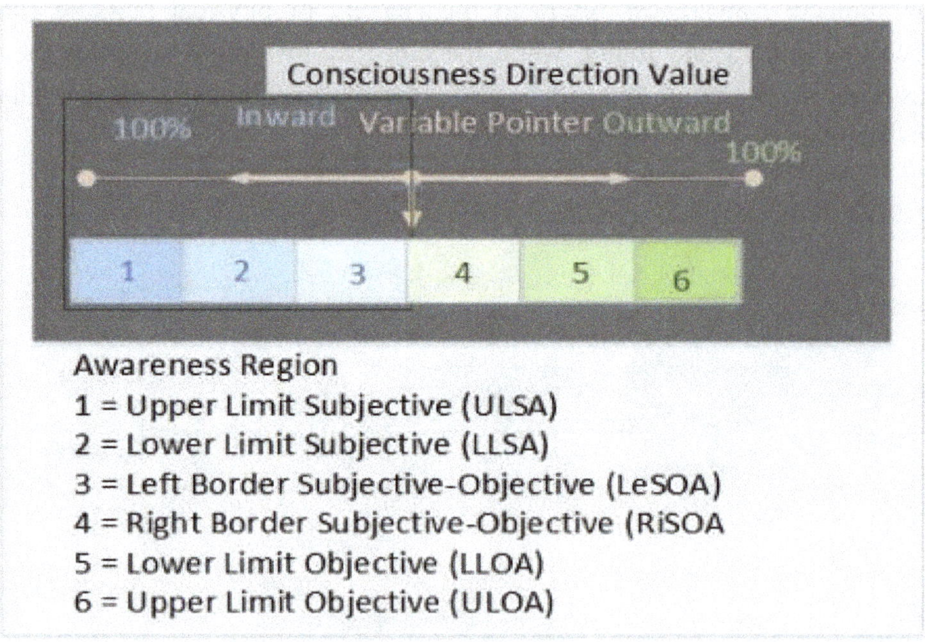

Figure 2. Regions of consciousness direction.

3.1.2. Synthetic pain description

In order to generate synthetic pain on the robot, we set shoulder joint restriction regions that should be avoided. People with a shoulder motor injury have specific joint regions which will evoke pain sensation whenever the shoulder moves into these areas. These joint regions are projected into the observer' shoulder joint and each restrictive joint regions constitutes a specific faulty joint value. Synthetic pain can then be generated when the robot joint moves into this region. Joint movement is monitored by the proprioceptive perception of the robot, which can subsequently be used by the robot mind to reason upon. For specific types of movement, for instance rotational movement for the shoulder joint, the pain level is determined by the current joint values with respect to the joint threshold value. This threshold value is set by the robot mind and its value is associated with the lowest fault joint value (see Figure 3).

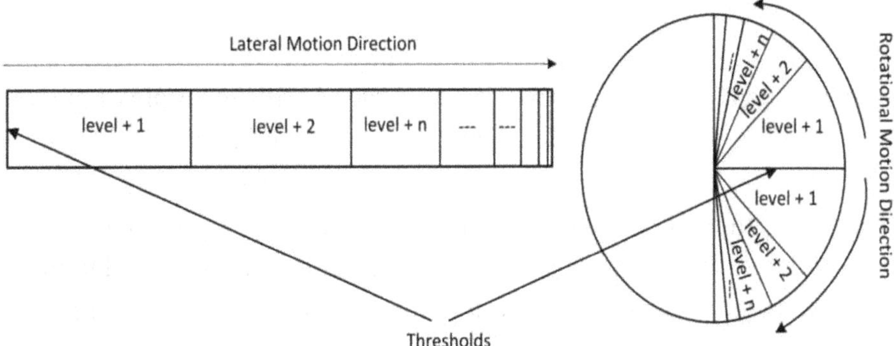

Figure 3. Synthetic pain generation.

Synthetic pain descriptions proposed by [1] have different applicable intensity level for each class (see Table 1).

Table 1. Synthetic pain description.

Categor	Synthetic pain	Description	Definition	Intensity Level
1	Proprioceptive	1.0	Potential hardware damage, as an alert signal	"None", "Slight"
2	Inflammatory reduction	2.1 2.2	Predicted robot hardware damage, real robot hardware damage	"None", "Slight" "Moderate", "Severe"
3	Sensory malfunction	3.1 3.2	Abnormal function of internal sensors, damage internal sensors	"None", "Slight" "Moderate", "Severe"

3.1.3. Robot mind

The robot mind in the framework utilises causal reasoning to draw conclusions from its perceptions which integrates the cause and effect relationship. This allows the framework to adapt to the world by predicting the robot's own future states through reasoning about the perceived/detected facts. Sequential pattern prediction is used to capture the behavior of the observed facts and then use them to predict the possible future conditions. The framework decision making utilizes covariance information obtained from sequence data so as to facilitate the causal reasoning process. The robot mind analyses the relationship amongst data covariance by making predictions of sequence data patterns obtained from robot's proprioceptive sensor (joint position sensor). The prediction process only takes place after several sequences of data so as to reduce biased analyses. There are two conditions of the state of the robot mind:

1. Constrained which represents a state where the CDV value is restricted to subjective awareness, region 1 (upper level). This state typically will force the robot to stop any physical activity on the hardware level.

2. Unconstrained which refers to a state where the CDV value is free to explore all the regions of the robot awareness (region 1 to region 6).

3.2. *Empathic actions generation and execution*

There are two stages that occur in the robot mind in the specific example of human shoulder pain: (1) The realization of the concept of artificial pain through synthetic pain classes integrated into the ASAF framework, and the utilization of robot body awareness to implement the fault detection as the primary source of synthetic pain activation; (2) the projection of the human shoulder motion into the robot arm motion using a projection process that allows the obtained information to be used to generate a corresponding synthetic pain in the robot and counter empathic responses. Stage 2 occurs at the first place as the observer robot projects the human shoulder motion into the robot's arm and simultaneously stage 1 occurs. Joint data is captured from the robot proprioceptive sensor attached to the shoulder joint and arranged into a sequence of data for pattern analyses. The robot mind analyses the relationship among data covariance by making predictions of sequence data patterns. The prediction process only takes place after several sequences of data so as to reduce biased analyses. Any decisions made from previous sequence predictions are reassessed with the current state, and the results are either kept as history for future prediction or amendment actions take place before placement proceeds. This cycle repeats only if current and predicted data are not classified in any of the restricted regions that refer to the painful joint settings. Once the reasoning indicates that the joint motions are heading towards or falls into these restricted joint regions, the robot mind will perform three consecutive actions:

1. Setting the robot awareness into constrained condition.
2. Modifying the CDV to shift robot's focus of attention to the subjective element, which is the robot shoulder.
3. Providing empathic response actions, such as alerting the human peer through verbal expressions and approaching the human peer for further assistance.

At any initial state, the robot mind specifies the awareness to a randomized style, which means that the attention may focus on one of among the sixth regions by randomly selecting the CDV. Once a selection is made, the robot mind is set to an unconstrained condition, allowing the robot to start visualizing and projecting the human shoulder motions. While the awareness is on the selected region and projection takes place, the robot mind at the same time monitors its proprioceptive sensor, joint arm sensors which physically project the human shoulder positions. The change of joint sensor readings produces the change in the pattern, and this situation is captured and used as the element of reasoning. As the joint moves, the robot's internal states are subjects to changes and the empathic action executions transforms the results into primitive actions for further execution.

4. Experimental design

The pilot experiment considers only a two-direction up and down rotational motion of the human's right shoulder. A set of pre-defined joint values which constitute the restricted joint values are "manually" specified on the robot. These joint values are associated with the painful regions of the human's shoulder which are supposed to be avoided. The experiment involves two NAO humanoid robots and a human peer. The scenario of experiment is a human peer and one NAO humanoid robot (mediator robot) are working together in a collaborative task, e.g. a hand pushing task, while the other NAO robot acts as an observer robot. The length of the rotation movement of the human shoulder follows the length of shoulder rotation of the mediator robot. We attach a red mark on the back side of the mediator robot, which will be recognized by the observer robot via its camera sensor.[1] During the experiment, the human's hand coincides with the mediator's hand, allowing both hands to move in parallel. Each human's shoulder rotation corresponds to the value of the mediator' shoulder joint position sensor, which is recorded in the mediator's Robot Mind (see Figure 4).

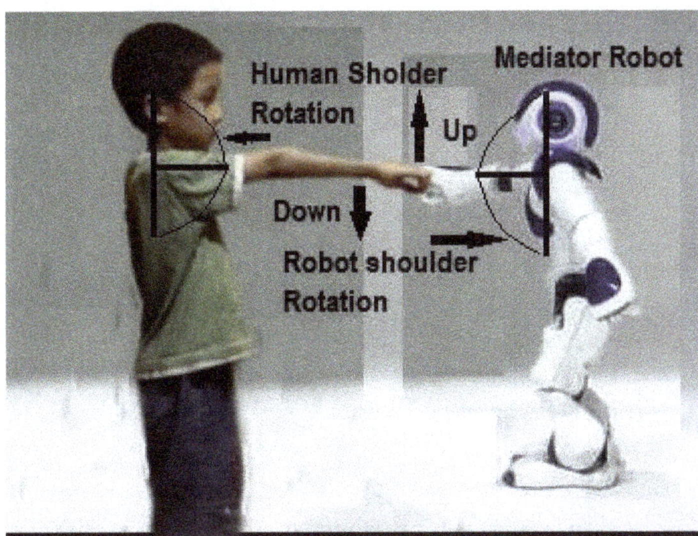

Figure 4. Human and mediator robot shoulder rotation mapping.

This recorded data is utilized for merely a comparison purpose in the data analyses which is presented in this section. The observer converts the visual representation using the geometric transformation (see Figure 5 and Figure 6).

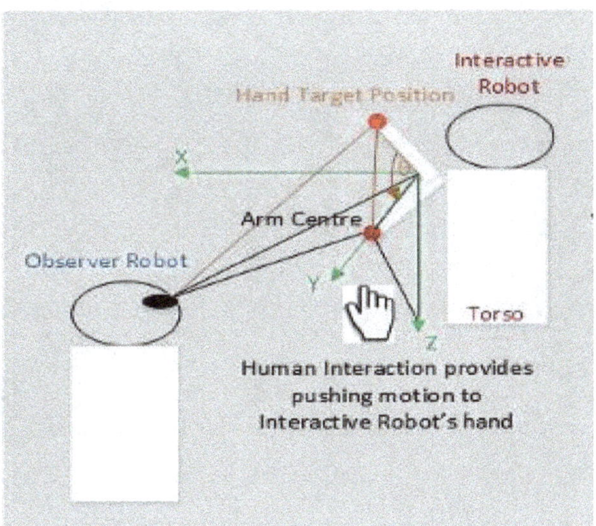

Figure 5. Experimental setup.

[1] The terms mediator and observer which refer to the mediator and observer robots will be used through the rest of the paper.

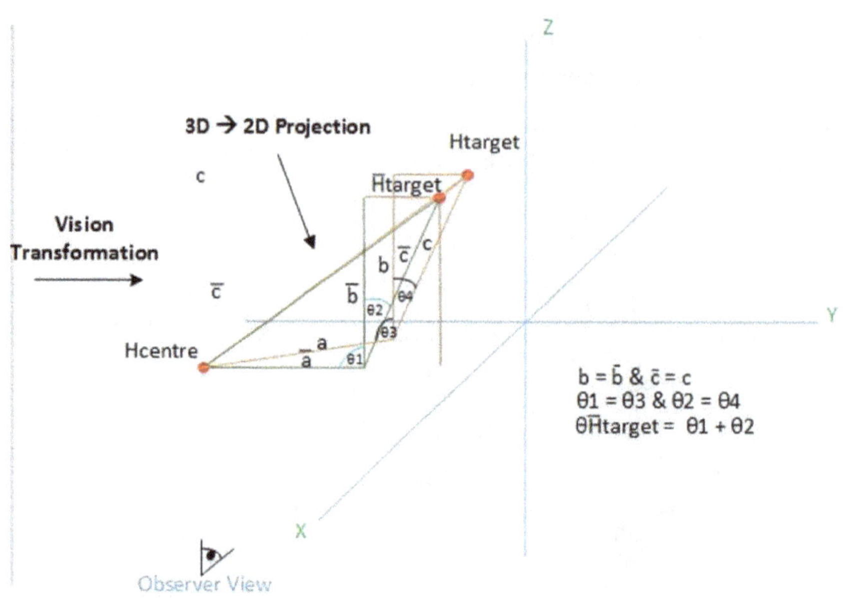

Figure 6. Geometric transformation.

The experiment is divided into two stages. Stage 1 serves as an initiation or calibration stage. Stage 2 is the projection stage which consists of self-reflection without awareness and empathic experiments. The poses of the two robots are shown in Figure 7 and Figure 8 shows the pose of human during interaction.

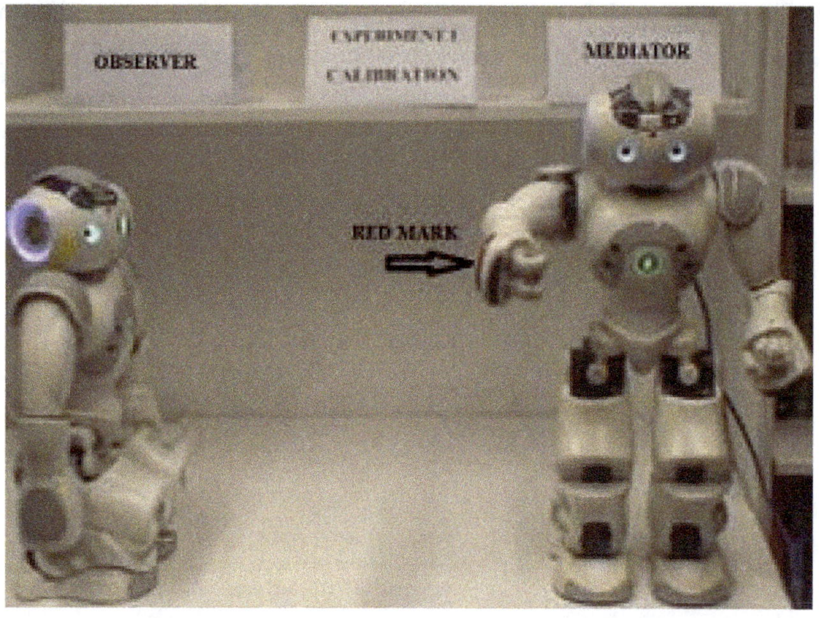

Figure 7. Initial pose of robot experiments.

During self-reflection experiment, the ASAF framework is deactivated in the observer. Instead, it only activates detection of faulty hardware region without anticipations' follow-up. The rest of experiment involves the implementation of a full functional ASAF framework.

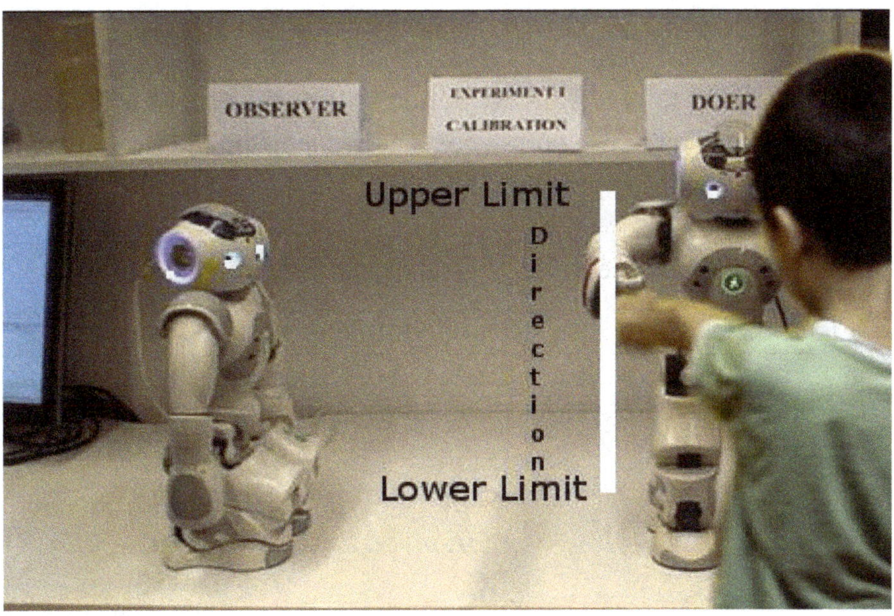

Figure 8. Experimental setting during interaction.

The kinds of synthetic pain and awareness region to be modelled during this experiment are shown in Table 2 and Table 3 respectively (See Figure 2 in Subsection 3.1 for details of each region).

Table 2. Consciousness region.

Consciouness Region		Robot Action	During Visitation
		Unconstrained	Constrained
Subjective	ULSA	Low Stiffness on Arm Joint	Increased Stiffness and Alert human peer
	LLSA	-	-
Subjective-Objective	LeSOA	-	-
	RiSOA	-	-
Objective	LLOA	-	-
	ULOA	-	-

Table 3. Synthetic pain experiment.

Synthetic Pain		Descriptions	Intensity Level
Proprioceptive	1.0	Modelled: "None"	Modelled: "Slight"
Inflammatory Reduction	2.1	Modelled: "None"	-
	2.2	-	-
Sensory Malfunctions	3.1	-	-
	3.2	-	-

5. Results and discussions

Three kinds of data: (1) Awareness region; (2) faulty joint region; (3) arm coordinate centre reference data, are collected in the initiation stage.

5.1. *Experiment results*

The awareness and faulty joint regions are defined before the experiment takes place, and stage 1 provides the shoulder shared reference point between the mediator and the human peer. These values are the same for the stage 2 of the experiment (see Table 4).

Table 4. Regions and data references.

Element	Region/Ordinate	Values
	ULSA	1
awareness region	LLSA	50
	LeSOA	51
	RiSOA	100
	LLOA	101
	ULOA	150
faulty joint region	1 Upper High-UH	−2.08313
	2 Upper Medium-UM	−1.58313
	3 Upper Low-UL	−1.38313
	4 Lower Low-LL	1.385669
	5 Lower Medium-LM	1.585669
	6 Lower High-LH	2.085669
shoulder mediator human shared reference	X	0.408
	Y	−0.155
	Y	0.186
	Time	154.98

Table 5. Self-Reflection direction.

Direction							
Up				Down			
Observer	Human Shoulder	Interval	Status	Observer	Human Shoulder	Interval	Status
−0.015	−0.01845	0	-	1.173	0.01845	0	-
−0.015	−0.01845	340	-	1.349	0.10742	762	-
−0.015	−0.01845	664	-	1.614	1.00941	1150	-
−0.422	−0.06439	991	-	-	-	-	-
−0.94	−0.43408	1469	-	-	-	-	-
−1.506	−1.21489	1992	-	-	-	-	-
−1.941	−1.63213	2530	-	-	-	-	-
	−1.63674	3064	-	-	-	-	-

The stage 2 experiment generates two sets of data, self-reflection data (Table 5) and empathic data (Table 6).

Table 7 provides additional data obtained from the empathy experiment. This data shows the changes in the embodiment elements that affect the internal state of the observer.

Table 6. Empathic experiment function.

	Observer			Human Shoulder		
	Interval	Data	Prediction	Interval	Data	Status
Up	12	1.214		891	0.01845	
	13	−0.291		2185	−0.21625	
	14	−0.777		2904	−0.55527	
	15	−1.165	−1.553	4849	−1.97268	
	16		−1.941	5522	−2.08567	
	17		−2.329	-	-	
	18		−2.717	-	-	
Down	12	0.242		509	0.01692	
	13	1.186		1240	0.35133	
	14	1.805		1890	1.33922	
	15	2.105	2.405	2537	1.83317	
	16		2.705	3186	2.08567	Not Exist
	17		3.005	-		
	18		3.305	-		

Table 7. Internal state.

Motion	CDV	Awareness		Status	Faulty Joint Region		Internal
		Region	Early Type		Real	Prediction	State
Down	131	6	ULOA		4		1
	33	2	LLSA		4		2
	17	1	ULSA	Unconstrained	6		3
	80	4	RiSOA		6 (2.105)	6 (2.405)	4
	110 to 3	5 to 1	LLOA	Constrained	6 (2.405)		5
Up	2	1	ULSA		4		6
	62	3	LeSOA		3		7
	116	5	LLOA	Unconstrained	3		8
	6	1	ULSA		3(−1.165)	2 (−1.553)	9
	126 to 6	6 to 1	ULSA	Constrained	1(−1.941)		10

5.2. *Analysis and discussion*

During the self-reflection experiment, the minimum sampling time required to capture incoming data, as shown in Figure 9(a) and Figure 9(b), is every 340 cycle of data. For the observer during upward motion direction, the first five sequences of data falls into Region 1 followed by Region 2 (data = −1.506, sequence = 1992), then Region 3 (data = −1.941, sequence = 2530). When data equals −1.506, the observer starts to experience Category 1 synthetic pain, which produces an alert signal (projecting the human shoulder would experience the same condition). However, the observer still captures incoming data which shifts to Region 3, causing the synthetic pain category to increase to Category 2 with the detail of 2.1. It can be seen that the sampling time tends to increase, from 327 to 478, 523 and finally 538 cycles of data as the joint falls into synthetic pain region. At the same time, during upward motion direction, the first six data sequence of human shoulder positions are classified into Region 1 (synthetic pain Category 1) and the final sequence falls into Region 3. This increasing sampling time occurs as more computation time is required by the observer to critically analyze and predict the plausible future internal state of the human shoulder position. During this upward motion direction, particularly in sequence 1992, the observer produces one false alarm, which generates Region 2 classification, while the human shoulder position is still in Region 1. However, both confirm that at sequence 2530, the internal state converges into Region 3. During the downward trend, the experiment lasts a short time, and the observer, unfortunately, misclassifies the internal state of the human shoulder position at sequence 1150. In this sequence, the observer internal state classifies Region 6 while the human shoulder position is Region 4. However, both of them share the same classification results, Region 4 which occurs at sequence 0 and 762. For the empathy experiment, the vision data comparison shown in Figure 10 and the empathic response experiment is shown Figure 11.

It can be seen from Figure 10, regeneration of the human shoulder data is similar, particularly during the downward trend, with a relatively low Δerror = 0.07751. A slight variant occurs during the upward trend with a considerable Δerror about 0.57492. These data discrepancies influence the reasoning process as any small fraction of data affects considerably prediction results.

Figure 11 shows, during the upward experiment, that the observer prediction starts at interval data 15 with the observer data is Region 3 (data = −1.165). However, prediction data at this time is Region 2 (data = −1.553) which still misclassifies the real data on the human shoulder (Region 1, data = −1.973, generated synthetic pain is Category 1.0). However, in the interval data 16, both observer prediction and human shoulder converge into Region 1 (observer data = −1.973, prediction data = −1.941 and human shoulder data = −2.086). This situation accurately is matched with the real data on the human shoulder position, and finally ends at Region 1 with synthetic pain Category 2, detail 2.1. The behavior of internal states of both robots during the downward experiment indicates a similar pattern. The observer prediction and real data nearly converge to the same pain region classification, Region 6, at interval data 15 with the observer data prediction is 2.405, observer data itself equals 2.105 and human shoulder data = 1.83317. Thus, it generates the kind of synthetic pain Category 2, details 2.1 forcing the robot to provide an alert signal. When the next interval data 16, the robot has already prepare an empathy response as the prediction data already shows an increase pattern of the observer data. The changes in the observer internal states show in Table 8.

Table 8. State of awareness, synthetic pain and empathy response generations.

Internal State	Awareness	Synthetic Pain		Empathy Response	
	Final Type	Categories	Intensity	Direct	Follow-Up
1	ULOA		-	-	-
2	LLSA		-	-	-
3	ULSA	No Pain	-	-	-
4	RiSOA		-	-	-
5	ULSA	1:0 Proprioceptive	"Slight"	painfully restricting	Approach the Scene
6	ULSA		-	-	-
7	LeSOA		-	-	-
8	LLOA	No Pain	-	-	-
9	ULSA		-	-	-
10	ULSA	1:0 Proprioceptive	"Slight"	right arm is mid	Alert Approach the Scene

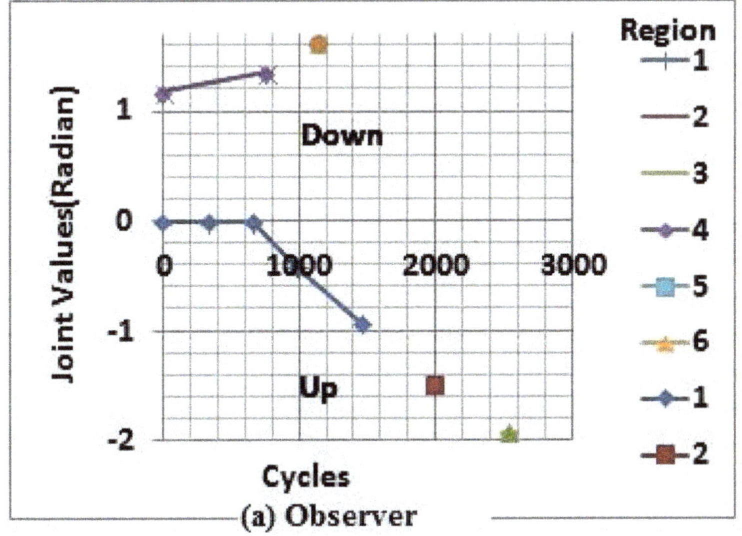

(a) Observer

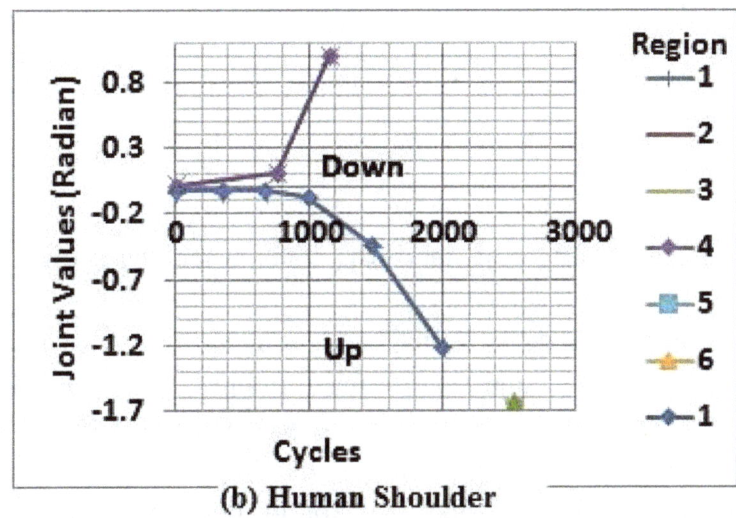

(b) Human Shoulder

Figure 9. Data mapping onto hardware faulty region.

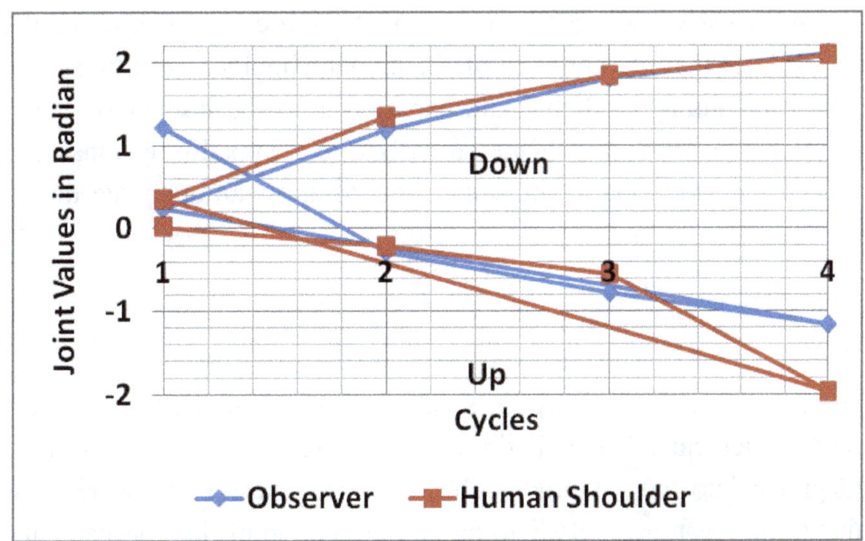

Figure 10. Empathy data conversion comparison.

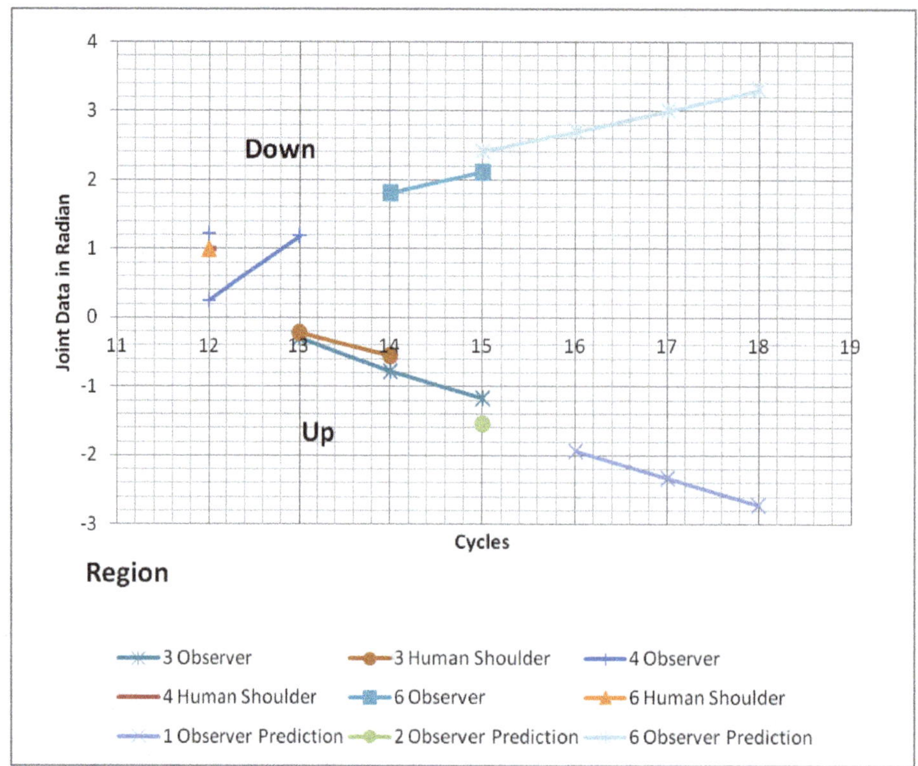

Figure 11. Empathy data mapping onto faulty region.

When the observer internal state is State 3, the awareness state switches to high priority subjective awareness, and the robot mind state is unconstrained. This state demonstrates that the robot mind may focus its attention on its embodiment aspects regardless of any synthetic pain being identified. The final awareness states for both, upward and downward experiments converge to high priority subjective awareness, forcing the robot attention to focus on the arm joint of the observer, and at the same time projecting the same situation on the human shoulder. A major difference occurs in the empathy response of the observer, in which during the upward experiment, direct impact of the projection forces the arm joint stiffness in a painful state as the observer prediction produces a false alarm at early stage of the experiment. While in the downward experiment, the observer accurately projects the internal state of the human shoulder, resulting in an accurate early alert information of an incoming synthetic pain experience on the human shoulder. This situation gives an advantage for the observer to provide an early direct empathy response by setting the arm joint stiffness to a medium level, and at the same time, to allow an adequate time for approaching the human peer and offer an assistance.

Conclusion

This paper implements robot empathy for synthetic pain by modelling robot self-awareness on subjective and objective elements. The embodiment of the consciousness feature through robot body part motions is integrated into the Adaptive Robot Self-Awareness Framework (ASAF) of a robot. We demonstrate that a robot can use ASAF, to build a projection of the internal state of agents apart from itself, and later on, to develop appropriate empathy responses. The projections allow the robot to simulate and experience the other robot's internal state, develop an accurate pain description, and generate appropriate empathy responses. Data transformation captured through robot vision determines the quality of projection process. The causal reasoning through sequential pattern prediction enables the robot's decision making to embrace the past, the current and the future considerations. This ability allows the robot to build expectations of the other agent's internal state. The observer's focus of attention switches as the reasoning process predicts the synthetic pain level that the human shoulder is experiencing.

Overall, the projection takes place accurately when both robots share a unified internal state. As the robot mind of the observer predicts that the element of body moves into the faulty joint region, the computation time increases and as a result, introduces data analyses discrepancies through a false alarm generation. This false projection occurs due three main causes: (i) Limited data to be used in sequence data prediction process decreases the quality of reasoning; (ii) the hardware discrepancies of the arm joint motor motion areas; (iii) there is a variable speed in hand movement of the human peer. The experiment also shows that robot awareness may revisit any of its consciousness regions under the unconstrained condition unless the robot mind switches to constrained condition. Utilization of the ASAF demonstrates a foreseeable application for empathy response towards synthetic pain for assistive robots application.

Building on this implementation and critical proof-of-concept work, future research will extend the pain acknowledgement and responses further by integrating sensor data across multiple sensors using more sophisticated data integration. Future works to carefully design experiments that evaluate other kinds of synthetic pain proposed in the paper. Experiments should be designed to accommodate the modelling of robot actions during the visitation of other regions existed in the ASAF framework. The pain activation mechanism will consider recognition of human pain through social cues, such as facial and verbal expressions. Furthermore, measuring the empathy response from human with disabilities would be our primary future study.

Acknowledgments

Our great appreciation to the Innovation and Entreprise Research Lab, the UTS Magic Lab, Faculty of Engineering and Information Technology, University of Technology Sydney UTS, Australia for experiment contributions. This work also marks the research collaboration between the UTS Magic Lab and the new established research collaboration project in the area of Cognitive and Social Robotics, Electrical Department, Faculty of Engineering, University of Hasanuddin UNHAS Makassar Indonesia. This work is integrated into The Advanced Artificial Intelligence Research Group (established in 2009).

References

1. Anshar M, Williams MA (2016) Evolving synthetic pain into an adaptive self-awareness framework for robots. *Bion Inspired Cognit Archit* 16: 8–18.
2. Helal A, Mokhtari M, Abdulrazak B (2008) The engineering handbook of smart technology for Aging, Disability, and Independence. *Wiley Online Library.*
3. Scassellati B (2002) Theory of mind for a humanoid robot. *Auton Robots* 12: 13–24.
4. Takeno J (2012) Creation of a conscious robot: Mirror image cognition and self-awareness. *Pan Stanford Publishing.*

5. Husserl E (1999) The essential husserl: Basic writings in transcendental phenomenology. *Stud Cont Thought* 54: 177–179.
6. Terrence F, Illah N, Dautenhahn K (2003) A survey of socially inter-active robots. *Rob Auton Syst J* 42: 143–166.
7. Feil-Seifer D, Matari MJ (2005) Defining socially assistive robotics. *Int Conf Rehabil Rob* 2005: 465–468.
8. Michel P, Gold K, Scassellati B (2004) Motion-based robotic self-recognition. *IEEE/RSJ Int Conf Intell Robots Syst* 3: 2763–2768.
9. Novianto R, Williams MA (2009) The role of attention in robot self-awareness. *Ro-man-the IEEE Int Symp Robot Hum Interact Commun* 175: 1047–1053.
10. Gorbenko A, Popov V, Sheka A (2012) Robot self-awareness: Exploration of internal states. *Appl Math Sci* 2012: 675–688.
11. Agha-Mohammad AA, Ure NK, How JP, et al. (2014) Health aware stochastic planning for persistent package delivery missions using quadrotors. *EEE/RSJ Int Conf Intell Robots Syst* 2014: 3389–3396.
12. Birlo M, Tapus A (2011) The crucial role of robot self-awareness in HRI. *Acm/IEEE Int Conf Human-robot Interact* 2011: 115–116.
13. Bongard J, Zykov V, Lipson H (2006) Resilient machines through continuous self-modeling. *Sci* 314: 1118–1121.
14. Marier JS, Rabbath CA, Lechevin N (2013) Health-aware coverage control with application to a team of small UAVs. *IEEE Trans Control Syst Technol* 21: 1719–1730.
15. Zagal JC, Lipson H (2009) Self-reflection in evolutionary robotics: Resilient adaptation with a minimum of physical exploration. *Conference Companion Genet Evolution Comput Conference: Late Break Paper* 2009: 2179–2188.
16. Lewis M (1991) Ways of knowing: Objective self-awareness or consciousness. *Biochem Rev* 11: 231–243.
17. Banissy MJ, Kanai R, Walsh V, et al. (2012) Inter-individual differences in empathy are reflected in human brain structure. *NeuroImage* 62: 2034–2039.
18. Cuff BMP, Brown SJ, Taylor L, et al. (2014) Empathy: A review of the concept. *Emotion Rev* 8: 144–153.
19. Goubert L, Craig, KD, Vervoort T, et al. (2005) Facing others in pain: The effects of empathy. *Pain* 118: 285–288.
20. Jackson PL, Rainville P, Decety J (2006) To what extent do we share the pain of others? Insight from the neural bases of pain empathy. *Pain* 125: 5–9.
21. Lamm C, Decety J, Singer T (2011) Meta-analytic evidence for common and distinct neural networks associated with directly experienced pain and empathy for pain. *NeuroImage* 54: 2492–2502.
22. Loggia ML, Mogil JS, Bushnell MC (2008) Empathy hurts: Compassion for another increases both sensory and affective components of pain perception. *Pain* 136: 168–176.
23. Singer T, Seymour B, O'Doherty J, et al. (2004) Empathy for pain involves the affective but not sensory components of pain. *Sci* 303: 1157–1162.
24. Meng J, Jackson T, Chen H, et al. (2013) Pain perception in the self and observation of others: An ERP investigation. *NeuroImage* 72: 164–173.
25. Woolf CJ (2010) What is this thing called pain? *J Clin Invest* 120: 3742–3744.
26. Mann WC (2005) Smart Technology for Aging, Disability and Independence: The State of the

Science. *Wiley-Interscience* 26: 75–77.

27. Harold A, Gerald-Jay S, Sussman J (1985) Structure and interpretation of computer programs. *MIT Press; McGraw-Hill* 74: 1167.
28. Baumgartner R, Gottlob G, Flesca S (2001) Visual Web Information Extraction with Lixto. *Int Conf on Vldb* 2001: 119–128.
29. Brachman RJ, Schmolze JG (1985) An overview of the KL-ONE Knowledge Representation System. *Cognit Sci* 9: 171–216.
30. Gottlob G (1992) Complexity Results for Nonmonotonic Logics. *J Logic Comput* 2: 397–425.
31. Gottlob G, Leone L, Scarcello F (2002) Hypertree decompositions and tractable queries. *Computer Syst Sci* 64: 579–627.
32. Levesque HJ (1984) Foundations of a functional approach to knowledge representation. *Artif Intell* 23: 155–212.
33. Levesque HJ (1984) A Logic of Implicit and Explicit Belief. *Natl Conf Artif Intell Austin* 1984: 198–202.
34. Nebel B (2011) On the compilability and expressive power of propositional planning formalisms. *J Art Intell Res* 12: 271–315.

8

Combined action observation and motor imagery therapy: a novel method for post-stroke motor rehabilitation

Jonathan R. Emerson*, Jack A. Binks, Matthew W. Scott, Ryan P. W. Kenny and Daniel L. Eaves*

School of Health and Social Care, Teesside University, Middlesbrough, UK

* **Correspondence:** Email: J.emerson@tees.ac.uk, d.eaves@tees.ac.uk;

Abstract: Cerebral vascular accidents (strokes) are a leading cause of motor deficiency in millions of people worldwide. While a complex range of biological systems is affected following a stroke, in this paper we focus primarily on impairments of the motor system and the recovery of motor skills. We briefly review research that has assessed two types of mental practice, which are currently recommended in stroke rehabilitation. Namely, action observation (AO) therapy and motor imagery (MI) training. We highlight the strengths and limitations in both techniques, before making the case for combined action observation and motor imagery (AO + MI) therapy as a potentially more effective method. This is based on a growing body of multimodal brain imaging research showing advantages for combined AO + MI instructions over the two separate methods of AO and MI. Finally, we offer a series of suggestions and considerations for how combined AO + MI therapy could be employed in neurorehabilitation.

Keywords: neurorehabilitation; mental practice; combined action observation and motor imagery; AO + MI; motor simulation; demonstrations; motor recovery; action representation; stroke; motor impairment

---

Abbreviations: AO: action observation; MI: motor imagery; AO + MI: combined action observation and motor imagery; fMRI: functional magnetic resonance imaging; EEG: electroencephalography; TMS: transcranial magnetic stimulation; BCI: brain computer interface; LSRT: layered stimulus response training

1. Introduction

Cerebral vascular accidents (strokes) are a leading cause of motor deficiency in millions of people worldwide [1]. Unfortunately, the number of people affected by stroke will inevitably rise as global life expectancy increases. The prevalence of motor deficits following a stroke can be up to 80% in a defined elderly population [2–3]. Only a small proportion of this group (approximately 20%) will partially recover from impaired motor ability, leaving approximately 50–60% who are left with some form of chronic motor deficiency [3–4]. Motor impairments are defined as the loss or restriction of function in the control of muscles, movements, or mobility [5]. Areas frequently affected are the hand, arm, face and leg, typically on one side of the body [1]. Motor impairments may involve disordered sensorimotor and proprioceptive control, which often result from an upper motor neuron lesion, as evidenced by intermittent or sustained involuntary muscle activations [6]. Hemiparesis or muscle weakness [7] is also commonly observed, resulting in altered movement patterns in both the contralateral and ipsilateral side (with respect to the side of the lesion, paretic or nonparetic [8]).

Encouragingly, there is strong evidence in cognitive neuroscience literature showing the brain can adapt or reorganise itself in response to sensory input, learning and experience [9]. This process is referred to as *neuroplasticity* [10], and can occur in both the healthy and impaired brain [11–12]. Following a stroke, neurorehabilitation aims to reduce motor deficits via neuroplasticity effects, typically through repetitive physical training, constraint-induced movement therapy, or physical therapy [13–15]. Several useful approaches highlighted in the literature also include: mirror box therapy, electrical stimulation (e.g., non-invasive brain stimulation or vagus nerve stimulation), fitness training, biofeedback and robotic interactions [16]. Given that everyday movements can be significantly impaired, particularly in the acute post-stroke phases, physical practice may not be possible or appropriate. To address this pertinent issue, a great deal of research has investigated the efficacy of mental practice techniques for enhancing neurorehabilitation instead [17].

In this paper our aim is not to provide a review of literature that is either exhaustive or fully systematic in nature. Instead, we provide a balanced and concise analysis and discussion of contemporary research examining the use of two mental practice techniques, namely, action observation (AO) and motor imagery (MI) in post-stroke rehabilitation. First, we briefly review some of the key studies investigating the benefits and limitations of using both AO and MI independently in stroke rehabilitation. We refer to the evidence supporting neuroplasticity effects, which are argued to underpin the rehabilitation process. We also address the practical and applied implications for the delivery of both AO and MI in clinical and home settings. Where possible we also make reference to published guidelines and recommendations for stroke rehabilitation.

We then review all available research to date that has investigated the effects of combined action observation and motor imagery (AO + MI) instructions, predominantly in healthy adults. This section covers a growing body of multimodal brain imaging research, and a collection of carefully designed behavioural studies. We give particular focus to the one study that has investigated combined AO + MI therapy in stroke rehabilitation [18]. While the main thrust of our argument is in favour of the advantages in this approach, we highlight the potential limitations of using combined AO + MI therapy with regards to a patient's cognitive ability and lesion location. To address some of these limitations, we suggest a method of carefully layering AO and MI practices over time, in line with the progressive nature of the rehabilitation process, to build toward a more complex and integrated form of AO + MI therapy, which could later be combined with physical rehabilitation.

Finally, we offer a series of suggestions and considerations for how combined AO + MI therapy could be incorporated into existing neurorehabilitation practice. The aim of this section is simply to provide a series of examples and scenarios to stimulate debate and discussion in the field about the suitability of AO + MI therapy in different contexts.

2. Neurorehabilitation via different forms of motor simulation

Action observation (AO) therapy and motor imagery (MI) training are two prominent mental practice techniques that have both been recommended as potentially effective intervention tools [19]. AO refers to the deliberate and structured observation of human movement [20], whereas MI is defined as "the mental representation of action without any [overt] concomitant body movement" [21]. The rationale for using these two methods is predicated on multimodal neuroimaging evidence, showing the brain areas involved in AO at least partially overlap with those involved during MI. Moreover, the brain regions activated during both AO and MI overlap extensively with those involved in motor execution [22]. On these grounds, Jeannerod's [23] influential hypothesis was that AO and MI can be regarded as two forms of motor simulation that are functionally equivalent to each other. Despite this early integrative account, it is surprising that both researchers and practitioners have largely employed either AO or MI methods in isolation from each other [24].

2.1. Action observation therapy

The efficacy of action observation (AO) therapy in neurorehabilitation is well grounded in neurophysiological research. Substantial evidence has confirmed that seeing an action can generate an internal representation of the observed action [25], which can prime execution of the same action [26]. The neuronal substrate for this has been termed the mirror neuron system [25]. On this basis, AO therapy involves the systematic observation of actions prior to execution [27]. For example, reaching, grasping, transporting and perhaps manipulating an object, before finally releasing the grip. Following each observed action, patients physically execute the same action and sessions are repeated daily. Research shows AO therapy can yield significant improvements in upper limb movement in ischaemic stroke patients, over a four week period, relative to both the baseline and a control group [28–29]. These improvements are typically retained for several months post intervention.

In particular, Ertelt et al.'s [28] functional magnetic resonance imaging (fMRI) study reported a significant rise in the neurophysiological activity recorded in premotor regions of the cortex. This increase was specifically in those stroke patients who were allocated to the AO therapy group, compared to those in the control groups. The brain regions exhibiting neuroplasticity effects included: the bilateral ventral premotor cortex, bilateral superior temporal gyrus, the supplementary motor area, and the contralateral supramarginal gyrus. Accordingly, those authors argued that the mirror neuron system's capacity to re-enact observed actions should be harnessed to promote rehabilitation in motor regions of the brain, and facilitate neuroplasticity effects [30]. Buccino [27] recently argued that future research should therefore consider how to combine AO therapy effectively with other methods in neurorehabilitation.

Live demonstrations are easily administered by practitioners in face-to-face clinical settings, wherein AO therapy would not normally not involve any particular skill on the patient's side. This assumption is based on substantial neurophysiological evidence showing that even passive action observation can activate an associated motor representation in the observer's brain [25]. To create home-based AO therapy would instead require a library of action videos. It would also be necessary for the patient to have both the access and capacity to engage with the technology that displays these videos within their home. Regardless of the location for delivery, however, a limitation in the current delivery method for AO therapy is that practitioners will rarely instruct a patient on either *how* they should observe the target action, or *what* features they should focus on. This is in contrast with MI training, which involves specific instructions for action content. For MI the vividness of the experience depends on each patient's ability to form and maintain the required motor simulation [31–32]. Moreover, while Gatti et al. [19] showed increased motor involvement for AO compared to MI, a number of studies have shown the reverse trend [24].

2.2. Motor imagery training

Motor imagery involves simulating the visual and kinaesthetic aspects of an action without any overt movement occurring [33]. This can be undertaken either from an internal, first person, perspective (as if performing the imagined movement from one's own point of view) or an external, third person, perspective (as if watching oneself making the movement form outside of the body). Furthermore, internal kinaesthetic imagery should be dissociated from internal visual imagery. This is on the basis that the former modulates corticospinal excitability at the supraspinal level, while the latter does not [34]. The kinaesthetic and first person internal perspective are also best measured using separate subscales in self-report questionnaires, reflecting the academic consensus for a more differentiated approach to assessing MI ability [35].

A large body of research shows MI training has the potential to improve motor abilities in neurorehabilitation [36], and that the neural reorganisation following MI training is similar to the changes following physical training [37–38]. In a landmark fMRI study into the neuroplasticity effects associated with MI training in stroke patients, Sharma et al. [39] reported three key findings. First, after subcortical stroke there was evidence for cortical neuroplasticity, both in terms of regional activation, and connectivity within distributed brain networks. These changes in network connectivity were observed most clearly during MI. Second, plasticity occurred in cortical areas that were remote from the subcortical infarct. Cortical changes were therefore not the result of local cortical injury, but a response to injury elsewhere in the motor system. Third, the changes in connectivity during MI correlated with motor function. A more recent study has also shown acute MI training not only modulates plasticity effects at the cortical level, but also further downstream at the level of spinal presynaptic inhibition, reflecting the sensitivity of the spinal circuitry to MI [40].

A systematic review by Zimmermann-Schlatter et al. [41] initially reported there was moderate evidence supporting the use of MI in conventional physiotherapy for stroke rehabilitation. They concluded MI is something easily learned, requires no physical effort and poses no harm to the patient. A more recent meta-analysis by Machado et al. [42] focused on randomized controlled trials that assessed imagery training effects. Those authors instead argued the evidence for imagery benefits in stroke rehabilitation is at best only mixed [36]. Despite contradictions like this in the evidence base, published guidelines from The American Heart Association, American Stroke

Association [43] and the Canadian Stroke Best Practice recommendations [44] all state MI should be included alongside physical practice to maximise stroke rehabilitation. Bovend'Eerdt and colleagues [45] have also provided an evidence-based guide for including MI in neurorehabilitation in a clinical setting. While these guides are constructive and informative, there are many areas of MI use in stroke rehabilitation that require further investigation.

For example, it is not yet clear what the optimal dosage for MI should be over the duration of a rehabilitation programme, and how this should be tailored to the individual. Previous efforts to define clinically optimal MI dosage effects on motor recovery include assessments for both twenty and sixty minute MI sessions, delivered three days a week for ten weeks [46]. Completing twenty minute sessions led to an increase in scores for the Action Research Arm Test (ARAT), while sixty minute sessions led to an increase in Fugl-Meyer Assessment (FMA) scores. Although these findings suggest MI can improve motor function, the assessment method should also be considered in terms of how the desired outcome is defined.

Another issue is that stroke patients can have difficulties in generating MI from verbal instructions in a clinical setting. In particular, cognitive impairments caused by a stroke can make verbal instructions and cues difficult to follow [47]. While it is not currently clear how existing approaches to MI training can avoid this problem, combined AO + MI therapy may offer potential solutions (discussed below). Future work must therefore further investigate the imagery training methods, delivery, format and scheduling best suited within stroke rehabilitation.

An intuitive advantage of MI is that this method is cost-free and can easily be incorporated throughout all stages of stroke recovery and existing physical rehabilitation programmes. Patients may also be able to practice MI independently between their physical therapy sessions. Furthermore, stroke patients can be encouraged to imagine performing actions or tasks that they are currently unable to physically achieve due to their impaired motor abilities.

Physical rehabilitation primarily focuses on the recovery of previously learned actions (i.e., motor re-learning) instead of training novel movements. It is crucial practitioners take the same approach in MI training. During physical practice, brain activity in healthy adults is typically more bilateral and diffuse across hemispheres when the task is novel compared to well-practiced [48]. In MI, this pattern of cortical activity is similarly more diffuse for imagery of un-practiced actions compared to imagery of familiar actions and, overall, cortical activity is more diffuse and bilateral for imagery compared to execution [49]. Accordingly, it can be difficult to learn novel actions via MI alone, as the task-related neural networks may be absent, unorganised [50], or damaged in the case of stroke patients. Research shows that cortical activity reduces in task specific brain regions as a function of physical practice and this effect can also occur, though to a lesser extent, using imagery [51]. Imagery based rehabilitation therapy must therefore incorporate actions that will encourage both the growth and refinement of these neural networks to support physical gains. Practitioners should also avoid making the MI task too challenging for the patient, considering both the severity of the stroke and the patient's motor repertoire prior to the stroke.

3. Combined action observation and motor imagery therapy

Traditionally, the two forms of motor simulation (that is, AO and MI) have been studied either in isolation from each other, or compared, in terms of their relative effectiveness in rehabilitation [19,24,47]. More recently, however, a growing number of studies has investigated the potential advantages of instructing combined action observation and motor imagery (AO + MI; [24,33]). This instruction involves imagining the kinaesthetic experience and sensations of action, while also observing a visual display of the same action at the same time [33]. Participants are normally instructed to synchronise their imagined action with the observed movement in real time. Despite the obvious need to verbally describe this task in the first instance, showing patients a visual representation of the target action could help to reduce the volume of instructions needed to cue imagery of the same action. This would therefore negate some of the problems inherent in stroke patient treatment, regarding their ability to understand and follow the verbal cues associated with traditional imagery training [47].

Multimodal brain imaging research now provides remarkably positive and consistent evidence showing combined AO + MI instructions can significantly increase the level of neurophysiological activation in cortico-motor regions of the brain, compared to either purely imagining or observing the same action [33]. This effect has been reliably demonstrated across the following neurophysiological measures: fMRI [52–55], electroencephalography (EEG; [56–59]) and transcranial magnetic stimulation (TMS; [60–65]). Given the main premise for undertaking both AO therapy and MI training is the increase in motor involvement compared to baseline and control conditions, it is striking that this facilitation in motor activity is significantly more pronounced, and in some cases in a super-additive way [55], for combined AO + MI instructions. Accordingly, this pattern of cortical activity in motor and motor-related regions of the brain more closely represents the motor system's involvement during physical execution [52]. In turn this would suggest clear advantages for combined AO + MI instructions in rehabilitation over separate AO and MI methods.

While those neurophysiological studies focused on healthy adult participants, the authors have regularly recommended combined AO + MI training for neurorehabilitation purposes. This is an intuitive suggestion that may hold promise for a range of brain injured patients, including those recovering from a stroke. The related behavioural research in a rehabilitation setting, however, is currently sparse. So far, a series of behavioural studies has shown significant advantages for combined AO + MI instructions in healthy adults. This was during balance training [66], instantaneous and automatic imitation [58,67–68], peak force development [69], target aiming [70], and accelerated rehabilitation post hip arthroplasty [71]. A recent study has also shown significantly greater modulations in movement kinematics for combined AO + MI instructions in Parkinson's disease patients, compared to AO instructions [72]. An open question is whether gains in similar tasks will also be possible in stroke patients. To our knowledge, Sun et al. [18] was the first, and remains the only experiment to investigate a combined AO + MI therapy intervention in stroke patients.

The study by Sun and colleagues [18] included ten right handed participants who all had a stroke lesion affecting their left hemisphere, resulting in impaired right arm function. All participants received the same conventional physical rehabilitation on a daily basis for four weeks, while undertaking five rounds of mental practice during this period. Patients were asked to imagine the effort and sensations of moving their right hand to grasp, lift, and insert a small peg into a hole on a board, before removing the peg from the hole. Half of the participants imagined this while they simultaneously observed the same action displayed on a screen (i.e., combined AO + MI therapy). In this condition, the observed action was intended as a visual guide to help refine and maintain the concurrently imagined action. The other half (control group) observed and then subsequently imagined the same action, that is, in a serial fashion, rather than in a combined way. For this group, the visual guide was intended as a method of priming the subsequently imagined action.

Sun et al. [18] reported significant improvements in two measures of motor ability: the FMA and pinch grip strength test. A clinically important improvement in FMA scores is defined as between 4.25 to 7.25 points [46]. In Sun et al.'s [18] study, both the combined AO + MI and the control group improved their FMA scores by a clinically important margin over the four week period (24.8 and 19.6, respectively). Indeed, the difference between the two groups at the end of the testing period could also be considered clinically meaningful, demonstrating combined AO + MI therapy can improve upper extremity motor function in post-stroke patients (see Table 1).

Table 1. Data adapted from the study published by Sun et al. [18]. Mean scores for the Fugl-Meyer Assessment, reported over a four week period for two post-stroke rehabilitation groups: action observation followed by motor imagery vs. combined action observation and motor imagery.

	Baseline	Week 1	Week 2	Week 3	Post-test	Change score
Action observation followed by motor imagery	14.8	19	24	29.6	34.4	19.6
Combined action observation and motor imagery	14.6	20.6	27.8	33	39.4	24.8
Between-group difference	0.2	1.6	3.8	3.4	5	5.2

Sun et al. [18] also reported EEG recordings over the primary sensorimotor cortex. Event-related desynchronization of the mu rhythm was greater in amplitude and duration for the combined AO + MI group, reflecting enhanced cortico-motor involvement in response to this training method. Although this study was both limited to a relatively small sample size, and did not include a strict control group, it does provide the first evidence indicating combined AO + MI therapy can facilitate neuroplasticity effects to support motor recovery within stroke patients more effectively than AO followed by MI.

One possibility, which now requires further investigation (for e.g., using structural modelling techniques), is that these changes for combined AO + MI therapy reflect a modulation of intracortical and subcortical excitatory mechanisms, through synaptic and cortical plasticity. In this context, the changes reported in Sun et al.'s [18] study are likely to be driven by mechanisms that more closely resemble those involved during physical practice of the same task, which in turn would be expected to produce gains that are greater in magnitude over and above those obtained using either AO or MI [47].

Overall, this growing body of multimodal neuroimaging evidence indicates that it is possible for healthy adults to co-represent both an observed and an imagined action simultaneously (termed 'dual-action' simulation [33,58]). Presumably, this is in the form of two parallel sensorimotor streams. A useful framework for conceptualising such dual-action simulation can be formulated on the basis of Cisek and Kalaska's [73] affordance competition hypothesis. Their model describes how multiple sensorimotor representations are maintained in parallel, as a set of action affordances.

Preparation for action would then involve different brain areas submitting their 'votes' to contribute toward the selection of available movement parameters, prior to movement execution. In the context of combined AO + MI therapy, concurrent representations involving an observed and an imagined action would be maintained simultaneously, and these two streams would either merge or compete, based on their content and relevance towards ongoing action plans [33,58,68,74]. While the efficacy of this dual-action simulation hypothesis is yet to be comprehensively explored both in the healthy brain, and the related motor behaviour, the application of this conceptual lens will likely offer novel approaches to rehabilitation of the injured brain.

3.1. Potential limitations of combined AO + MI therapy

An important point when considering combined AO + MI therapy in stroke patients is that some (though not all) of the limitations that currently apply to the use of MI could also apply to combined AO + MI therapy. The primary issue concerns whether a stroke patient is indeed capable of engaging in imagery at all. Several studies have shown mental imagery is multifaceted, involving a number of different cognitive functions and brain areas [31]. Visual compared to motor imagery for instance involves activations in different neuronal subsystems. There is also sufficient evidence for individual differences underlying imagery ability, based on differences in brain structure [35].

As mentioned earlier, there is currently mixed support for the efficacy of MI training in stroke rehabilitation. One explanation for the discrepancies in the literature may be the lack of control for MI ability. The key issue is that the particular location of damage in a patient's brain may prevent successful MI performance, and this may account for the absence of an MI-based treatment effect [75]. Research has established that impairments in parietal lobe function, either through stroke [76] or inhibitory brain stimulation in healthy participants [77–78] significantly reduces MI ability. Moreover, Oostra et al.'s [76] study highlighted the importance of an intact fronto-parietal network for MI, and the crucial role of the basal ganglia and premotor cortex when performing MI tasks. This was on the basis of their finding that low scores on a self-report MI vividness scale were associated with lesions in the left putamen, left ventral premotor cortex and long association fibres linking parieto-occipital regions with the dorsolateral premotor and prefrontal areas. Poor temporal congruence was otherwise linked to lesions in the more rostrally located white matter of the superior corona radiate [76].

In support of these findings, McInnes et al.'s [75] recent review and meta-analysis found broad evidence showing patients with parietal lobe damage were most impaired on their ability to perform MI. Damage to specific brain structures such as the parietal lobe, frontal lobe and basal ganglia consistently showed impairment in MI ability. Accordingly, McInnes and colleagues concluded that MI-based neurorehabilitation may not be efficacious in all patient populations.

While this conclusion is well grounded in terms of the limits inherent in a patient's imagery ability, as determined by the nature of the damage experienced in specific brain regions, the patient's rehabilitation outcomes may also be limited by virtue of traditional imagery training methods themselves. Neuroplasticity, or rewiring of motor networks, is the intended aim for the rehabilitation process, which ultimately strives to improve movement recovery rates [75]. The question remains, therefore, to what extent can combined AO + MI therapy help restore lost motor function in damaged brain regions, compared to traditional MI training methods? An increasingly persuasive rationale is that rehabilitation practitioners should attempt to capitalise on the significant increase in motor involvement associated with using combined AO + MI therapy, for the purpose of facilitating neuroplasticity.

A further challenge in stroke rehabilitation relates to the associated cognitive impairment. It is not within the scope of this article to review the extant literature on this substantial topic, but consideration of this evidence does have a strong bearing on the potential effectiveness of any modality for rehabilitation. Approximately 50% of stroke survivors are left with some form of cognitive impairment [79]. The affected cognitive domains are typically: attention and attention span, concentration, memory and decision making [80]. An important consideration for the use of combined AO + MI therapy in stroke rehabilitation therefore is the possible cognitive abilities participants might need to engage in this protocol.

Eaves et al. [58] recently showed that when healthy adult participants observed and concurrently imagined performing the same action there was a specific increase in the electrophysiological activity recorded over the rostral prefrontal cortex. Combined AO + MI methods may therefore come at an additional challenge to the user, in terms of the cognitive demands associated with supervisory control [58]. For stroke survivors, it will therefore be crucial to initially assess whether they are capable of undertaking AO + MI, in light of any cognitive impairments they may be experiencing.The preliminary evidence from Sun et al. [18] is that the stroke patients in their study were at least capable of achieving motor proficiency gains through combined AO + MI therapy, despite these additional cognitive demands. If patients can follow AO + MI instructions, then a fruitful avenue for future research is to investigate whether this method facilitates neural reorganisation effects in motor and motor-related areas, as well as in prefrontal regions. This suggestion is based on Jackson et al.'s [38] work, which similarly found neural reorganisation in prefrontal regions that correlated with increased physical performance following imagery combined with physical practice.

In summary, there are converging lines of evidence indicating combined AO + MI instructions may be more beneficial than the traditional approach of using AO and MI independently. This evidence comes from multimodal imaging studies, which show increased motor involvement for combined AO + MI instructions relative to the two individual techniques; as well as behavioural studies showing improvements in physical execution. Careful consideration should be given, however, to the potential constraints inherent in post-stroke brain function (on an individual patient basis), because this could impact the effectiveness of combined AO + MI therapy, in much the same way as it can impact the effectiveness of other therapies. There is now a rich opportunity for future research to investigate the extent to which combined AO + MI therapy could perhaps mitigate against these constraints, compared to other therapies, in clinical populations. One approach could be to examine neuroplasticity effects over time in the structural and functional brain mechanisms underpinning combined AO + MI instructions.

3.2. Integrating combined action observation and motor imagery therapy with existing methods

In this final section, we offer a series of proposals and considerations for how combined AO + MI therapy could be employed in neurorehabilitation. Our suggestions are intended primarily as illustrations to help stimulate debate and discussion in the field about the suitability of AO + MI therapy in different contexts.

From a practitioner's perspective, the key features of combined AO + MI therapy are that this method is essentially cost-free and does not require specialist delivery. Instead, implementation requires a simple change to clinical practice. As a matter of course, stroke rehabilitation practitioners regularly provide visual demonstrations of the actions they intend their patient to perform. As part of this process, it is less common for a practitioner to advise their patient on exactly *how* they should pay their attention and *what* features of the action they should focus on. Combined AO + MI instructions represent a straight forward way to formalise this important part of the rehabilitation programme. The recent review paper by Eaves et al. [33] suggested a number of critical considerations when using this technique in stroke rehabilitation, particularly from a research viewpoint. Here we make additional suggestions from a practical perspective on how to administer this technique.

Action observation is arguably more familiar to patients and demands less cognitive input compared to motor imagery. This argument is based on the idea that although AO can involve active attention (for example, when there is intention to imitate the observed action), it can also be passive in nature, operating predominantly on the basis of automatic processing mechanisms [81]. On the other hand, MI is largely a voluntary, purposeful and directed activity. It may therefore be more useful to focus on basic AO therapy in the early stages of rehabilitation. As the patient's ability and engagement in the task increases over time, it may be useful to gradually introduce the imagery component. To achieve this, it would be necessary to provide some basic training in how to engage in motor imagery. A number of protocols exist for structuring and priming the relevant imagery components, including the model for Physical, Environment, Task, Timing, Learning, Emotion, and Perspective (PETTLEP; [82]) imagery training. A technique that may then specifically help to bridge the gap between traditional AO therapy and traditional imagery training is Layered Stimulus Response Training (LSRT; [83]).

Based on bioinformational theory [84–85], LSRT is intended to help individuals more easily generate and control their imagery experience by breaking down the different elements of an image, before bringing them together again in layers that can become increasingly complex [31]. From this perspective, it would be useful to first introduce a visual demonstration of the action, which is later accompanied by specific instructions to imagine performing carefully selected action features, such as the velocity, the trajectory or the goal of the action, which are synchronised with the on-line display. Prior to this exercise, and through individual consultation, participants would identify the action features they find most vivid and accessible through their imagery. As their ability in this task increases, the same visual display would be used repeatedly, upon which it is possible to layer imagery content with additional action features that are increasingly more complex and vivid. While this can all be achieved as part of existing face-to-face provision, further opportunities arise through the incorporation of technology.

The use of simple smartphone apps aimed at health-related outcomes have increased both in health professionals and the general public [86]. Smartphones are invaluable for the education and management of health conditions [87] and, specifically within stroke patients, for providing: education, exercises, functional skills training, daily living activities, and assistive device tutorials [88–90]. Moreover, the National Clinical Guidelines for Stroke also encourage the use of smartphones within stroke care [91].

Apps can easily display interactive videos and pictures of actions that provide an opportunity to further implement and explore the effectiveness of combined AO + MI therapy in rehabilitative practice. This could either be in the presence of rehabilitation professionals, or independently while patients are alone, as long as the patient has the capacity to engage with this technology independently. App developers would therefore need to work closely with clinicians, researchers and stroke patients to refine the contents of the actions displayed and the tasks involved, so they are: 1) adaptable and cater for individual differences in ability for patients with various impairments following cerebral vascular accidents; 2) carefully regulated and integrated with accurate information and evidence based research; and 3) have the ability to collect data and provide feedback.

In addition to traditional rehabilitation methods, imagery instructions can also be employed when using more sophisticated methods, such as brain computer interface (BCI) technology. The aim of a BCI is to foster neuroplasticity through manipulation or self-regulation of neurophysiological activity facilitating motor recovery. This could be achieved through neurofeedback mechanisms that incorporate MI instructions. Using this approach, it is possible to control the movements of an on-screen cursor by recording the neural activity, for example, over the patient's motor cortex, while they imagine executing an action [92]. In a recent meta-analysis, Cervera et al. [93] showed evidence for BCI-induced functional and structural neuroplasticity at a subclinical level. Of the nine studies included in their review, which involved 235 stroke survivors in total, the motor improvements following BCI training exceeded the minimal clinically important difference, when quantified using the upper limb FMA tool. The summary effect size was also reported as ranging from medium to large.

A successful BCI setup depends on the user's ability to voluntarily control their own neural activity. Neuper et al. [59] was the first to investigate if the input signals required for effective BCI can be enhanced by combined AO + MI instructions. Using EEG methods, those authors showed AO + MI instructions produced significantly greater modulations of sensorimotor rhythms. This was when participants imagined performing a reach-grasp action while also observing visual feedback representing the same action, which was controlled using their own BCI input. This was compared to when participants purely imagined this task. This subtle but important change in protocol was therefore recommended as a more advantageous method for successful BCI. Given the recommendations in Cervera at al.'s [93] meta-analysis for future BCI research to engage with knowledge and understanding in the field of MI research, we would further recommend extending this to the literature investigating combined AO + MI methods. In doing so, it will be important to acknowledge the potential limits of these methods, which relate to a patient's capacity to engage with the technology, with respect to their level of cognitive and imagery ability.

4. Conclusion

There is now convincing evidence that combined AO + MI instructions elicit increased activity in motor regions of the brain, compared to either AO or MI independently. On these grounds, combined AO + MI therapy, in conjunction with physical practice, is recommended as a potentially more effective tool for practitioners in rehabilitation settings. While preliminary research indicates combined AO + MI therapy can be administered to stroke patients to directly impact neuroplasticity and motor outcomes [18], high quality research is now required to further validate this result. For practitioners, it is free and relatively easy to incorporate into their existing practice. It also represents an opportunity to prescribe useful home based training, which would be in addition to their one-to-one therapy sessions. Future research must now establish if this approach can help to improve motor recovery rates and facilitate independent rehabilitation. It is also important that future research establishes the best methods of delivery for combined AO + MI therapy, and how this should be tailored to the participant's ability and needs, while also exploring how this approach can be integrated with new technology that is both affordable and widely available.

References

1. Warlow CP, van Gijn J, Dennis MS, et al. (2008) *Stroke: Practical Management* (3rd ed.), Oxford: Blackwell Publishing.
2. Barker WH, Mullooly JP (1997) Stroke in a defined elderly population, 1967–1985. A less lethal and disabling but no less common disease. *Stroke* 28: 284–290.
3. Hendricks HT, van Limbeek J, Geurts AC, et al. (2002) Motor recovery after stroke: a systematic review of the literature. *Arch Phys Med Rehabil* 83: 1629–1637.
4. De Vries S, Mulder T (2007) Motor imagery and stroke rehabilitation: a critical discussion. *J Rehabil Med* 39: 5–13.
5. Wade DT (1992). *Measurement in Neurological Rehabilitation*, Oxford: Oxford University Press.
6. Pandyan AD, Gregoric M, Barnes MP, et al. (2005) Spasticity: clinical perceptions, neurological realities and meaningful measurement. *Disabil Rehabil* 27: 2–6.
7. Andrews AW, Bohannon RW (1989) Decreased shoulder range of motion on paretic side after stroke. *Phys Ther* 69: 768–772.
8. Meskers CG, Koppe PA, Konijnenbelt MH, et. al. (2005) Kinematic alterations in the ipsilateral shoulder of patients with hemiplegia due to stroke. *Am J Phys Med Rehabil* 84: 97–105.
9. Chan DYL, Chan CCH, Au DKS (2006) Motor relearning programme for stroke patients: a randomized controlled trial. *Clin Rehabil* 20: 191–200.
10. Rossini PM, Calautti C, Pauri F, et al. (2003) Post-stroke plastic reorganisation in the adult brain. *Lancet Neurol* 2: 493–502.
11. Hubbard IJ, Parsons MW, Neilson C, et al. (2009) Task-specific training evidence for and translation to clinical practice. *Occup Ther Int* 16: 175–189.
12. Arya KN, Pandian S, Verma R, et al. (2011) Movement therapy induced neural reorganization and motor recovery in stroke: a review. *J Bodyw Mov Ther* 15: 528–537.
13. Aichner F, Adelwöhrer C, Haring HP (2002) Rehabilitation approaches to stroke, In: Fleischhacker WW, Brooks DJ, *Stroke-vascular Diseases*, Vienna: Springer, 59–73.
14. Byl N, Roderick J, Mohamed O, et al. (2003) Effectiveness of sensory and motor rehabilitation of the upper limb following the principles of neuroplasticity: patients stable poststroke. *Neurorehabil Neural Repair* 17: 176–191.
15. Jang SH, Kim YH, Cho SH, et al. (2003) Cortical reorganization induced by task-oriented training in chronic hemiplegic stroke patients. *Neuroreport* 14: 137–141.
16. Langhorne P, Coupar F, Pollock A (2009) Motor recovery after stroke: a systematic review. *Lancet Neurol* 8: 741–754.
17. Park SW, Kim JH, Yang, YJ (2018) Mental practice for upper limb rehabilitation after stroke: a systematic review and meta-analysis. *Int J Rehabil Res* 41: 197–203.

18. Sun Y, Wei W, Luo Z, et al. (2016) Improving motor imagery practice with synchronous action observation in stroke patients. *Top Stroke Rehabil* 23: 245–253.
19. Gatti R, Tettamanti A, Gough PM, et al. (2013) Action observation versus motor imagery in learning a complex motor task: a short review of literature and a kinematics study. *Neurosci Lett* 540: 37–42.
20. Neuman B, Gray R (2013) A direct comparison of the effects of imagery and action observation on hitting performance. *Movement Sport Sci: Sci Motricité* 79: 11–21.
21. Guillot A, Collet C (2008) Construction of the motor imagery integrative model in sport: a review and theoretical investigation of motor imagery use. *Int Rev Sport Exer P* 1: 31–44.
22. Hardwick RM, Caspers S, Eickhoff SB, et al. (2018) Neural Correlates of Action: Comparing Meta-Analyses of Imagery, Observation, and Execution. *Neurosci Biobehav Rev* 94: 31–44.
23. Jeannerod M (2006) *Motor Cognition*, Oxford: Oxford University Press.
24. Vogt S, Di Rienzo F, Collet C, et al. (2013) Multiple roles of motor imagery during action observation. *Front Hum Neurosci* 7: 807.
25. Rizzolatti G, Sinigaglia C (2010) The functional role of the parieto-frontal mirror circuit: interpretations and misinterpretations. *Nat Rev Neurosci* 11: 264–274.
26. Vogt S, Thomaschke R (2007) From visuo-motor interactions to imitation learning: behavioural and brain imaging studies. *J Sports Sci* 25: 497–517.
27. Buccino G (2014) Action observation treatment: a novel tool in neurorehabilitation. *Philos Trans R Soc Lond B Biol Sci* 369: 20130185.
28. Ertelt D, Small S, Solodkin A, et al. (2007) Action observation has a positive impact on rehabilitation of motor deficits after stroke. *Neuroimage* 36: 164–173.
29. Franceschini M, Ceravolo MG, Agosti M, et al. (2012) Clinical relevance of action observation in upper-limb stroke rehabilitation: a possible role in recovery of functional dexterity. A randomized clinical trial. *Neurorehabil Neural Repair* 26: 456–462.
30. Zhang JJQ, Fong KNK, Welage N, et al. (2018) The activation of the mirror neuron system during action observation and action execution with mirror visual feedback in stroke: a systematic review. *Neural Plast* 2018: 2321045.
31. Cumming J, Eaves DL (2018) The nature, measurement, and development of imagery ability. *Imagin Cog Pers* 37: 375–393.
32. Eaves DL, Emerson JR, Binks JA, et al. (2018) Imagery ability: the individual difference gradient and novel training methods (Commentary on Kraeutner et al. (2018)) *Eur J Neurosci* 47: 1219–1220.
33. Eaves DL, Riach M, Holmes PS, et al. (2016) Motor imagery during action observation: A brief review of evidence, theory and future research opportunities. *Front Neurosci* 10: 514.
34. Stinear CM, Byblow WD, Steyvers M, et al. (2006) Kinesthetic, but not visual, motor imagery modulates corticomotor excitability. *Exp Brain Res* 168: 157–164.
35. De Vries S, Tepper M, Feenstra W, et al. (2013) Motor imagery ability in stroke patients: the relationship between implicit and explicit motor imagery measures. *Front Hum Neurosci* 7: 790.
36. Braun S, Kleynen M, van Heel T, et al. (2013) The effects of mental practice in neurological rehabilitation; a systematic review and meta-analysis. *Front Hum Neurosci* 7: 390.
37. Pascual-Leone A, Nguyet D, Cohen LG, et al. (1995) Modulation of muscle responses evoked by transcranial magnetic stimulation during the acquisition of new fine motor skills. *J Neurophysiol* 74: 1037–1045.

38. Jackson PL, Lafleur MF, Malouin F, et al. (2003) Functional cerebral reorganization following motor sequence learning through mental practice with motor imagery. *Neuroimage* 20: 1171–1180.
39. Sharma N, Baron JC, Rowe JB (2009) Motor imagery after stroke: relating outcome to motor network connectivity. *Ann Neurol: Official J American Neurol Assoc Child Neurol Soc* 66: 604–616.
40. Grosprêtre S, Lebon F, Papaxanthis C, et al. (2018) Spinal plasticity with motor imagery practice. *J Physiol.*
41. Zimmermann-Schlatter A, Schuster C, Puhan MA, et al. (2008) Efficacy of motor imagery in post-stroke rehabilitation: a systematic review. *J Neuroeng Rehabil* 5: 8.
42. Machado S, Lattari E, de Sa AS, et al. (2015) Is mental practice an effective adjunct therapeutic strategy for upper limb motor restoration after stroke? A systematic review and meta-analysis. *CNS Neurol Disord Drug Targets* 14: 567–575.
43. Winstein CJ, Stein J, Arena R, et al. (2016) Guidelines for adult stroke rehabilitation and recovery: a guideline for healthcare professionals from the American Heart Association/American Stroke Association. *Stroke* 47: e98–e169.
44. Hebert D, Lindsay MP, McIntyre A, et al. (2016) Canadian stroke best practice recommendations: stroke rehabilitation practice guidelines, update 2015. *Int J Stroke* 11: 459–484.
45. Bovend'Eerdt TJ, Dawes H, Sackley C, et al. (2012) Practical research-based guidance for motor imagery practice in neurorehabilitation. *Disabil Rehabil* 34: 2192–2200.
46. Page SJ, Fulk GD, Boyne P (2012) Clinically important differences for the upper-extremity Fugl-Meyer scale in people with minimal to moderate impairment due to chronic stroke. *Phys Ther* 92: 791–798.
47. Tani M, Ono Y, Matsubara M, et al. (2018). Action observation facilitates motor cortical activity in patients with stroke and hemiplegia. *Neurosci Res* 133: 7–14.
48. Burianová H, Marstaller L, Sowman P, et al. (2013) Multimodal functional imaging of motor imagery using a novel paradigm. *Neuroimage* 71: 50–58.
49. Kraeutner SN, McWhinney SR, Solomon JP, et al. (2018) Experience modulates motor imagery-based brain activity. *Eur J Neurosci* 47: 1221–1229.
50. Bar RJ, DeSouza JF (2016) Tracking plasticity: effects of long-term rehearsal in expert dancers encoding music to movement. *PloS One* 11: e0147731.
51. Lacourse MG, Orr EL, Cramer SC, et al. (2005) Brain activation during execution and motor imagery of novel and skilled sequential hand movements. *Neuroimage* 27: 505–519.
52. Macuga KL, Frey SH (2012) Neural representations involved in observed, imagined, and imitated actions are dissociable and hierarchically organized. *Neuroimage* 59: 2798–2807.
53. Nedelko V, Hassa T, Hamzei F, et al. (2012) Action imagery combined with action observation activates more corticomotor regions than action observation alone. *J Neurol Phys Ther* 36: 182–188.
54. Villiger M, Estévez N, Hepp-Reymond MC, et al. (2013) Enhanced activation of motor execution networks using action observation combined with imagination of lower limb movements. *PLoS One* 8: e72403.
55. Taube W, Mouthon M, Leukel C, et al. (2015) Brain activity during observation and motor imagery of different balance tasks: an fMRI study. *Cortex* 64: 102–114.

56. Bian Y, Qi H, Zhao L, et al. (2018) Improvements in event-related desynchronization and classification performance of motor imagery using instructive dynamic guidance and complex tasks. *Comput Biol Med* 96: 266–273.
57. Berends HI, Wolkorte R, Ijzerman MJ, et al. (2013) Differential cortical activation during observation and observation-and-imagination. *Exp Brain Res* 229: 337–345.
58. Eaves DL, Behmer LP, Vogt S (2016) EEG and behavioural correlates of different forms of motor imagery during action observation in rhythmical actions. *Brain Cogn* 106: 90–103.
59. Neuper C, Scherer R, Wriessnegger S, et al. (2009) Motor imagery and action observation: modulation of sensorimotor brain rhythms during mental control of a brain-computer interface. *Clin Neurophysiol* 120: 239–247.
60. Mouthon A, Ruffieux J, Wälchli M, et al. (2015) Task-dependent changes of corticospinal excitability during observation and motor imagery of balance tasks. *Neuroscience* 303: 535–543.
61. Sakamoto M, Muraoka T, Mizuguchi N, et al. (2009) Combining observation and imagery of an action enhances human corticospinal excitability. *Neurosci Res* 65: 23–27.
62. Tsukazaki I, Uehara K, Morishita T, et al. (2012) Effect of observation combined with motor imagery of a skilled hand-motor task on motor cortical excitability: difference between novice and expert. *Neurosci Lett* 518: 96–100.
63. Wright DJ, Williams J, Holmes PS (2014) Combined action observation and imagery facilitates corticospinal excitability. *Front Hum Neurosci* 8: 951.
64. Wright DJ, McCormick SA, Williams J, et al. (2016) Viewing instructions accompanying action observation modulate corticospinal excitability. *Front Hum Neurosci* 10: 17.
65. Wright DJ, Wood G, Eaves DL, et al. (2018) Corticospinal excitability is facilitated by combined action observation and motor imagery of a basketball free throw. *Psychol Sport Exerc* 39: 114–121.
66. Taube W, Lorch M, Zeiter S, et al. (2014) Non-physical practice improves task performance in an unstable, perturbed environment: motor imagery and observational balance training. *Front Hum Neurosci* 8: 972.
67. Bek J, Poliakoff E, Marshall H, et al. (2016) Enhancing voluntary imitation through attention and motor imagery. *Exp Brain Res* 234: 1819–1828.
68. Eaves DL, Haythornthwaite L, Vogt S (2014) Motor imagery during action observation modulates automatic imitation effects in rhythmical actions. *Front Hum Neurosci* 8: 28.
69. Scott M, Taylor S, Chesterton P, et al. (2018) Motor imagery during action observation increases eccentric hamstring force: an acute non-physical intervention. *Disabil Rehabil* 40: 1443–1451.
70. Romano-Smith S, Wood G, Wright DJ, et al. (2018) Simultaneous and alternate action observation and motor imagery combinations improve aiming performance. *Psychol Sport Exerc* 38: 100–106.
71. Marusic U, Giordani B, Moffat SD, et al. (2018) Computerized cognitive training during physical inactivity improves executive functioning in older adults. *Aging Neuropsychol Cogn* 25: 49–69.
72. Bek J, Gowen E, Vogt S, et al. (2018) Combined action observation and motor imagery influences hand movement amplitude in Parkinson's disease. *Parkinsonism Relat Disord*.
73. Cisek P, Kalaska JF (2010) Neural mechanisms for interacting with a world full of action choices. *Annu Rev Neurosci* 33: 269–298.

74. Eaves DL, Turgeon M, Vogt S (2012) Automatic imitation in rhythmical actions: kinematic fidelity and the effects of compatibility, delay, and visual monitoring. *PLoS One* 7: e46728.
75. McInnes K, Friesen C, Boe S (2016) Specific brain lesions impair explicit motor imagery ability: a systematic review of the evidence. *Arch Phys Med Rehabil* 97: 478–489.
76. Oostra KM, Van Bladel A, Vanhoonacker AC, et al. (2016) Damage to fronto-parietal networks impairs motor imagery ability after stroke: a voxel-based lesion symptom mapping study. *Front Behav Neurosci* 10: 5.
77. Evans C, Edwards MG, Taylor LJ, et al. (2016) Perceptual decisions regarding object manipulation are selectively impaired in apraxia or when tDCS is applied over the left IPL. *Neuropsychologia* 86: 153–166.
78. Kraeutner SN, Keeler LT, Boe SG (2016) Motor imagery-based skill acquisition disrupted following rTMS of the inferior parietal lobule. *Exp Brain Res* 234: 397–407.
79. Pinter MM, Brainin M (2012) Rehabilitation after stroke in older people. *Maturitas* 71: 104–108.
80. Pinter MM (2015) Rehabilitation in Stroke Patients: Focusing on the Future. *Hamdan Medical J*, 8: 321–330.
81. Heyes C (2011) Automatic imitation. *Psychol Bull* 137: 463–483.
82. Holmes PS, Collins DJ (2001) The PETTLEP approach to motor imagery: a functional equivalence model for sport psychologists. *J Appl Sport Psychol* 13: 60–83.
83. Cumming J, Cooley SJ, Anuar N, et al. (2017) Developing imagery ability effectively: a guide to layered stimulus response training. *J Sport Psychol Action* 8: 23–33.
84. Lang PJ (1977) Imagery in therapy: an information processing analysis of fear. *Behav Ther* 8: 862–886.
85. Lang PJ (1979) A bio-informational theory of emotional imagery. *Psychophysiology* 16: 495–512.
86. Ventola CL (2014) Mobile devices and apps for health care professionals: uses and benefits. *Pharmacy Theraputics* 39: 356–364.
87. Mosa AS, Yoo I, Sheets L (2012) A systematic review of healthcare applications for smartphones. *BMC Med Inform Decis Mak* 12: 67.
88. Sureshkumar K, Murthy GV, Munuswamy S, et al. (2015) 'Care for Stroke', a web-based, smartphone-enabled educational intervention for management of physical disabilities following stroke: feasibility in the Indian context. *BMJ Innov* 1: 127–136.
89. Goodney A, Jung J, Needham S, et al. (2012) Dr Droid: assisting stroke rehabilitation using mobile phones, *International Conference on Mobile Computing, Applications and Services*, Berlin, Heidelberg: Springer, 231–242.
90. Carr JH, Shepherd RB (2012) An excellent initiative. *J Physiother* 58: 134–135.
91. Intercollegiate Stroke Working Party (2012) *National Clinical Guideline for Stroke*, 4th edition, London: Royal College of Physicians.
92. Wolpaw JR, Birbaumer N, McFarland DJ, et al. (2002) Brain-computer interfaces for communication and control. *Clin Neurophysiol* 113: 767–791.
93. Cervera MA, Soekadar SR, Ushiba J, et al. (2018) Brain-computer interfaces for post-stroke motor rehabilitation: a meta-analysis. *Ann Clin Transl Neurol* 5: 651–663.

9

Special Issue: Alzheimer's disease

Khue Vu Nguyen[1,2,*]

[1] Department of Medicine, Biochemical Genetics and Metabolism, The Mitochondrial and Metabolic Disease Center, School of Medicine, University of California, San Diego, Building CTF, Room C-103, 214 Dickinson Street, San Diego, CA 92103-8467, USA

[2] Department of Pediatrics, University of California, San Diego, School of Medicine, San Diego, La Jolla, CA 92093, USA

* **Correspondence:** Email: kvn006@ucsd.edu;

Abstract: More than 45 million people worldwide have Alzheimer's disease (AD), a deterioration of memory and other cognitive domains that leads to death within 3 to 9 years after diagnosis. The principal risk factor for AD is age. As the aging population increases, the prevalence will approach 131 million cases worldwide in 2050. AD is therefore a global problem creating a rapidly growing epidemic and becoming a major threat to healthcare in our societies. It has been more than 20 years since it was first proposed that the neurodegeneration in AD may be caused by deposition of amyloid-β (Aβ) peptides in plaques in brain tissue. According to the amyloid hypothesis, accumulation of Aβ peptides, resulting from a chronic imbalance between Aβ production and Aβ clearance in the brain, is the primary influence driving AD pathogenesis. Current available medications appear to be able to produce moderate symptomatic benefits but not to stop disease progression. The search for biomarkers as well as novel therapeutic approaches for AD has been a major focus of research. Recent findings, however, show that neuronal-injury biomarkers are independent of Aβ suggesting epigenetic modifications, gene-gene and/or gene-environment interactions in the disease etiology, and calling for reconsideration of the pathological cascade and assessment of alternative therapeutic strategies. In addition, recent research results regarding the expression of the β-amyloid precursor protein (*APP*) gene resulting in the presence of various APP-mRNA isoforms and their quantification, especially for identifying the most abundant one that may decisive for the normal status or disease risk, have been reported. As such, a more complete understanding of AD pathogenesis will likely require greater insights into the physiological function of the β-amyloid precursor protein (APP).

Keywords: Alzheimer's disease; Amyloid-β (Aβ) peptides; Neurofibrillary tangles (NFTs); β-amyloid precursor protein (APP); Familial AD (FAD); Sporadic AD (SAD); Epigenetic modifications; gene-gene and/or gene-environment interactions

1. Introduction

It is with great pleasure to introduce a special issue, namely "Alzheimer's disease", which is scheduled to appear this year in AIMS Neuroscience. I cordially invite authors to contribute their excellent works to this exciting forum. Submissions are now open and will be fully considered for publication.

Alzheimer's disease (AD) is renowned as the most prevalent multifactorial neurodegenerative disorder in today's world. It is the most common cause of dementia in the elderly, affecting about 46.8 million persons worldwide, and will reach a height of 74.7 million in 2030 and 131.5 million in 2050 [1]. In AD, a deterioration of memory and other cognitive domains that leads to death within 3 to 9 years after diagnosis. Owing to the dramatic increase in the population as the year and age progresses, AD is not only considered to be life threatening but also an economic and social burden to the health-care system. Since 1992, the amyloid cascade hypothesis has played a prominent role in explaining the etiology AD. It proposes that the deposition of amyloid-β (Aβ) peptides, resulting from a chronic imbalance between Aβ production and Aβ clearance, is the initial pathological event in AD leading to the formation of extracellular senile plaques (SPs) and then to intracellular neurofibrillary tangles (NFTs) of hyperphosphorylated tau proteins, neuronal cell death and, ultimately, dementia [2]. Aβ peptides are natural products of metabolism consisting of 36 to 43 amino acids. Monomers of $Aβ_{40}$ are much more prevalent than the aggregation-prone and damaging $Aβ_{42}$ species. Aβ peptides originate from proteolysis of the β-amyloid precursor protein (APP) by sequential enzymatic action of beta-site amyloid precursor protein-cleaving enzyme 1 (BACE-1), a β-secretase, and γ-secretase, a protein complex with presenilin 1 at its catalytic core [3]. AD is currently classified by age at onset and genetic status [4]. Sporadic AD (SAD) is characterized by late age at onset (onset age >65 years) and accounts for ~99% of AD cases. Familial AD (FAD) accounting for ~1% of cases, is characterized by early age at onset (onset age <65 years) and a genetic component [4]. In these cases, mutations in the *APP* gene, and the *presenilin* (*PS*) genes *PS1* and *PS2* are known to be associated with FAD.

2. Biomarkers

Advances in research have been translated into several drug candidates with disease-modifying potential, many of which are now being evaluated in clinical trials [5]. Studies in transgenic mouse models of AD suggest that the majority of these types of disease-modifying drugs may be most effective early on in the process of Aβ aggregation, and be less effective in later stages when there is severe plaque pathology and neurodegeneration [6]. However, the current diagnostic criteria from the National Institute of Neurological and Communicative Disorders and Stroke and the Alzheimer's Disease and Related Disorders Association (NINCDS-ADRDA) that are used to identify patients with AD who have overt dementia correspond to neuropathologically advanced disease. Consequently, early recognition of the disease needs to be improved. Indeed, it is estimated that interventions that could delay the clinical onset of dementia by 1 year would reduce the prevalence in 2050 by 9 million cases [6]. Several multimodal core biomarkers candidates derived from structural, functional and metabolic neuroimaging, and from neurochemistry and genetic studies of AD have been investigated but their values in pivotal efficacy studies for AD are still limited [6]. Examples of genetic analysis in biomarker research include testing for *PS1, PS2,* and *APP* mutations; however, as *PS1*, *PS2*, or *APP* mutations are rare, screening for these mutations currently has to be organized on an ad hoc basis. In addition, over the last decades, the apolipoprotein E gene (*APOE*) with three variants referred as *APOE* ε2, ε3 and ε4 alleles, has been irrefutably recognized as a major risk factor for SAD. Unlike *APP, PS1, and PS2* mutations that are fully penetrant (causal), *APOE* ε4 allele is the most important genetic risk factor for SAD. Only about 20–25% of the general population carries one or more ε4 alleles, whereas 50–65% of people with AD are ε4 carriers. The presence of at least one ε4 allele has ben associated with reduced age at onset rather than increases in the lifetime risk of developing AD. Homozygous ε4 allele carriers develop AD up to 10 years earlier than individuals who do not have this allele. Nonetheless, *APOE* ε4 does not account for all genetic variation in AD. The use of *APOE* as a diagnostic or predictive factor in clinical practice is therefore not warranted. Recent works have demonstrated a rare functional variant (R47H) in triggering receptor expressed on myeloid cells 2 gene (*TREM2*), encoding TREM2 transmembrane glycoprotein, increase susceptibility to SAD, with an odds ratio similar to that of the *APOE* ε4 allele [7,8]. Emerging evidence has demonstrated that TREM2 could suppress inflammatory response by repression of microglia-mediated cytokine production and secretion, which may prevent inflammation-induced bystander damage of neurons. Proteolytic processing of TREM2 results in release of a soluble, ectodomain-containing TREM2 fragment (sTREM2) that is detectable in cerebrospinal fluid (CSF) and serum. Changes in the levels of AD-related proteins in CSF, such as $A\beta_{42}$ and tau, reflect the presence and progression of AD pathology in the brain. Studies of SAD and autosomal-dominant AD populations found that sTREM2 levels were increased in the CSF of AD patients and that sTREM2 levels were positively correlated with levels of tau and phosphorylated tau (p-tau); however, no robust correlation between sTREM2 and $A\beta_{42.}$ This suggests that sTREM2 levels increase in association with neuronal damage resulting from an inflammatory process in AD rather than with the appearance of Aβ plaques per se. Then, much work remains to both validate the relationship between sTREM2 and AD and understand the mechanism underlying a potential relationship between TREM2 and neuronal toxicity. Although several studies indicate that elevated sTREM2 levels may mark the transition from preclinical AD to symptomatic AD, some studies have reported contrary findings of either decreased or unchanged CSF sTREM2 levels in AD patient populations. In addition, although most of studies support the hypothesis that inflammation is present as a pathogenetic force in the process of AD, it still remains unclear whether inflammation is a causative factor or just a consequence of this disease. Understanding the role of TREM2 in regulating the response of the innate immune system to Aβ and/or tau pathology may lead to the discovery of novel biomarkers and therapeutic strategies. Finally, up to present, none of the imaging, genetic or biochemical markers has been sufficiently qualified as a surrogate for the actual NINCDS-ADRDA. There is a growing need for biomarkers of AD pathology to improve drug development related to the disorder. Indeed, biomarkers are needed to monitor drug safety, to identify individuals who are most likely to respond to specific treatments, to stratify pre-symptomatic patients and to quantify the benefits of treatments [6].

3. Treatment strategies

Up to now, six broad therapeutic strategies based on Aβ biology have been proposed [5,9]. First, one could attempt to partially inhibit either of the two proteases, β- and γ-secretase, that generate Aβ from APP. Second, one could attempt to prevent the oligomerization of Aβ or enhance its clearance from the cerebral cortex. The third broad approach is an anti-inflammatory strategy based on the observation that a cellular inflammatory response in the cerebral cortex is elicited by the progressive accumulation of Aβ. The fourth approach is based on modulating cholesterol homeostasis. The fifth strategy is based on the observation that Aβ aggregation is, in part, dependent on the metal ions Cu^{2+} and Zn^{2+}. The sixth broad amyloid-based strategy is to prevent the synaptotoxic and neurodegenerative effects putatively triggered by Aβ accumulation. Numerous approaches have been contemplated, including the use of compounds with antioxidant, neuroprotective, and/or neurotrophic properties, but again, no slowing of cognitive decline has been documented in human to date. Thus, for now, clinically validated treatments for AD remain confined to symptomatic interventions such as treatment with acetylcholinesterase inhibitors such as donepezil, rivastigmine, galantamine, huperzine-A, and memantine (a partial antagonist of N-methyl-D-aspartate receptor, NMDAR), and drugs that ameliorate behavioral disturbances such as antidepressants, sleeping tablets, tranquilizers [5,9].

4. Future directions

Although the amyloid cascade hypothesis has been dominated the field for more than 20 years, and offered a broad framework to explain AD pathogenesis, it is currently lacking in detail, and certain observations do not fit easily with the simplest version of the hypothesis [9,10]. The most frequently voiced objection is that the number of amyloid deposits in the brain does not correlate well with the degree of cognitive impairment that the patient experienced in life. Furthermore, over recent years, data have illustrated that reciprocal interactions between APP and its various metabolites, including Aβ, can powerfully regulate key neuronal functions including cell excitability, synaptic transmission and neural plasticity [11]. As a consequence, perturbation of some of these activities may contribute to AD pathogenesis and neurodegeneration in an Aβ-dependent or Aβ-independent manner, and therefore (a) SPs and NFTs may be developed independently and able to interact with each other, and thereby promoting the AD neuropathological cascade, and (b) SPs and NFTs may be the products rather than causes of neurodegeneration in AD [11]. We are entering an era in which the unitary view of AD as a single sequential pathological pathway with Aβ considered as the only initial and causal event is likely to be progressively replaced by a more complex picture in which AD is considered as a multi-parameter pathology that is subtended by several partly independent pathology processes. In this disease, neuronal injury could be caused by different factors, with various possible sequences of pathological events. In contrast to monogenic disease, SAD exhibits numerous non-Mendelian anomalies that suggest epigenetic modifications, gene-gene and/or gene-environment interactions in the disease etiology. Compared to genetic causes, epigenetic factors are probably much more suited to explain the observed anomalies in SAD as aberrant epigenetic patterns may be acquired during many developmental stages. The epigenome is particularly susceptible to deregulation during early embryonal and neonatal development, puberty and especially old age, which is the most important known risk factor for AD [11–13]. Indeed, mutations in FAD represent a very small percentage (~1%), and ~99% of cases are SAD [4]. Multiple studies conducted to determine disease-causative loci have revealed that AD is highly complex and heterogeneous in nature. Therefore, non-genetic factors, such as epigenetic modifications, gene-gene and/or gene-environment interactions may also be causative and currently the subject of intense research [11–13]. As such, it is important to continue to investigate the normal function of APP. Understanding its physiological function will not only provide insights into the pathogenesis of AD but may also prove vital in the development of an effective therapy. Recently, reports on epigenetic regulation of alternative splicing of *APP* gene resulting in the presence of various APP-mRNA isoforms and their quantification, especially for identifying the most abundant one that may decisive for the normal status or disease risk, have been described [14–17]. These findings may provide new directions for the research in neurodevelopmental and neurodegenerative disorders in which the *APP* gene is involved in the pathogenesis of diseases such as autism [18,19], fragile X syndrome [19], amyotrophic lateral sclerosis [20], multiple sclerosis [21], and AD [10,11,19], and may pave the way for new strategies applicable to rational antisense drugs design [22].

In conclusion, it is clear that APP undergoes complex regulation and is important for neuronal and synaptic function in both central and peripheral nervous systems. This may involve the APP extracellular domain, the APP intracellular domain, the Aβ sequence or, indeed, cross communication among these motifs [11]. Then, *APP*, a house keeping gene [23], and endogenous ligand (http://www.genenames.org/genefamilies/EnDOLIG), is an important molecular hub at the center of interacting pathways and acts as a permissive factor for various neurodevelopmental and neural circuit processes [24], altered APP processing may affect brain function through a host of altered cellular and molecular events occurring in neurodevelopmental and neurodegenerative disorders such as autism, fragile X syndrome, and AD. As such, a more complete understanding of AD pathogenesis will likely require greater insights into the physiological function of APP.

References

1. World Alzheimer Report 2015.
2. Hardy JA, Higgin GA (1992) Alzheimer's disease: the amyloid cascade hypothesis. *Science* 256: 184–185.
3. Haass C, Selkoe DJ (2007) Soluble protein oligomers in neurodegeneration: lessons from the Alzheimer's amyloid beta-peptide. *Nat Rev Mol Cell Biol* 8: 101–112.
4. Bettens K, Sleegers K, Van Broeckhoven C (2010) Current status on Alzheimer's disease molecular genetics: from past, to present, to future. *Hum Mol Genet* 19: R4–R11.
5. Klafki HW (2006) Therapeutic approaches to Alzheimer's disease. *Brain* 129: 2840–2855.
6. Hampel H, Frank R, Broich K, et al. (2010) Biomarkers for Alzheimer's disease: academic, industry and regulatory perspectives. *Nat Rev* 9: 560–574.
7. Jiang T, Yu JT, Zhu XC, et al. (2013) TREM2 in Alzheimer's disease. *Mol Neurobiol* 48: 180–185.
8. Ulrich JD, Ulland TK, Colonna M, et al. (2017) Elucidating the role of TREM2 in Alzheimer's disease. *Neuron* 94: 237-248.
9. Hardy J, Selkoe DJ (2002) The amyloid hypothesis of Alzheimer's disease: progress and problems on the road to therapeutics. *Science* 297: 353–356.
10. Chetelat G (2013) Aβ-independent processes-rethinking preclinical AD. *Nat Rev Neurol* 9: 123–124.
11. Nguyen KV (2015) The human β-amyloid precursor protein: biomolecular and epigenetic aspects. *BioMol Concepts* 6: 11–32.
12. Wang SC, Oelze B, Schumacher A (2008) Age-specific epigenetic drift in late-onset Alzheimer's disease. *PLoS One* 3: e2698.
13. Combarros O, Cortina-Borja M, Smith AD, et al. (2009) Epistasis in sporadic Alzheimer's disease. *Neurobiol Aging* 30: 1333–1349.
14. Nguyen KV (2014) Epigenetic regulation in amyloid precursor protein and the Lesch-Nyhan syndrome. *Biochem Biophys Res Commun* 446: 1091–1095.
15. Nguyen KV (2015) Epigenetic regulation in amyloid precursor protein with genomic rearrangements and the Lesch-Nyhan syndrome. *Nucleosides Nucleotides Nucleic Acids* 34: 674–690.
16. Nguyen KV, Nyhan WL (2017) Quantification of various APP-mRNA isoforms and epistasis in Lesch-Nyhan disease. *Neurosci Lett* 643: 52–58.
17. Nguyen KV, Leydiker K, Wang R, et al. (2017) A neurodevelopmental disorder with a nonsense mutation in the Ox-2 antigen domain of the amyloid precursor protein (*APP*) gene. *Nucleosides Nucleotides Nucleic Acids* 36: 317–327.

18. Ray B, Long JM, Sokol DK, et al. (2011) Increased secreted amyloid precursor protein-α (sAPPα) in severe autism: proposal of a specific, anabolic pathway and putative biomarker. *PLoS One* 6: e20405.
19. Sokol DK, Maloney B, Long JM, et al. (2011) Autism, Alzheimer's disease, and fragile X, APP, FMRP, and mGluR5 are molecular links. *Neurology* 76: 1344–1352.
20. Bryson JB, Hobbs C, Parsons MJ, et al. (2012) Amyloid precursor protein (APP) contributes to pathology in the SOD^{G93A} mouse model of amyotrophic lateral sclerosis. *Hum Mol Genet* 21: 3871–3882.
21. Matias-Guiu JA, Oreja-Guevara C, Cabrera-Martin MN, et al. (2016) Amyloid proteins and their role in multiple sclerosis. Considerations in the use of amyloid-PET imaging. *Front Neurol* 7: 53.
22. Saonere JA (2011) Antisense therapy, a magic bullet for the treatment of various diseases: present and future prospects. *J Med Genet Genomics* 3: 77–83.
23. Sabaum JM, Weidermann A, Lemaire HG, et al. (1988) The promoter of Alzheimer's disease amyloid A4 precursor gene. *EMBO J* 7: 2807–2813.
24. Nicolas M, Hassan BA (2014) Amyloid precursor protein and neural development. Development 141: 2543–2548.

10

Volitional down-regulation of the primary auditory cortex via directed attention mediated by real-time fMRI neurofeedback

Matthew S. Sherwood[1,*], Jason G. Parker[2], Emily E. Diller[2,3], Subhashini Ganapathy[1,4], Kevin Bennett[5] and Jeremy T. Nelson[6]

[1] Department of Biomedical, Industrial & Human Factors Engineering, Wright State University, Dayton, OH, USA

[2] Department of Radiology and Imaging Sciences, Indiana University School of Medicine, Indiana University, IN, USA

[3] School of Health Sciences, Purdue University, West Lafayette, IN, USA

[4] Department of Trauma Care, Boonshoft School of Medicine, Wright State University, Dayton, OH, USA

[5] Department of Psychology, Wright State University, Dayton, OH, USA

[6] Department of Defense Hearing Center of Excellence, JBSA-Lackland, USA

* **Correspondence:** Email: matt.sherwood@wright.edu;

Abstract: The present work assessed the efficacy of training volitional down-regulation of the primary auditory cortex (A1) based on real-time functional magnetic resonance imaging neurofeedback (fMRI-NFT). A1 has been shown to be hyperactive in chronic tinnitus patients, and has been implicated as a potential source for the tinnitus percept. 27 healthy volunteers with normal hearing underwent 5 fMRI-NFT sessions: 18 received real neurofeedback and 9 sham neurofeedback. Each session was composed of a simple auditory fMRI followed by 2 runs of A1 fMRI-NFT. The auditory fMRI alternated periods of no auditory with periods of white noise stimulation at 90 dB. A1 activity, defined from a region using the activity during the preceding auditory run, was continuously updated during fMRI-NFT using a simple bar plot, and was accompanied by white noise (90 dB) stimulation for the duration of the scan. Each fMRI-NFT run alternated "relax" periods with "lower" periods. Subjects were instructed to watch the bar during the relax condition and actively reduce the bar by decreasing A1 activation during the lower condition. Average A1 de-activation, representative of the ability to volitionally down-regulate A1, was extracted from each fMRI-NFT run. A1 de-activation was found to increase significantly across training and to be higher in those receiving real neurofeedback. A1 de-activation in sessions 2 and 5 were found to be significantly greater than session 1 in only the group receiving real neurofeedback. The most successful subjects reportedly adopted mindfulness tasks associated with directed attention. For the first time, fMRI-NFT has been applied to teach volitional control of A1 de-activation magnitude over more than 1 session. These are important findings for therapeutic development as the magnitude of A1 activity is altered in tinnitus populations and it is unlikely a single fMRI-NFT session will reverse the effects of tinnitus.

Keywords: fMRI; neurofeedback; neuromodulation; primary auditory cortex; attention; tinnitus

1. Introduction

Advances in acquisition techniques, computational power, and algorithms have revolutionized the speed in which functional Magnetic Resonance Imaging (fMRI) data can be measured and processed. This acceleration has led to real-time fMRI, where fMRI data (*i.e.,* blood-oxygen-level-dependent [BOLD] signals) can be processed faster than it is collected. There are currently four domains where real-time fMRI is being implemented: Intraoperative surgical guidance [1], brain-computer interfaces [2,3], adapting stimuli for current brain states [4], and neurofeedback training [5].

Neurofeedback training (NFT), although not the original focus of real-time fMRI, is a growing field of research where BOLD signals are presented using visual or auditory stimuli during data acquisition so the subject may learn to modulate the signals at will (*i.e.,* closed-loop endogenous neuromodulation). This technique differs from traditional fMRI where individuals respond to exogenous stimuli without being informed of the timing and location of induced brain activity (*i.e.,* open-loop neuromodulation), as well as exogenous neuromodulation techniques like transcranial direct current stimulation (tDCS) or pharmacotherapy. Information regarding the activity of a specific brain region is presented to the subject in real-time during fMRI-NFT. Through the implementation of mental strategies, individuals learn to self-regulate the BOLD signal and, therefore, brain activity as these are tightly coupled through neurovascular mechanisms [6–8]. Researchers have shown that people can learn volitional control over the BOLD signal measured from numerous brain regions including the anterior cingulate cortex (ACC) [9], amygdala [10], anterior insula [11,12], auditory and attention related networks [13], bilateral rostrolateral prefrontal cortex [14], left dorsolateral prefrontal cortex [15–17], motor cortices [18–20], primary auditory cortex [21–23], regions associated with emotional network [24,25], right inferior frontal gyrus [26], and visual cortices [27,28].

The efficacy of fMRI-NFT in altering behavior was demonstrated for the first time in 2015 [29]. Since, fMRI-NFT has been demonstrated across a broad range of medical applications. In one study, participants suffering from schizophrenia were able to learn control over the BOLD signal measured from the left and right insula [30]. In another study, an experimental group of participants diagnosed with Parkinson's disease exhibited significant clinical and functional improvements which were not observed from a control group of patients who received sham feedback [31]. Other studies have demonstrated potential applications for people suffering from major depression [32] and chronic tinnitus [21]. One group of researchers combined fMRI-NFT with TMS and found that endogenous neuromodulation of the ventral premotor cortex helps decrease intracortical inhibition measured from TMS. This application may enhance facilitation of stroke victims [18]. Overall, this trend represents the wide range of medical applications of fMRI-NFT but also the specificity of training required for each application.

In several previous studies, control groups who received sham BOLD signals lacked the differences in activity observed from those who received true feedback [9–11,13,14,20,26,27,29,31,33,34], implicating neuromodulation or behavioral training strategies affecting global arousal are not effective. Additionally, control groups which received identical instructions and the same period of training but no feedback on the current level of brain activity did not exhibit similar results as the experimental groups who were given neurofeedback [11,14,24,29,32]. These findings suggest the experiential effects are attributable to real-time fMRI-induced learning rather than other learning or nonspecific changes. Therefore, specific training regimens must be developed which target specific neurophysiological systems to obtain the desired effects. The results from the control groups in Decharms et al. [29] further indicate behavioral training, practice, sensory feedback, and biofeedback alone do not produce effects that are equivalent to those obtained with control groups who receive NFT from real-time fMRI. The exact mechanism translating neuromodulation into behavioral effects are still unknown. One postulation is the brain network responsible for the behavior is reinforced when one actively regulates neural activity in one or more of these regions. Such reinforcement results in the engagement of neuroplastic mechanisms causing the network to execute more efficiently. This theory coincides with other neuromodulation training techniques such as EEG-based neurofeedback where individuals are trained to control frequency bands of electrical signals measured from the local regions of the scalp [35–37]. Another hypothesis is that participants who learn appropriate mental strategies to modulate the BOLD signal will recruit task related brain networks more readily than others when processing stimuli [16].

In this work, we investigated the use of fMRI-NFT to teach volitional down-regulation of A1 during binaural auditory stimulation using directed attention strategies. It is not currently known whether individuals are capable of down-regulating A1 in the presence of auditory stimulation. However, two previous studies indicate that volitional down-regulation of A1 activation is achievable. In the one study, twenty-two healthy participants were divided into two equal groups completing the same tasks: one group received neurofeedback and the other group did not. All participants underwent multiple sessions consisting of five neurofeedback blocks. During neurofeedback, participants were asked to increase the activated volume in the primary and secondary auditory cortex from auditory stimulation. The change in activated volume was indicated at the end of each neurofeedback block only for the experimental group. This study found that participants receiving neurofeedback were successful in increasing the activated volume in the primary and secondary auditory cortex using fMRI-NFT; those not receiving neurofeedback were unsuccessful and did not exhibit any trends of habituation to the noise in the fMRI data [23]. In the other study, six participants with chronic tinnitus underwent 4 runs of fMRI-NFT conducted in a single session. It was reported that tinnitus patients were able to volitionally increase A1 activation. However, the study was not controlled so this finding could not be necessarily attributable to fMRI-NFT [21]. The second indicates that fMRI-NFT can train volitional down-regulation. In one uncontrolled study, schizophrenia patients were successfully able to learn volitional down-regulation of the superior temporal gyrus over four fMRI-NFT sessions [38]. In another controlled study, a group of 16 healthy females learned to down-regulate activation of the amygdala in the presence of aversive scenes using one fMRI-NFT session[39]. We used these findings to hypothesize that an experimental group receiving real neurofeedback will have greater volitional control over A1 de-activation than a control group receiving sham feedback.

2. Methods

2.1. Participants

Healthy volunteers were recruited from Wright State University and the surrounding community. Prior to being enrolled, each potential participant completed a telephone screening to qualify for the study. Forty-seven (47) participants meeting the inclusion/exclusion criteria were recruited (no contraindication to MRI procedures, between the ages of 18 and 50, right handed, no unstable medical or mental illness, no history of neurologic disorders, no hearing loss > 40 dB). These participants were selected at random from the qualifying group. The study was approved by Wright State University's Institutional Review Board (IRB) and the Air Force Medical Support Agency Surgeon General's Research Oversight Committee; informed consent was obtained prior to the execution of any experimental procedures. Participants eligible for compensation received equal remuneration.

Participants were randomly assigned to one of two groups and were blinded to the assigned group. The experimental group (EXP) received real feedback regarding activity in A1 during closed-loop endogenous neuromodulation. The control group (CON) was supplied with sham feedback yoked from a random participant in the experimental group matched for training time. Nineteen (19) participants voluntarily withdrew or were withdrawn from the study due to excessive motion, absenteeism/tardiness, or software/hardware issues limiting the completion of study procedures. The MRI data for a single participant was corrupted. This resulted in a final group of eighteen (18) EXP participants (mean age 23.2 +/− 1.1, 11 males) and nine (9) CON participants (mean age 24.4 +/− 2.5, 4 males).

2.2. Experimental design

All participants first completed a consent visit. After obtaining informed consent, the participants completed a MRI screening form. Next, a short hearing test was conducted to verify normal hearing (no frequency > 40 dB on a standard audiogram; Shoebox Audiometry, Ontario, Canada). This test is a simple self-applied test that has been clinically validated [40,41]. Following the consent visit, the subjects completed five fMRI-NFT sessions. All MRI procedures were conducted on a 3 Tesla (T) MRI (Discovery 750 W, GE Healthcare, Madison, WI) using a 24-channel head coil. These five sessions were executed within 21 days (EXP: 14.61 +/− 0.71 days; CON: 12.44 +/− 1.59) with only one per day.

2.2.1. fMRI-NFT

We performed fMRI-NFT across five sessions for each participant. Prior to entering the MRI environment, MRI screening forms were reviewed by a registered MRI technician. Female participants were required to take a urine dipstick pregnancy test. Once entering the MRI, the participants first inserted MRI-compatible ear plugs (MagnaCoil, Magnacoustics Inc., Atlantic

Beach, NY) capable of providing communication and auditory stimulation (Genesis Ultra, Magnacoustics Inc., Atlantic Beach, NY). Next, the participants were positioned supine on the MRI table, their head was padded to restrict motion, and the upper part of the 24-channel head coil was attached. Using a laser, the nasion was landmarked relative to the MRI. The landmarked position was moved to the center of the MRI bore.

Once positioned, the fMRI-NFT procedures began (Figure 1). Each fMRI-NFT session consisted of a single run of bilateral auditory stimulation which was used to individually and functionally localize A1. This scan is referred to as the "functional localizer". Two runs of closed-loop endogenous neuromodulation followed the functional localizer. A structural MRI was performed between the functional localizer and closed-loop endogenous neuromodulation runs. The structural MRI was acquired using an 3D brain volume imaging (BRAVO) pulse sequence which acquires images using an inversion recovery prepared fast spoiled gradient-echo (FSPGR). The structural images were acquired using a 256 × 256 element matrix, 172 slices oriented in the same plane as the functional scans, 1 mm^3 isotropic voxels, 0.8 phase field of view factor, TI/TE = 450/3.224 ms, a flip angle of 13°, and an auto-calibrated reconstruction for cartesian sampling with a phase acceleration factor of 2.0. The left and right A1 were manually identified using anatomical markers and an activation map produced from the functional localizer. Once identified, a region-of-interest (ROI) was selected from the voxels in the left and right A1 most robustly activated during the functional localizer. The BOLD signals from this ROI were used to generate the subsequent neurofeedback.

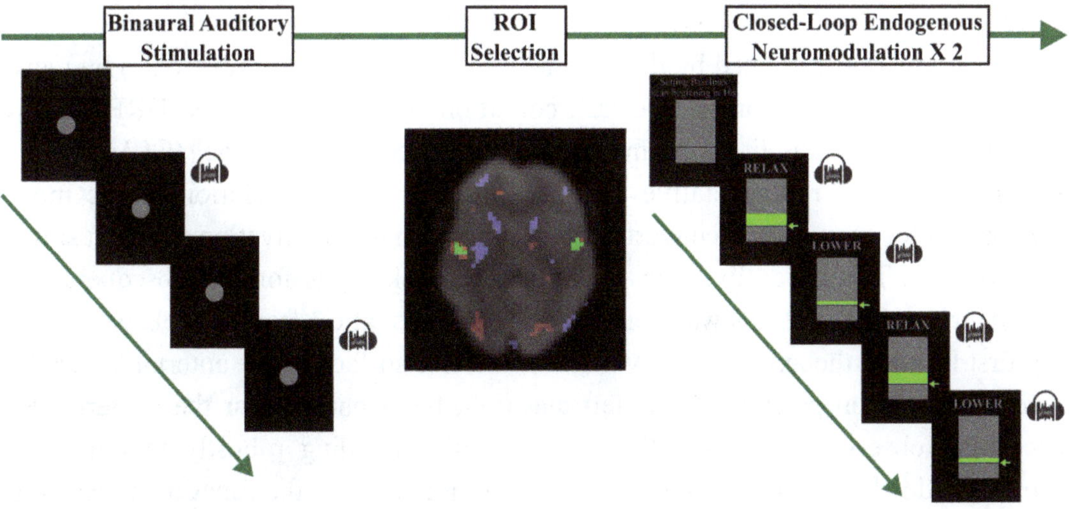

Figure 1. Overview of each fMRI-NFT session. Each session began by acquiring BOLD data during a blocked binaural auditory stimulation paradigm. Next, a region-of-interest for subsequent neurofeedback was selected from activated voxels in the right and left A1. Finally, two runs of closed-loop endogenous neuromodulation were executed to train A1 down-regulation.

2.2.2. Binaural auditory stimulation

A single run of binaural auditory stimulation was executed to identify A1 using a boxcar design with eight (8) repetitions of OFF and ON blocks. The auditory stimuli were 10 kHz lowpass filtered white noise with a 6 dB roll-off and a 0.5 s fade-in (Audacity 2.1.3, www.audacity.org). The duration of each block was 20 s, and the first block began after the acquisition of four (4) dummy volumes and one (1) software preparation volume. Binaural auditory stimulation was delivered via the headphones only during ON blocks and controlled via a stimulus presentation software (Presentation, Neurobehavioral Systems, Inc., Berkeley, CA). Auditory stimulation consisted of 10 kHz lowpass filtered white noise presented at 90 dB, previously shown to be effective at producing a BOLD response [21]. The participants were not required to respond in any way during the scan, however they were instructed to remain awake and to focus on a round fixation dot presented in gray with a black background on a MRI-compatible display (SensaVue, Invivo, Gainesville, FL). FMRI data were acquired using a gradient-recalled-echo (GRE) sequence sensitive to the BOLD signal. This sequence acquired data using the following parameters: 64×64 element matrix, 41 slices oriented parallel to the AC-PC plane, $3.5 \times 3.5 \times 3$ mm^3 voxels size, 0.5 mm slice gap, TR/TE = 2000/20 ms, and a flip angle of 90° with fat suppression enabled. In previous data collections, these parameters have been shown to reduce susceptibility artifacts which can be significant at high field strengths such as 3T.

2.2.3. ROI selection

Immediately following acquisition, the BOLD data were pre-processed using custom MATLAB and C++ software. The pre-processing included standard spatial filtering (3D, 5-point Gaussian low-pass kernel, full-width half-maximum of 7 mm), motion correction (corrected to the first volume using a rigid-body 3-parameter model) and temporal filtering (5-point Gaussian low-pass kernel, sigma of 3 s) processing functions [42].

An activation map was created by defining a single explanatory variable (EV) by convolving a boxcar model containing 20 s control and task conditions with a pre-defined HRF [43]. Next, the BOLD data at each voxel was fit to the model using a general linear model (GLM) by applying a weight of +1 to the EV, representative of activation (positive correlation to the model). The resulting β parameter maps were converted to t statistic maps (activation maps) using standard statistical transforms. The region in A1 in which the feedback signal for the subsequent closed-loop endogenous neuromodulation runs was derived from this activation map. Voxels were added to the A1 ROI by first locating the axial slice in which the inferior surface of the anterior ventricle horns is visible. Finally, activation patterns on the left and right hemispheres near the posterior end of the lateral sulci were observed. Voxels within this region responding robustly to binaural auditory stimulation were added to the ROI to complete the determination of the functional localizer.

2.2.4. Closed-loop endogenous neuromodulation

Two runs of closed-loop endogenous neuromodulation were completed following the functional localizer. BOLD data was acquired using the same scan parameters as described for the functional localizer. Four dummy volumes and one software preparation volume were acquired first. Then, eight volumes were acquired to determine a baseline BOLD signal value for the selected A1 ROI. During the acquisition of the baseline volumes, a countdown was displayed on the screen, however there was no auditory stimulation during either the eight baseline volumes or the five preparatory volumes. In the subsequent scanning for the experimental group, a feedback signal was computed and displayed to the participants from real-time analysis of BOLD data. This real-time analysis was implemented in custom MATLAB and C++ software, and included standard spatial filtering

(3D, 5-point Gaussian low-pass kernel, full-width half-maximum of 7 mm) and motion-correction (corrected to the first volume of the functional localizer using a rigid-body 3-parameter model) processing functions [42]. This custom software further compared the average BOLD signal in the voxels selected from the functional localizer at baseline to that of the current volume to derive the percent signal change. The current feedback signal was determined by temporally-filtering (5-point Gaussian low-pass kernel consisting of only past components, sigma of 3 s) the percent BOLD signal change with the feedback signals from previous volumes. This feedback signal was presented to the participants using a thermometer-style bar plot within an average of 750 ms from the end of acquisition of a complete volume (~500 ms for reconstruction and DICOM writing/reading, ~250 ms for data processing and display). The thermometer plot contained a running average of the previous four values and a running task minimum. For participants in the control group, the feedback signal was yoked from a random EXP participant with experimental progress matched. Both runs from each session were duplicated from the same EXP participant but the EXP participant was selected randomly each session.

After baseline, six repetitions of 30 s relax and lower blocks were completed in a boxcar-design. Both blocks were accompanied with binaural auditory stimulation using the same continuous noise from the functional localizer. During relax, every participant was instructed to relax and clear their mind, resulting in an increase in the feedback signal. They were also instructed to keep their eyes open. Participants were instructed to lower the feedback signal during lower blocks by performing a mindfulness task wherein they should decrease brain activity associated with auditory input. A list of four example mindfulness tasks was provided, giving the participants a few starting points (mindful meditation, thinking about a hobby, doing a mentally engaging task such as math, or thinking about other senses). Through training, participants learned mindfulness tasks that are most successful in regulating A1. Task instructions indicating the current block (relax or lower) were supplied above the thermometer plot.

Participants were then removed from the MRI and escorted out of the MRI room. Participants were then informally interviewed by the experimenter.

2.3. Data analysis

The BOLD data acquired from each closed-loop endogenous neuromodulation run was processed using the FMRIB Software Library (FSL) [44,45] on a 72-core Rocks Cluster Distribution (www.rocksclusters.org) high-performance computing system capable of running 120 threads in parallel. First, individual (first-level) analyses were conducted on each of the 4D fMRI data sets. Prior to the individual analyses, *t* pre-processing was performed using standard techniques. These consisted of applying a high-pass temporal filter (Gaussian-weighted least-squares straight line fitting, cut-off = 60 s) to each voxel, correcting for motion by registering each volume to the center volume of the data set (rigid-body 12-parameter model) [46], creating a brain mask from the first volume and applying to each subsequent volume [47], spatial filtering on each volume using Gaussian convolution (full-width half-maximum of 5.625 mm), and removing low-frequency trends using a local fit of a straight line across time at each voxel with Gaussian weighting within the line to create a smooth response.

Next, individual analyses were conducted on each of the 4D fMRI data sets. A single EV was defined by convolving a boxcar model containing 30 s relax and lower conditions with a HRF (modeled by a gamma function; phase offset = 0 s, standard deviation = 3 s, mean lag = 6 s). The temporal derivative of the original waveform was added to the result. The temporal filter used in pre-processing was applied to the model. The data set was fit to the model using a GLM with prewhitening by applying a weight of −1 to the EV, representative of de-activation during closed-loop endogenous neuromodulation. *Z* statistic maps were created using standard statistical transforms to convert the β parameter maps. A clustering method allowed us to account for false positives due to multiple comparisons. This method considers adjacent voxels with a z statistic of 2.3 or greater to be a cluster. The significance of each cluster was estimated and compared to a threshold of $p < 0.05$ using Gaussian Random Field theory. The significance of voxels that either did not pass the significance level threshold or do not belong to a cluster were set to zero. A mean image of the data set was registered to the individual's high-resolution structural image by estimating motion from a boundary-based registration method including a fieldmap-based distortion correction [48], then further registered to the MNI-152 T1-weighted 2 mm template provided in FSL [49,50] using a 12-parameter model. The z statistic maps were converted to standard space using the transform responsible for morphing the mean image of each data set to the template to co-register all volumes. A similar process was performed on the BOLD data acquired during the auditory localizer, but a temporal filter with a cut-off of 40 s and a boxcar model with 20 s conditions were used.

2.3.1. ROI-based analysis

The target ROI coordinates in each fMRI-NFT session were converted to a binary mask. Since the ROI was determined from the first volume of the functional localizer, motion was corrected in the functional localizer data by registering each volume to the first volume using the method described above and a mean image was created. Next, the mean image of each neuromodulation run was registered to the mean image of the associated functional localizer using a rigid-body 12-parameter model. The transform responsible for morphing the mean image of each neuromodulation run was applied to the associated ROI mask. Volitional down-regulation of A1 was assessed in both groups by masking the de-activation map (*i.e.,* decreased BOLD signal during the lower condition compared with the relax condition) from above with the registered ROI mask. A mixed factor ANOVA (between-subjects factor: Group; within-subjects factors: Session and run) was performed on the neuromodulation performance metric using SPSS (IBM SPSS statistics version 24.0, IBM Corp., Amonk, New York).

2.3.2. Whole brain analysis

Group (second level) analyses were performed in FSL using to conduct a voxel-wise 2 × 2 (between subject factor: Group; within-subjects factor: Session) mixed factor ANOVA in FSL. Run 1 from the first fMRI-NFT session and run 2 from the last fMRI-NFT session were included to assess the overall change in A1 de-activation. Prior to running this analysis, each individual de-activation map was masked to remove activated voxels. This enabled us to assess only changes in de-activation, as the results of the ANOVA are bi-directional. The 2 × 2 ANOVA analysis assumed the covariance between measures within-subject follow a compound symmetric structure (equal variance and intra-subject correlations being equal). This assumption is valid as the data was acquired in close proximity and regularly sampled. Two contrasts were created to identify voxels more de-active during the fifth training session than the first session and a larger change in de-activation from the first to fifth training session (5–1) for the EXP group than the CON group. *Z* statistic maps, created by transforming the resulting β parameter maps using standard statistical transforms, were thresholded using the clustering method outlined above with a *z* statistic threshold of 1.96. Furthermore, β parameter estimates from each of these contrasts underwent separate *F* tests to explore the main effect of session and the session by group interaction. This analysis lacked the degrees of freedom necessary to include the main effect of group and, therefore, this contrast was not included. *Z* statistic images were created from *F* statistic images using standard statistical transformations. This group analysis was repeated using the auditory localizer from sessions 1 and 5.

3. Results

Using an independent samples *t*-test, the mean age for each the EXP group was found to not significantly differ from the CON group ($t_{25} = 1.447$, $p = 0.160$, two-tailed). Equal variances were assumed as Levene's test was not significant ($F_{1.25} = 3.832$, $p = 0.062$). Furthermore, the training time, calculated as the separation between the first and last neurofeedback session, did not significantly differ between the EXP and CON groups ($t_{25} = -0.522$, $p = 0.606$, two-tailed). Equal variances were assumed as Levene's test was not significant ($F_{1.25} = 1.278$, $p = 0.269$).

3.1. ROI-based analysis

A mixed factor ANOVA evaluated the size (overall average = 1490 mm^3) of the functionally-defined ROI across sessions and groups (Figure 2). The size of the ROIs did not significantly differ between sessions or groups ($p = 0.567$, $p = 0.108$, respectively, two-tailed). Furthermore, the interaction of session by group was not significant in the ROI size ($p = 0.713$, two-tailed). Although the ROIs for the CON group were not used during neurofeedback, these ROIs were utilized for post-processing to compute A1 de-activation. The average size of each ROI across groups and sessions was 1490 $mm^3 \pm 283.15$ mm^3. Furthermore, the 3D coordinates of the center of mass (COM) or each ROI was computed from the standard-space transformed ROI per session and hemisphere. A total of six 5 × 2 mixed factor ANOVAs evaluated the COM location for each dimension and hemisphere across sessions and groups. The main effect of session was significant for only the z-dimension in the right hemisphere ($F_{4,100} = 5.098$, $p = 0.001$). Bonferroni-corrected *post hoc* comparisons revealed the z-location at session 2 varied significantly from sessions 1 and 4 ($p = 0.003$ and $p = 0.002$, respectively). The main effect of session was not significant for any of the other dimensions/hemispheres ($p > 0.05$). The main effects of group and the group by session interactions were not significant ($p > 0.05$) for all three dimensions and both hemispheres, suggesting the location of the selected ROIs were consistent across groups and the small variation in the right z-dimension did not vary differently between groups.

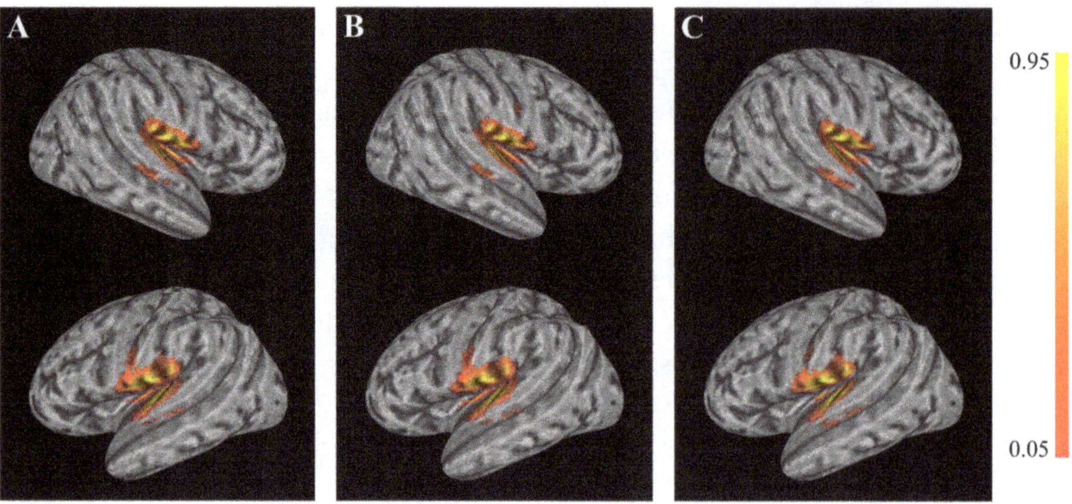

Figure 2. The probability of voxel inclusion during fMRI-NFT for: (A) both EXP and CON groups; (B) EXP group only; (C) CON group only. ROIs were transformed to standard space using the same transformation responsible for morphing the fMRI data to standard space. Yellow voxels were included most frequently in the functionally-defined ROIs while red voxels were selected less frequently.

The effects of group, session, and run on A1 de-activation during closed-loop endogenous neuromodulation were evaluated using a mixed factor ANOVA. A1 de-activation is representative of an individual's ability to volitionally down-regulate A1. The results of the tests of between-subjects effects (Table 1) revealed a significant main effect of group (p = 0.029, one-tailed). One-tailed statistics are reported (the a priori hypothesis was that A1 de-activation would be greater in the EXP group). The ANOVA analysis included Mauchly's Test of Sphericity which determined that the variances of the differences between all possible pairs of within-subject conditions were not significant for the main effect of session (p = 0.160, two-tailed) or the interaction of session and run (p = 0.776, two-tailed). This test could not be conducted on the main effect of run because there is only a single difference to compute and, therefore, no comparison to be made. These results validate the assumption of sphericity, which was used to assess the results of the within-subjects tests henceforth. The results of the within-subjects testing (Table 2) identify a significant main effect of session (Figure 3; p = 0.0175, one-tailed). One-tailed statistics are reported (the a priori hypothesis was that A1 de-activation would increase with training). The main effect of run was not significant (p = 0.283, one-tailed). The interaction effects of session by group, run by group, session by run, and session by group and run were not significant (p = 0.225, p = 0.175, p = 0.070, and p = 0.218, respectively).

Table 1. A1 de-activation ANOVA between-subjects test results. Power was computed using an alpha of 0.05. Highlighted rows indicate significance at or below p = 0.05.

Source	Type III Sum of Squares	df	Mean Square	F	Sig. (one-tailed)	Partial Eta Squared	Observed Power
Intercept	22.381	1	22.381	6.073	0.011	0.195	0.659
Group	14.524	1	14.524	3.941	0.029	0.136	0.480
Error	92.135	25	3.685				

Table 2. A1 de-activation ANOVA within-subjects test results. Power was computed using an alpha of 0.05. Highlighted rows indicate significance at or below $p = 0.05$.

Factor	Type III Sum of Squares	df	Mean Square	F	Sig. (one-tailed)	Partial Eta Squared	Observed Power
Session	59.395	4	14.849	2.702	0.0175	0.098	0.731
Session* Group	20.447	4	5.112	0.930	0.225	0.036	0.286
Run	0.933	1	0.933	0.338	0.283	0.013	0.087
Run* Group	2.506	1	2.506	0.908	0.175	0.035	0.150
Session* Run	11.377	4	2.844	1.772	0.070	0.066	0.524
Session* Run* Group	6.121	4	1.530	0.953	0.218	0.037	0.292

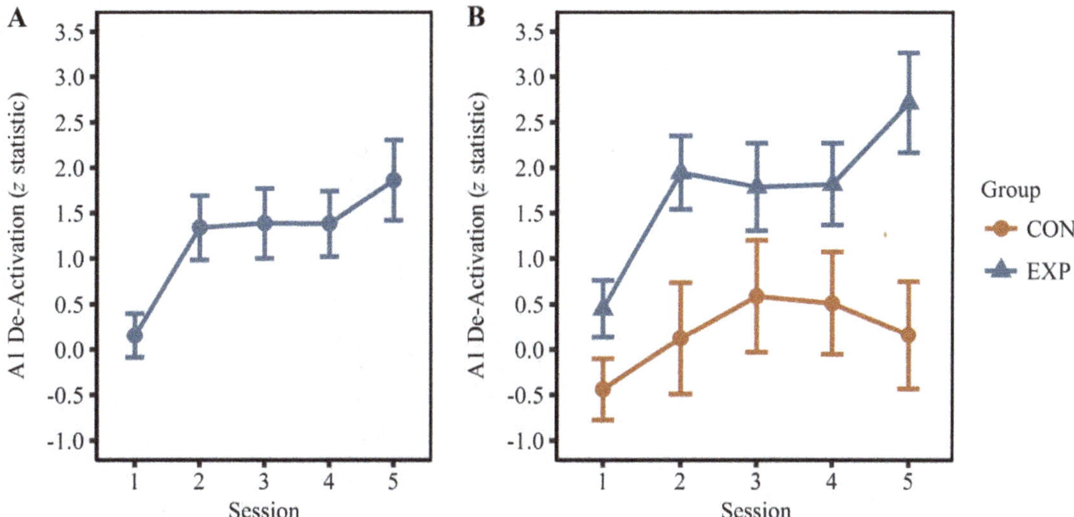

Figure 3. A1 de-activation during closed-loop endogenous neuromodulation. (A) A1 de-activation averaged across groups and runs for each session. The main effect of session was found to be significant ($p = 0.0175$). (B) A1 de-activation averaged across runs separated by group and session. The *post hoc* pairwise comparisons did not reveal any significant differences for the CON group, however sessions 2 ($p = 0.038$) and 5 ($p = 0.0165$) were found to be significantly greater than session 1 for the EXP group.

Post hoc, Bonferroni-corrected pairwise comparisons were conducted on the session by group interaction. These results revealed no significant difference between session 1 and 5 for the CON group ($p > 0.05$; Table 3); however, a significant difference between these sessions was identified in the EXP group ($p = 0.0165$, one-tailed). There was also a significant difference between sessions 1 and 2 for the EXP group ($p = 0.038$, one-tailed). Furthermore, the EXP group was found to have significantly greater A1 de-activation than the CON groups on session 2 ($p = 0.031$, one-tailed) and 5 ($p = 0.021$, one-tailed) as identified in Table 4.

Table 3. A1 de-activation *post hoc* pairwise comparison results for session by group. Statistical significances were computed using Bonferroni correction for multiple comparisons. Highlighted rows indicate significance at or below $p = 0.05$. The reported statistical significance is one-tailed due to the *a priori* hypotheses.

Group	(I) Session	(J) Session	Mean Difference (I–J)	Std. Error	Sig. (one-tailed)
CON	1	2	−0.563	0.730	1.000
		3	−1.024	0.802	1.000
		4	−0.949	0.813	1.000
		5	−0.597	0.978	1.000
	2	3	−0.461	0.719	1.000
		4	−0.386	0.828	1.000
		5	−0.034	0.829	1.000
	3	4	0.076	0.742	1.000
		5	0.427	0.739	1.000
	4	5	0.352	0.571	1.000
EXP	1	2	−1.496	0.516	0.038
		3	−1.339	0.567	0.132
		4	−1.369	0.575	0.125
		5	−2.266	0.692	0.0165
	2	3	0.157	0.509	1.000
		4	0.126	0.586	1.000
		5	−0.770	0.586	1.000
	3	4	−0.030	0.525	1.000
		5	−0.927	0.523	0.441
	4	5	−0.897	0.404	0.178

Table 4. A1 de-activation *post hoc* pairwise comparison results for group by session. Statistical significances were computed using Bonferroni correction for multiple comparisons. Highlighted rows indicate significance at or below $p = 0.05$. The reported statistical significance is one-tailed due to the *a priori* hypotheses.

Session	(I) Group	(J) Group	Mean Difference (I–J)	Std. Error	Sig. (one-tailed)
1	EXP	CON	0.888	0.585	0.071
2	EXP	CON	1.821	0.931	0.031
3	EXP	CON	1.203	1.121	0.147
4	EXP	CON	1.309	1.007	0.103
5	EXP	CON	2.557	1.194	0.021

3.2. Whole brain analysis

A 2 × 2 (group by session) mixed factor ANOVA was performed on the BOLD data from the session 1 run 1 and session 5 run 2 closed-loop endogenous neuromodulation runs using FSL. The *F* test revealed a significant ($z > 1.96$) main effect of session on de-activation magnitude during closed-loop endogenous neuromodulation in several regions throughout the brain (Figure 4; Table 5).

Increased de-activation was observed across training in auditory regions (superior temporal gyrus, transverse temporal gyrus, and insula) limited to the right hemisphere. In contrast, increased de-activation in attention-related regions (medial frontal gyrus, superior frontal gyrus, and middle frontal gyrus) were observed in the left hemisphere. However, bilateral changes in the anterior cingulate and caudate were observed.

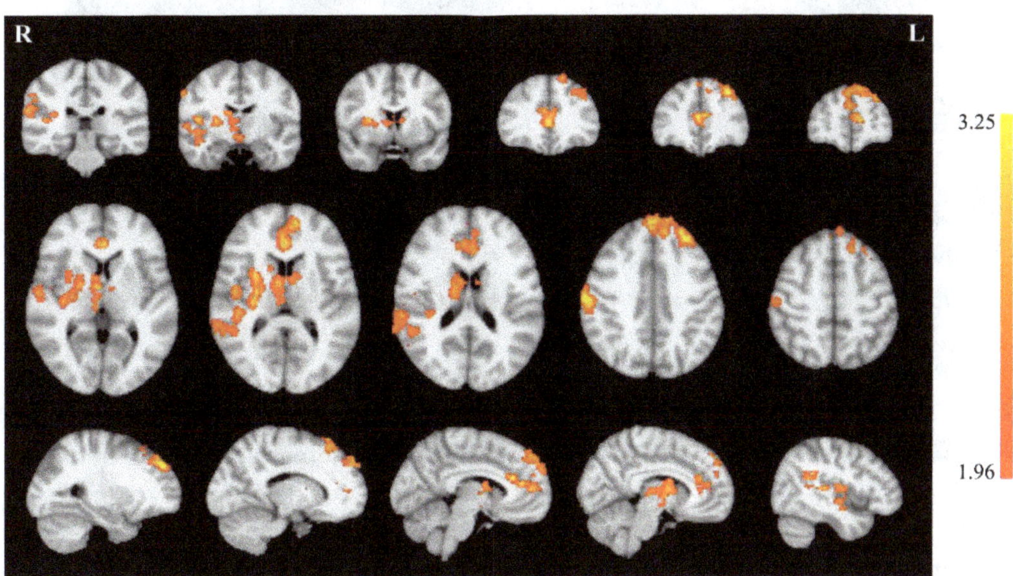

Figure 4. *F* test results for the main effect of session indicate increased de-activation during neurofeedback across training for several brain regions. Coronal slices (top row) are displayed at MNI coordinates y = −30, −10, 6, 34, 40 and 52 mm (left to right). Axial slices (middle row) are displayed at MNI coordinates z = 4, 10, 18, 40, and 52 mm (left to right). Sagittal slices (bottom row) are displayed at MNI coordinates y = −26, −14, −6, 8, and 44 mm (left to right).

Table 5. Local maxima for the *F* test results for the main effect of session. Coordinates are specified in MNI space.

	Coordinates		
Z statistic	X (mm)	Y (mm)	Z (mm)
3.82	62	−16	42
3.55	−26	46	38
3.4	−32	40	40
3.36	54	−42	24
3.33	2	38	12
3.3	60	−36	24
3.22	4	54	40
3.15	30	−20	12
3.15	0	34	6
3.14	28	6	10
3.14	−40	28	22

Additional pairwise comparisons revealed a large increase in de-activation magnitude for the EXP group (Figure 5, top row; Table 6). This was apparent in both magnitude and extent. Increases in de-activation magnitude were also observed in the CON group (Figure 5, bottom row; Table 7), however these effects were smaller and more focal than in the EXP group.

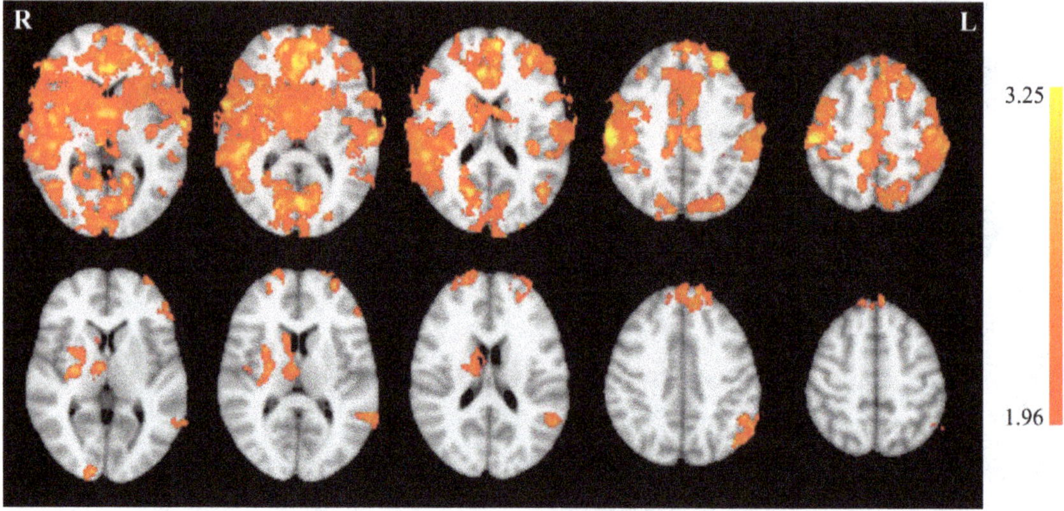

Figure 5. Increasing de-activation across training by group. The EXP group (top row) demonstrated a larger increase in de-activation across training than the CON group (bottom row) in both magnitude and extent. Axial slices (middle row) are displayed at MNI coordinates z = 4, 10, 18, 40, and 52 mm (left to right).

Table 6. Local maxima for increased de-activation across training for the EXP group. Coordinates are specified in MNI space.

		Coordinates	
Z statistic	X (mm)	Y (mm)	Z (mm)
4.31	10	−86	4
3.97	62	−18	42
3.86	−66	−12	4
3.85	34	18	−22
3.83	−14	104	18
3.74	−12	−58	68

An additional 2 × 2 (group by session) mixed factor ANOVA was performed on the BOLD data using the session 1 and 5 auditory localizer using FSL. The *F* test revealed a significant ($z > 1.96$) main effect of session on activation magnitude during auditory stimulation in the right inferior frontal gyrus and bilaterally in the superior temporal gyrus (Figure 6). The contrast identifying voxels with significantly greater activation in session 1 compared to session 5 was assessed to clarify the directionality. This contrast identified the regions in the right inferior frontal gyrus and bilateral superior temporal gyrus, implying activation in these regions significantly decreased with training. However, there were no significant findings in the *F* test for the session by group interaction and, thus, these changes were not found to vary significantly between groups and, thus, suggests the differences in neurofeedback performance cannot be explained by variations in the auditory localizer.

Table 7. Cluster maxima for increased de-activation across training for the CON group. Coordinates are specified in MNI space.

		Coordinates	
Z statistic	X (mm)	Y (mm)	Z (mm)
3.45	−45	−54	28
3.4	−56	−32	−16
3.33	28	−12	8
3.23	−20	64	24
3.23	−52	46	−10
3.17	22	−98	−8

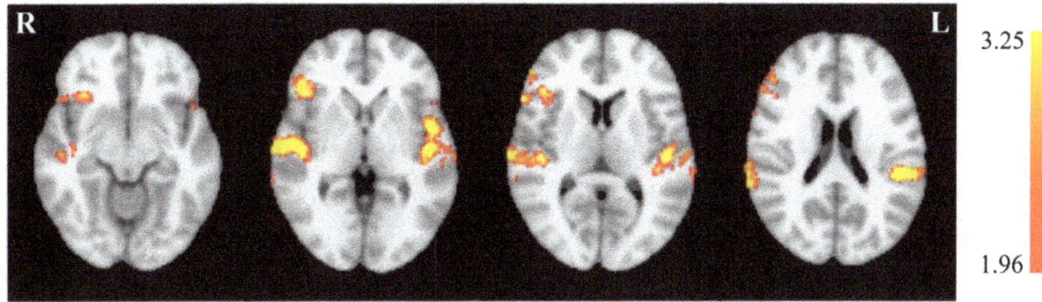

Figure 6. *F* test results for the main effect of session indicate decreased activation during auditory stimulation across training bilaterally in the superior temporal gyrus and in the right inferior frontal gyrus. Axial slices are displayed at MNI coordinates y = −10, 0, 8 and 20 mm (left to right).

4. Discussion

Training self-regulation of brain activity from fMRI-NFT has shown promise in a broad range of applications such as the improvement of human performance [15,16,27] and a variety of medical applications including recovery from stroke [18,20], major depression [32,51], Parkinson's disease [31], and chronic pain [29]. Of the techniques currently being explored, endogenous neuromodulation techniques [6,44,52] have the advantages of no known side effects and may be translated to exercises that could be performed at home without the use of sophisticated equipment and trained professionals [11,32]. Real-time functional magnetic resonance imaging [53,54] has seen a dramatic rise in interest since its advent in 1995, with a large portion of research dedicated to its application for training endogenous neuromodulation. In this technique, termed closed-loop endogenous neuromodulation, the BOLD signal is measured from a specific region of the brain, processed, and presented to the subject in real-time. Through training, subjects develop self-directed mental processing techniques that regulate this signal.

The present study found evidence for successful down-regulation of A1 using fMRI-NFT. The experimental group attempted down-regulation with the aid of real information regarding the current BOLD signals in A1 while the control group was supplied sham feedback yoked from a random participant in the experimental group and matched for training progress. In both groups, the bilateral A1 was identified both anatomically and functionally using an activation map produced during binaural continuous noise stimulation at each of the five training sessions. The results indicate an overall increase in the ability to volitionally decrease A1 activity across training. The most successful participants reported focusing on breathing during "lower" conditions during neurofeedback. A1 de-activation was not found to be significantly different at the first session between the experimental and control groups. However, the ability to volitionally decrease A1 activity was observed to be significantly greater for the experimental group compared to the control group at sessions two and five. Furthermore, self-control over A1 de-activation between the first and last training session was significantly increased in the experimental group. There was also a significant increase between the first and second training session signifying a rapid effect of neurofeedback training on A1 de-activation. These effects were not observed in the control group.

Interestingly, attempting volitional down-regulation of the auditory cortex resulted in a right-lateralized increase of de-activation in the occipital cortex (Figure 3). Asymmetry in the auditory system is well-documented (*i.e.,* "right ear advantage"), thought to be largely due to language processing regions contained in the left hemisphere. Typically, right ear advantage would be observed in the left hemisphere, as the sensory tracts largely decussate so that right ear information is almost entirely processed in the left hemisphere. However, due to the assessment of de-activation in the present study, the right ear advantage might reflect the right-lateralized results. There is a potential for handedness to also play a role similar to the right ear advantage, with similar logic regarding results apparent in de-activation. Additionally, habituation to the noise could be a contributing factor, though unlikely as habituation would have manifested as decreased activation in auditory regions equally apparent in both lower and relax conditions of the neurofeedback training. However, since this result arouse in both groups on average (main effect of session), our study lacks the control group necessary to disregard the potential of these effects as a result from habituation.

Our results add to a growing body of research that demonstrates the success of fMRI-NFT in teaching individuals to self-regulate localized brain activity. A previous controlled study indicates healthy individuals can learn to control the activated cortical volume in the primary and secondary auditory cortex using fMRI-NFT [23]. A second previous study indicated that control over the magnitude of A1 activation is also achievable however not necessarily attributable to fMRI-NFT [21]. The results above add to these previous studies by indicating fMRI-NFT aids control over the magnitude of A1 de-activation. In addition, this result shows that 60 min of distributed fMRI-NFT is adequate to train volitional A1 down-regulation, but significant observable effects are prevalent after only 24 min of training.

Our findings are important in the search for a possible treatment and/or therapy for tinnitus. Tinnitus, the phantom perception of sound, is often a symptom of an underlying condition such as age-related hearing loss, ear injury, or a circulatory system disorder. The phantom noise is highly variable in laterality, pulsatility, percept (pitch, intensity), and duration. Furthermore, a central mechanism has been implied as the percept remains following the complete resection of the auditory nerve [55] and acoustic tumors [56]. Tinnitus has been associated with hyperactivity in the auditory cortex in response to auditory stimulation [57,58] and at rest [59–62]. Additionally, altered attentional processes has been implicated as the source of the percept [58,63]. Only one previous study has investigated fMRI-NFT as a possible treatment for tinnitus [21]. In their study, four 4 min closed-loop endogenous neuromodulation runs to train up-regulation of A1 activation were completed in a single training session. The behavioral assessments were conducted before and after the single fMRI-NFT session. Their study indicates the promise of fMRI-NFT in treating tinnitus, but only included six participants and did not offer a control group. Furthermore, the researchers did not perform any statistical analysis on the behavioral data. Our study is unique for two reasons. First, we employed fMRI-NFT to reduce A1 activity which, as the literature suggests, is hyperactive in tinnitus populations. Second, A1 activity was reduced by directing attention away from the auditory cortex. This is important since it has been suggested that over-attention is drawn toward auditory processing in tinnitus populations.

5. Conclusion

The results presented in this work align with previous findings which indicate fMRI-NFT can be used to teach participants to voluntarily control the auditory cortex. However, the results of the presented work add to the previous findings by indicating volitional down-regulation of the auditory cortex is achievable in the presence of continuous noise using fMRI neurofeedback. This has not been previously reported. Tinnitus can cause severe impairments and can even limit the ability to perform daily functions. The financial burden associated with tinnitus is extensive. The number of U.S. veterans receiving service-connected disability for tinnitus exceeded all other disorders including post-traumatic stress disorder, hearing loss, and major depression [Annual Benefits Report Fiscal Year 2014, U.S. Department of Veterans Affairs]. The tinnitus percept is attributed to a central mechanism. Also, tinnitus has been associated with hyperactivity in the auditory cortex and abnormal attentional processes (theorized to cause the tinnitus percept). The results presented suggest attempting down-regulation of the auditory cortex may be a possible treatment for tinnitus by decreasing hyperactivity of the primary auditory cortex and directing attention away from auditory processing. Future work is necessary to study these procedures in a cohort of tinnitus patients but should also assess changes in activation associated with volitional down-regulation of the auditory cortex.

Acknowledgements

This material is based on research sponsored by the U.S. Air Force under agreement number FA8650-16-2-6702. The views expressed are those of the authors and do not reflect the official views or policy of the Department of Defense and its Components. The U.S. Government is authorized to reproduce and distribute reprints for Governmental purposes notwithstanding any copyright notation thereon. The voluntary, fully informed consent of the subjects used in this research was obtained as required by 32 CFR 219 and DODI 3216.02_AFI 40-402.

References

1. Hirsch J, Ruge MI, Kim KH, et al. (2000) An integrated functional magnetic resonance imaging procedure for preoperative mapping of cortical areas associated with tactile, motor, language, and visual functions. *Neurosurgery* 47: 711–722.
2. Yoo SS, Fairneny T, Chen NK, et al. (2004) Brain computer interface using fMRI: Spatial navigation by thoughts. *Neuroreport* 15: 1591–1595.
3. Sorger B, Reithler J, Dahmen B, et al. (2012) A real-time fMRI-based spelling device immediately enabling robust motor-independent communication. *Curr Biol* 22: 1333–1338.
4. Yoo JJ, Hinds O, Ofen N, et al. (2012) When the brain is prepared to learn: Enhancing human learning using real-time fMRI. *Neuroimage* 59: 846–852.
5. Weiskopf N, Veit R, Erb M, et al. (2003) Physiological self-regulation of regional brain activity using real-time functional magnetic resonance imaging (fMRI): Methodology and exemplary data. *Neuroimage* 19: 577–586.
6. Mak JN, Wolpaw JR (2009) Clinical applications of brain-computer interfaces: Current state and future prospects. *IEEE Rev Biomed Eng* 2: 187–199.
7. Logothetis NK, Pauls J, Augath M, et al. (2001) Neurophysiological investigation of the basis of the fMRI signal. *Nature* 412: 150–157.
8. Longden TA, Dabertrand F, Koide M, et al. (2017) Capillary K^+-sensing initiates retrograde hyperpolarization to increase local cerebral blood flow. *Nat Neurosci* 20: 717–726.
9. Hamilton JP, Glover GH, Hsu JJ, et al. (2011) Modulation of subgenual anterior cingulate cortex activity with real-time neurofeedback. *Hum Brain Mapp* 32: 22–31.
10. Zotev V, Krueger F, Phillips R, et al. (2011) Self-regulation of amygdala activation using real-time fMRI neurofeedback. *PLoS One* 6: e24522.
11. Caria A, Veit R, Sitaram R, et al. (2007) Regulation of anterior insular cortex activity using real-time fMRI. *Neuroimage* 35: 1238–1246.
12. Veit R, Singh V, Sitaram R, et al. (2012) Using real-time fMRI to learn voluntary regulation of the anterior insula in the presence of threat-related stimuli. *Soc Cogn Affect Neurosci* 7: 623–634.
13. Lee JH, Kim J, Yoo SS (2012) Real-time fMRI-based neurofeedback reinforces causality of attention networks. *Neurosci Res* 72: 347–354.
14. Mccaig RG, Dixon M, Keramatian K, et al. (2011) Improved modulation of rostrolateral prefrontal cortex using real-time fMRI training and meta-cognitive awareness. *Neuroimage* 55: 1298–1305.
15. Zhang G, Yao L, Zhang H, et al. (2013) Improved working memory performance through self-regulation of dorsal lateral prefrontal cortex activation using real-time fMRI. *PLoS One* 8: e73735.
16. Sherwood MS, Kane JH, Weisend MP, et al. (2016) Enhanced control of dorsolateral prefrontal cortex neurophysiology with real-time functional magnetic resonance imaging (rt-fMRI) neurofeedback training and working memory practice. *Neuroimage* 124: 214–223.
17. Sherwood MS, Weisend MP, Kane JH, et al. (2016) Combining real-time fMRI neurofeedback training of the DLPFC with N-Back practice results in neuroplastic effects confined to the neurofeedback target region. *Front Behav Neurosci* 10: 1–9.
18. Sitaram R, Veit R, Stevens B, et al. (2012) Acquired control of ventral premotor cortex activity by feedback training: An exploratory real-time fMRI and TMS study. *Neurorehabil Neural Repair* 26: 256–265.

19. Berman BD, Horovitz SG, Venkataraman G, et al. (2012) Self-modulation of primary motor cortex activity with motor and motor imagery tasks using real-time fMRI-based neurofeedback. *Neuroimage* 59: 917–925.
20. Chiew M, Laconte SM, Graham SJ (2012) Investigation of fMRI neurofeedback of differential primary motor cortex activity using kinesthetic motor imagery. *Neuroimage* 61: 21–31.
21. Haller S, Birbaumer N, Veit R (2010) Real-time fMRI feedback training may improve chronic tinnitus. *Eur Radiol* 20: 696–703.
22. Haller S, Kopel R, Jhooti P, et al. (2013) Dynamic reconfiguration of human brain functional networks through neurofeedback. *Neuroimage* 81: 243–252.
23. Yoo SS, O'Leary HM, Fairneny T, et al. (2006) Increasing cortical activity in auditory areas through neurofeedback functional magnetic resonance imaging. *Neuroreport* 17: 1273–1278.
24. Johnston S, Linden DE, Healy D, et al. (2011) Upregulation of emotion areas through neurofeedback with a focus on positive mood. *Cognit Affective Behav Neurosci* 11: 44–51.
25. Johnston SJ, Boehm SG, Healy D, et al. (2010) Neurofeedback: A promising tool for the self-regulation of emotion networks. *Neuroimage* 49: 1066–1072.
26. Rota G, Sitaram R, Veit R, et al. (2010) Self-regulation of regional cortical activity using real-time fMRI: The right inferior frontal gyrus and linguistic processing. *Hum Brain Mapp* 30: 1605–1614.
27. Scharnowski F, Hutton C, Josephs O, et al. (2012) Improving visual perception through neurofeedback. *J Neurosci* 32: 17830–17841.
28. Shibata K, Kawato M (2011) Perceptual learning incepted by decoded fmri neurofeedback without stimulus presentation. *Science* 334: 1413–1415.
29. Decharms RC, Maeda F, Glover GH, et al. (2005) Control over brain activation and pain learned by using real-time functional MRI. *Proc Natl Acad Sci U S A* 102: 18626–18631.
30. Ruiz S, Lee S, Soekadar SR, et al. (2013) Acquired self-control of insula cortex modulates emotion recognition and brain network connectivity in schizophrenia. *Hum Brain Mapp* 34: 200–212.
31. Subramanian L, Hindle JV, Johnston S, et al. (2011) Real-time functional magnetic resonance imaging neurofeedback for treatment of Parkinson's disease. *J Neurosci* 31: 16309–16317.
32. Linden DEJ, Habes I, Johnston SJ, et al. (2012) Real-time self-regulation of emotion networks in patients with depression. *PLoS One* 7: e38115.
33. Decharms RC, Christoff K, Glover GH, et al. (2004) Learned regulation of spatially localized brain activation using real-time fMRI. *Neuroimage* 21: 436–443.
34. Yoo SS, Lee JH, O'Leary H, et al. (2008) Neurofeedback fMRI-mediated learning and consolidation of regional brain activation during motor imagery. *Int J Imaging Syst Technol* 18: 69–78.
35. Birbaumer N, Cohen LG (2007) Brain-computer interfaces: Communication and restoration of movement in paralysis. *J Physiol* 579: 621–636.
36. Daly JJ, Wolpaw JR (2008) Brain-computer interfaces in neurological rehabilitation. *Lancet Neurol* 7: 1032–1043.
37. Ros T, Munneke MAM, Ruge D, et al. (2010) Endogenous control of waking brain rhythms induces neuroplasticity in humans. *Eur J Neurosci* 31: 770–778.
38. Orlov ND, Giampietro V, O'Daly O, et al. (2018) Real-time fMRI neurofeedback to down-regulate superior temporal gyrus activity in patients with schizophrenia and auditory hallucinations: A proof-of-concept study. *Transl Psychiatry* 8: 46.
39. Paret C, Kluetsch R, Ruf M, et al. (2014) Down-regulation of amygdala activation with real-time fMRI neurofeedback in a healthy female sample. *Front Behav Neurosci* 8: 299.

40. Saliba J, Al-Reefi M, Carriere JS, et al. (2016) Accuracy of mobile-based audiometry in the evaluation of hearing loss in quiet and noisy environments. *Otolaryngol Neck Surg* 156: 706–711.
41. Thompson GP, Sladen DP, Borst BJ, et al. (2015) Accuracy of a tablet audiometer for measuring behavioral hearing thresholds in a clinical population. *Otolaryngol Neck Surg* 153: 838–842.
42. Worsley KJ, Friston KJ (1995) Analysis of fMRI time-series revisited—again. *Neuroimage* 2: 173–181.
43. Ashby F Gregory (2011) *Statistical analysis of fMRI data.* MIT press.
44. Smith SM, Jenkinson M, Woolrich MW, et al. (2004) Advances in functional and structural MR image analysis and implementation as FSL. *Math Brain Imaging* 23: S208–S219.
45. Woolrich MW, Jbabdi S, Patenaude B, et al. (2009) Bayesian analysis of neuroimaging data in FSL. *Math Brain Imaging* 45: S173–S186.
46. Jenkinson M, Bannister P, Brady M, et al. (2002) Improved optimization for the robust and accurate linear registration and motion correction of brain images. *Neuroimage* 17: 825–841.
47. Smith SM (2002) Fast robust automated brain extraction. *Hum Brain Mapp* 17: 143–155.
48. Greve DN, Fischl B (2009) Accurate and robust brain image alignment using boundary-based registration. *Neuroimage* 48: 63–72.
49. Collins DL, Holmes CJ, Peters TM, et al. (2004) Automatic 3-D model-based neuroanatomical segmentation. *Hum Brain Mapp* 3: 190–208.
50. Mazziotta J, Toga A, Evans A, et al. (2002) A probabilistic atlas and reference system for the human brain: International Consortium for Brain Mapping (ICBM). *Brain Mapp Methods* 356: 1293–1322.
51. Young KD, Zotev V, Phillips R, et al. (2014) Real-time fMRI neurofeedback training of amygdala activity in patients with major depressive disorder. *PLoS One* 9: e88785.
52. Sulzer J, Haller S, Scharnowski F, et al. (2013) Real-time fMRI neurofeedback: Progress and challenges. *Neuroimage* 76: 386–399.
53. Cox RW, Jesmanowicz A, Hyde JS (1995) Real-time functional magnetic resonance imaging. *Magn Reson Med* 33: 230–236.
54. Weiskopf N, Sitaram R, Josephs O, et al. (2007) Real-time functional magnetic resonance imaging: Methods and applications. *Proc Int Sch Magn Reson Brain Funct* 25: 989–1003.
55. Folmer RL, Griest S, Martin W (2001) Chronic tinnitus as phantom auditory pain. *Otolaryngol—Head Neck Surg* 124: 394–400.
56. Berliner KI, Shelton C, Hitselberger WE, et al. (1992) Acoustic tumors: Effect of surgical removal on tinnitus. *Otol Neurotol* 13: 13.
57. Gu JW, Halpin CF, Nam EC, et al. (2010) Tinnitus, diminished sound-level tolerance, and elevated auditory activity in humans with clinically normal hearing sensitivity. *J Neurophysiol* 104: 3361–3370.
58. Seydellgreenwald A, Leaver AM, Turesky TK, et al. (2012) Functional MRI evidence for a role of ventral prefrontal cortex in tinnitus. *Brain Ress* 1485: 22–39.
59. Wang H, Tian J, Yin D, et al. (2001) Regional glucose metabolic increases in left auditory cortex in tinnitus patients: A preliminary study with positron emission tomography. *Chin Med J* 114: 848–851.
60. Langguth B, Eichhammer P, Kreutzer A, et al. (2006) The impact of auditory cortex activity on characterizing and treating patients with chronic tinnitus—first results from a PET study. *Acta Otolaryngol* 126: 84–88.

61. Schecklmann M, Landgrebe M, Poeppl TB, et al. (2013) Neural correlates of tinnitus duration and Distress: A positron emission tomography study. *Hum Brain Mapp* 34: 233–240.
62. Geven LI, de Kleine E, Willemsen ATM, et al. (2014) Asymmetry in primary auditory cortex activity in tinnitus patients and controls. *Neuroscience* 256: 117–125.
63. Kim SG, Ogawa S (2012) Biophysical and physiological origins of blood oxygenation level-dependent fMRI signals. *J Cereb Blood Flow Metab* 32: 1188–1206.

11

The reflexive imagery task: An experimental paradigm for neuroimaging

Hyein Cho[1], Wei Dou[1], Zaviera Reyes[1], Mark W. Geisler[1] and Ezequiel Morsella[1,2,*]

[1] Department of Psychology, San Francisco State University, CA, USA
[2] Department of Neurology, University of California, San Francisco, CA, USA

* **Correspondence:** Email: morsella@sfsu.edu;

Abstract: High-level cognitions can be triggered into consciousness through the presentation of external stimuli and the activation of certain action sets. These activations arise in a manner that is involuntary, systematic and nontrivial. For example, in the Reflexive Imagery Task (RIT), subjects are presented with visual objects and instructed to not think of the names of the objects. Involuntary subvocalizations arise on roughly 80% of the trials. We review the findings from this paradigm, discuss neural findings that are relevant to the RIT, and present new data that further corroborate the reliability and robustness of the RIT, a paradigm that could be coupled with neuroimaging technologies. We developed an RIT variant in which two, non-focal objects are presented simultaneously. In previous RITs, visual objects were presented only one at a time, in the center of the screen, and subjects were instructed to focus on the center of the screen, where these objects were presented. Replicating the RIT effect, involuntary subvocalizations still occurred on a high proportion of trials ($M = 0.78$). An RIT effect arose for both objects on a considerable proportion of the trials ($M = 0.35$). These findings were replicated in a second experiment having a different sample of subjects. Our findings are relevant to many subfields of neuroscience (e.g., the study of high-level mental processes, attention, imagery and action control).

Keywords: consciousness; cognitive control; involuntary processing; reflexive imagery task; stimulus control

1. Introduction

Understanding the mechanisms underlying "entry into consciousness" ("entry", for short [1,2]) remains one of the most challenging puzzles in science [3]. Entry is influenced by various processes, including those that are voluntary (e.g., choosing to think about certain things) or attention-based (see review in Most et al. [4]). Recent research has begun to illuminate the nature of the various kinds of mechanisms underlying entry that is involuntary. This form of entry can arise from the salience, motion, novelty or incentive/emotional quality of the stimulus [9]. Involuntary entry can be of percepts, urges [10] or even high-level cognitions. Regarding high-level cognitions, their involuntary entry can arise as a consequence of the activation of *action sets*, the topic of the present project. An action set would be "when perceiving *X*, then do *Y*" [11]; for example, "when I see a mailbox, I must deposit the letter that I am carrying". Regarding action sets, Ach [11] speaks of the example in which, after activating the action set to "add things" and being presented with the numbers five and three, there is the involuntary entry of the *conscious content*[1] "eight". In this way, entry of high-level conscious contents can arise from the activation of action sets ("set-based entry", for short). Theorists (e.g., Freud [12]; Helmholtz [13]; James [14]; N. E. Miller [15]; Wegner [16]) have proposed that, during such entry, one is conscious of the product (e.g., the phonological form "eight") of sophisticated and unintentional processes, but not of the processes themselves, a view that has recurred in the history of psychology (e.g., [17,18]).[2]

These conclusions suggest that, in a neuroimaging study, if the experimenter controls the activation of set and the stimulus conditions, then entry could be controlled externally and predictably, in ways that are not trivial and that involve high-level contents. Such a study on entry could employ the Reflexive Imagery Task (RIT [23]), which we review, along with the relevant neural findings, in the next section. We conclude our review with the presentation of new data which further corroborate the reliability and robustness of the paradigm.

1.1. *Reflexive Imagery Task*

The RIT (see review in Bhangal et al. [24]) is based on a rich research tradition, stemming from the experimental approaches of Ach [11], Stroop [25], Wegner [16], and Gollwitzer [26]. The paradigm was developed to investigate experimentally the involuntary entry of high-level conscious contents. In the initial, most basic version of the task [23], subjects are instructed to not subvocalize

---

[1] A "conscious content" is anything that one is aware of [5]; for example, it might be a color, an urge or a spontaneous autobiographical memory. The "conscious field" is all that one is aware of at one moment in time, which is the combination of all activated conscious contents [6–8].

[2] Theorists have posited that conscious contents arise involuntarily because of the "encapsulated" nature of the generation of most conscious contents [10,19]. This encapsulation is evident in perception and also in the generation of action-related urges. In certain stimulus environments, these urges (e.g., to inhale while holding one's breath while underwater) are triggered in a predictable and insuppressible manner [20]. The urges cannot be modulated or turned off voluntarily, even when doing so would be adaptive [20,21]. The action-related urges are externally-triggered and encapsulated from volitional processes. As noted by Bargh and Morsella [22], these action-related inclinations can be *behaviorally suppressed*, but they often cannot be *mentally suppressed*.

(i.e., say in their head but not aloud) the names of objects (e.g., line drawings from Snodgrass & Vanderwart [27]). In Allen et al. [23], subjects were presented before each trial with the instruction, "Don't Think of the Name of the Object" before an object was presented for 4 s, during which time subjects indicated by button press if they happened to subvocalize the name of the object. On the majority of the trials (86% in Allen et al. [23]; 87% in Cho et al. [28]; 73% in Merrick et al. [29]), subjects fail to suppress such subvocalizations. To illustrate the basic version of the RIT effect, momentarily, we will present to you, the reader, an object enclosed within parentheses. Your task is to *not* subvocalize (i.e., "say in one's head") the name of the object. Here is the stimulus (▲). When presented with these instructions (which induce a certain action set) and then presented with this stimulus, most people cannot suppress the conscious experience of the phonological form of the word "triangle".

It is important to appreciate that this RIT effect requires the process of object naming, a sophisticated, multi-stage process in which only one of tens of thousands of phonological representations is selected for production in response to a stimulus (e.g., CAT yields /k/, /œ/, /t/; Levelt [30]). After the presentation of the stimulus, the RIT effect arises after a few moments (M = 1,451.27 ms [SD = 611.42] in Allen et al. [23]; M = 2,323.91 ms [SD = 1,183.01] in Cho et al. [28]; M = 1,745.97 ms [SD = 620.86] in Merrick et al. [29]). There are more complex versions of the task. For example, in one study, RIT effects arose even though the involuntary effect involved a word-manipulation task similar to the childhood game of pig Latin (e.g., "CAR" becomes "AR-CAY"). In this variant of the RIT [31], subjects were instructed to not transform stimulus words according to the rule. Nevertheless, involuntary transformations still arose on more than 40% of the trials. This set-based effect is noteworthy because the involuntary transformation of the word stimulus requires symbol manipulation, a complex operation which is known to be associated with frontal cortex [32].[3]

1.2. *Validity of subjects' self-reports*

The evidence suggests that the RIT effect is both robust and reliable. However, some important questions remain concerning the validity of the effect. For instance, one major criticism is that the paradigm relies on the technique of self-report. Self-reports can be inaccurate as a result of (a) inaccurate memories of fleeting conscious contents that lead to incorrect self-reports [33]; (b) subjects basing their reports on a strategy of how to comport oneself during an experiment (see discussion in Morsella et al. [34]). Evidence from neuroimaging studies suggests that subjects are not confabulating about the occurrence of these mental events. In these studies, subjects must report about the occurrence of involuntary conscious contents [35–39]. Strong behavioral evidence for subjects' self-reports stems from one variant of the RIT. In this variant [40], subjects indicated by button press the basic RIT effect but, in addition, they had to press another button if the involuntary subvocalization rhymed with a word held in mind. Accurate performance (> 80% mean accuracy

---

[3] In another complex version of the task [29], subjects were presented with a single, focal object and instructed to (a) not subvocalize the name of the visual object; (b) not subvocalize the number of letters in the object name. On a considerable proportion of the trials (0.30 [SE = 0.04]), subjects reported experiencing both kinds of imagery. Importantly, the occurrence of both involuntary thoughts reflects the involvement of two very different kinds of unintentional cognitive processes: *object naming* versus *letter counting*. Each of these processes is quite sophisticated and high-level, yielding outputs (e.g., the phonological forms "sun" and "three") that are not direct reflections of external stimuli.

across trials) on this rhyming task provided evidence that subjects experience involuntary subvocalizations of the name of the object, for detecting a rhyme requires the retrieval of either the whole object name or, at minimum, the coda of the object name.

1.3. Evidence that the effect resembles a reflex

Empirical evidence and theory, including Wegner's [41] model of *ironic processing*[4] (see discussion of relationship between Wegner's [41] model and the RIT in Bhangal et al. [24]) suggest that, for subjects, the effect "just happens". The effect does not seem to be an artifact of high-level strategic processes. Supporting this view, in one version of the RIT, subjects reported on the majority of trials that the involuntary subvocalizations felt "immediate" [42]. Separate evidence supports the notion that the effect is not an artifact of strategic processes. First, on many trials, the effect arises too quickly to be caused by strategic processing [23,28]. Second, the RIT effect still arises under conditions of cognitive load, in which it is difficult for subjects to implement strategic processing [28]. Third, the effect habituates (i.e., is less likely to arise) after repeated presentation of the same stimulus object, which suggests that the RIT effect is activated in a reflex-like manner [43]. Last, the nature of the subvocalizations is influenced systematically by stimulus dimensions such as word frequency [42]. Such an artifact of experimental demand would require for subjects to know the ways in which word frequency should influence latencies in an object-naming experiment.

It is important to note that the RIT is "reflex-like", but is not a true reflex. A true reflex

[4] Ironic effects arise when one is more likely to think about a given thing when attempting to not think about that thing. Wegner [41] proposes that these effects arise from an interaction between two distinct processes. One process is an *operating* process, which is associated with the conscious intention to maintain a particular mental state. This process actively scans mental contents (e.g., thoughts, sensations) that can help maintain the desired mental state (e.g., to be calm). This process tends to be effortful, capacity-limited and consciously mediated [41]. The other mechanism is an "ironic" *monitoring* process that automatically scans activated mental contents to detect contents signaling the failure to establish the desired mental state. When the monitor detects contents that signify failed control of the operating mechanism, it increases the likelihood that the particular content will enter consciousness, so that the operating mechanism can then process the content and change its own operations accordingly. The ironic monitor mechanism is usually unconscious, autonomous and requires little mental effort. Harmony between the two kinds of processes fails when the goal in mental control is to *not* activate a particular mental content (e.g., content *X*), because (a) the operating process can bring only goal-related contents into consciousness and cannot actively exclude contents; (b) the ironic monitor will reflexively bring into consciousness mental contents (e.g., content *X*) that are incongruent with the goal. Hence, there will be the automatic activation of content *X* in consciousness (for reviews of ironic processing and thought suppression, see [16,46]). One difference between the involuntary subvocalization that constitutes the RIT effect and the kinds of effects that have been obtained in most experiments concerning ironic processing is that, in the latter, subjects are presented with a verbal description (e.g., verbal instructions such as "*Do not think of white bears*"), and then the subjects experience involuntary perceptuo-semantic imagery. In the RIT, however, the stimuli are visual and it is the involuntary imagery that is phonological in nature. One could state that the RIT involves the opposite direction of activation of that found in the classic studies on ironic processing.

possesses a magnitude that reflects the intensity of the stimulus, as in the case of the startle reflex. The RIT does not have this property. Instead, the RIT depends on the activation of high-level, involuntary sets.

1.4. *The importance of set in set-based entry*

It is important to note that, in the basic version of the RIT, it is unlikely that subjects would experience the phonological representations of the names of the objects that are perceived visually without the activation of the action set. The activation of the action set is somehow initiated by the instruction to not think of the name of the object. With this in mind, it is important to point out that, in Allen et al. [23], there was an *Incidental Naming* condition in which subjects were not provided with the "do not think" instruction that leads to ironic effects [41]. Instead, the condition involved no explicit instructions regarding naming or not naming. For this condition, involuntary subvocalization of the object names still arose on 99% of the trials (range = 80% to 100%). The effect was comparable even on the very first trial (31 [97%] out of 32 first trials). The Incidental Naming condition served to evaluate subjects' spontaneous subvocalization rates in response to the stimuli when having no obvious action set toward the stimuli. Of course, simply mentioning to subjects the possibility of naming will increase the likelihood of subvocalization, which is a limitation of this condition.[5]

1.5. *Neural correlates of the RIT effect*

Investigations on the neural correlates of cognitive control, phonological processing and involuntary cognitions (including ironic processing; see Footnote 4), suggest that, in the basic RIT effect, there might be the recruitment of at least three distinct neural mechanisms: Those associated with (*1*) the action set to not subvocalize the name of the object; (*2*) the detection of a discrepancy between desired performance and the involuntary effect; (*3*) the phonological representation of the object name.

Regarding 1, neuroimaging studies suggest that the action set to perform a simple action (such as to *not* subvocalize an object name or to follow another simple rule of behavior) involves prefrontal cortex [32,47,48] (see evidence from neurophysiological studies involving monkeys in 47). For example, in ironic processing, the effortful, *operating* process (see Footnote 4)

---

[5] Two other findings complement the Incidental Naming condition. First, subvocalizations toward the visual objects in an RIT [44] arose even when subjects, before being presented with a visual object, performed a block of trials of a task involving another, very different kind of action set (e.g., the Stroop task [17]). Second, the kind of involuntary entry into consciousness found in the RIT arises in tasks that lack any kind of negative instruction to not perform some kind of mental operation. For example, involuntary entry of contents into consciousness arises for ambiguous objects (e.g., Necker cube). In one experiment [45], subjects were instructed to hold in mind, for as long as possible, one way of perceiving an ambiguous object (e.g., Necker cube). Importantly, subjects were never told to *not* think about alternative ways in which the object could be perceived. Involuntary "perceptual reversals" involving involuntary entry into consciousness of the rivalrous percept for a given object, occurred on around 80% of the trials, with roughly three such reversals per 30-second trial.

involves the dorsolateral prefrontal cortex [37,49]. This was observed in a study involving functional magnetic resonance (fMRI) imaging [37].

The RIT effect involves the detection of undesired conscious content, resulting, in part, from the activation of set and stimulus conditions (for an electroencephalography study on thought suppression, see [50]). Studies employing fMRI have revealed that such detection has been associated with the activities of the anterior cingulate cortex [37,39,49], a region that has been associated with cognitive control [51], including cognitive conflict [52], the detection of error-prone processing [an fMRI study 53] and more inclusively, any form of inefficient processing [54] (the region is located on the medial surface of the frontal lobe and interconnected with many motor areas). Inefficient processing includes both error-prone and conflict-related processes (see [55–57] for discussions of the role of the anterior cingulate cortex, lateral prefrontal cortex and hippocampus in the suppression, not of involuntary subvocalizations, but of undesired memory retrieval. These studies [55–57] are based on data from fMRI).

Regarding 3, controversy continues to surround the identification of the neural correlates of the phonological representations that are activated by heard, spoken speech (e.g., [58,59]) (see relevant data from transcranial magnetic stimulation in 59). Thus, at this stage of understanding, strong claims cannot be made regarding the neural correlates of subvocalized speech (see discussion in Buchsbaum [60]; Buchsbaum & D'Esposito [61]). Nevertheless, investigations in neuropsychology and neuroimaging (e.g., fMRI) [62] suggest that the neural correlates of phonological representations involve the left superior temporal cortex (including the superior temporal gyrus and sulcus) and a medley of other regions (supramarginal gyrus, inferior frontal gyrus, precentral gyrus [62–65]).

Buchsbaum [60] concludes that the subvocalization of speech is often associated with activations in both (a) motor-related regions in frontal cortex, such as the inferior frontal gyrus (for phonological planning) and the precentral gyrus (for motor programming); (b) perception-related regions that are associated with speech perception (e.g., superior temporal sulcus). Accordingly, Scott [66] presents evidence that, during the act of subvocalization, corollary discharge provides the conscious sensory content of one's inner speech [67]. In an electroencephalography study by Ford et al. [67], mismatches involving one's intended speech and what one actually hears oneself utter aloud are associated with decreased functional synchrony (a kind of communication) between frontal and temporal lobes.

It should be pointed out that it remains controversial whether the subvocalization of speech requires the activation of motor-related regions or whether subvocalized speech and other forms of auditory imagery can arise without these activations [58,59,61,68]. Thus, today there is no conclusive evidence that, for example, lesions to motor areas associated with speech production eradicate the capacity for subvocalizing or other kinds of verbal imagery [69–72]. For some evidence of a necessary, causal role of motor areas in speech perception, see Schomers, Kirilina, Weigand, Bajbouj and Pulvermüller [59].

In summary, it is clear that much is known about the neural correlates of many of the component processes underlying the RIT effect. Hence, the RIT is a rich and fecund experimental paradigm for hypothesis-testing research studies in the field of neuroscience.

1.6. *Replication and extension of the RIT*

For this review of the RIT, we took the opportunity to complement previous findings with new data that further corroborate the reliability and robustness of the paradigm. In previous RITs, involuntary entry arose from the processing of one single, focal stimulus, one that was in the center of the subjects' visual field and was the focus of visual attention. No RIT variant to date has presented an array of stimuli and had the subject not focus on one of the objects. There is always the possibility that subjects, when presented with such a complex stimulus scene, in which more than one visual object is presented, may not experience any RIT effect or, at the least, may be much less likely to experience the effect on a given trial. This leads to the question, would an RIT effect still arise if (a) more than one stimulus object is presented simultaneously; (b) the stimuli in the task are not as focal as those of previous studies? Can the RIT effect survive in a multi-stimulus scenario? Would the effect arise on a large proportion (> 0.70) of the trials, as was found in previous studies (e.g., 0.86 in Allen et al. [23]; 0.87 in Cho et al. [28]; and 0.73 in Merrick et al. [29])? If so, then this would corroborate that the RIT effect is both a robust and reliable phenomenon, one capable of arising in stimulus scenes that resemble everyday scenarios more than those of previous RITs.

To begin to investigate these questions, we developed a variant of the RIT in which, on each trial, two stimuli (visual objects) were presented (6 s) as a pair, with one stimulus being presented on the left side of the computer screen and one stimulus being presented on the right side of the screen (Figure 1). On each trial, subjects were instructed to focus on the fixation cross presented on the center of the screen and to not think of the names of any of the objects. Subjects indicated by button press if they happened to think of the name of any of the objects. Subjects pressed one button if they thought of the name of the object on the left, and they pressed another button if they thought of the name of the object on the right. If, during the duration of the trial, subjects thought of the name of any of the objects more than once, then they pressed the corresponding button each time that they experienced the thought. Unlike in previous studies, we examined the occurrence and latencies of all button presses. With this variant of the RIT, we took the opportunity to examine (a) whether the RIT effect still arises under so complex a circumstance, which is more complicated than that of previous studies; (b) whether subjects, on a given trial, experienced more than one involuntary subvocalization; (c) on a trial-by-trial basis, the latencies of the first subvocalization and rates of occurrence of all subsequent subvocalizations; (d) whether, because of the nature of reading (which is left to right), the spatial location (i.e., left versus right) of the object influenced the nature of our dependent measures.[6]

If more than one thought is triggered in this experimental context, then this is quite noteworthy, because it would be one of the first demonstrations of entry of more than one thought arising from external control. In addition, finding an RIT effect with our variant would corroborate the view that the RIT effect in other paradigms is not solely an artifact of subjects focusing on the critical stimulus. Moreover, if the RIT effect arises for each of the two objects presented on a given trial, then this

[6] Because prior RIT research [73] suggests that the valence of a stimulus (that is, positive versus negative valence) might, under some circumstances, influence the nature of the RIT effect, and because our stimuli stem in large part from the stimulus set used by Pugh et al. [73], we took the opportunity to have an equal number of objects that fall within the continua of positive valence and negative valence, with each stimulus array having an equal number of objects from each continuum. Because (a) the valence-related data have no bearing on the question here under investigation; (b) the influence of valence on RIT effects is far from straightforward (see discussion in Cho [23]), and (c) at least at this stage of understanding, such valence effects are not worthy of report, we will not discuss the matter of stimulus valence any further. For additional information about the nature of the valence of the stimuli and of potential valence effects, see [73].

would suggest that it is not the case that subjects' responding to one object hinders the ability of a response to the other object. This could occur if the involuntary subvocalization on a trial depletes the cognitive resources that are necessary for the involuntary subvocalization of the name of another object, at least during the 6 s span. To date, no RIT has taxed to this extent the processes involved in involuntary subvocalization.

Of import, our research project is the kind of incremental, *cumulative, theory-driven* research that leaders in the field of experimental psychology have recently encouraged [74,75]. Moreover, the phenomenon at hand (the RIT effect and ironic processing) is a robust, multifaceted and reliable phenomenon that has been investigated for years, yielding the kind of programmatic research that is incremental and important for progress in the fields of psychological science and neuroscience [75]. In addition, the paradigm is perfectly suited for scanner-based neuroimaging research, because the task involves a simple procedure for presenting stimuli (e.g., a black-and-white line drawing), and because the dependent measure (the occurrence of involuntary mental imagery) does not require complicated movements on the part of the subject. Last, our task also provides a way of examining the mechanisms underlying entry into consciousness, one of the greatest enigmas in science [3,76,77]. The phenomenon of involuntary entry is of interest to many subfields within neuroscience, including consciousness, attention, self-regulation, psychopathology, mental imagery and mind wandering.

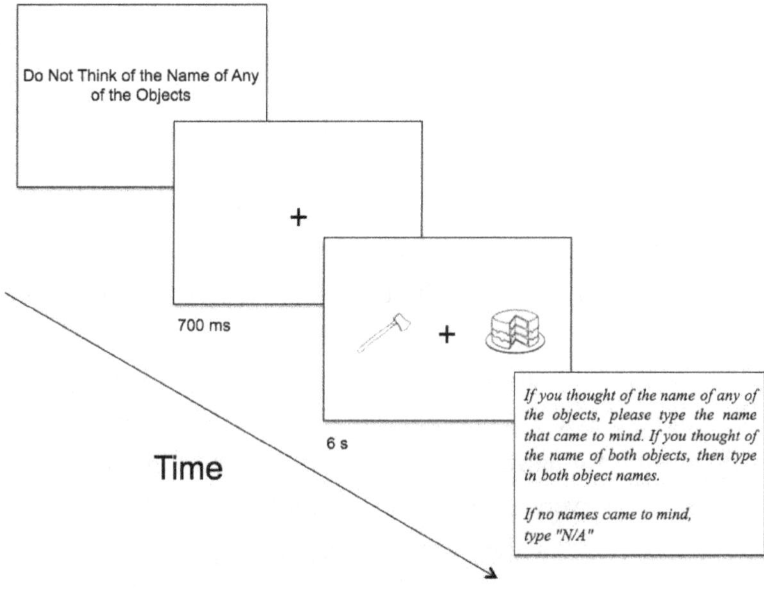

Figure 1. Schematic depiction of a trial (not drawn to scale).

2. Method

2.1. Subjects

San Francisco State University students (n = 45; 37 females; M_{Age} = 23.90 years; SD_{Age} = 7.17 years) participated for course credit. The involvement of human subjects in our project was approved by the Institutional Review Board at San Francisco State University.

2.2. *Stimuli and apparatus*

Stimuli were presented on an Apple iMac computer monitor (50.8 cm) with a viewing distance of approximately 48 cm. Stimulus presentation and data recording were controlled by PsyScope software [78]. Subjects inputted their responses to questions and instructions by computer keyboard. All questions and instructions were written in black 36-point Helvetica font; all fonts and images were displayed in black hue on a light gray background. The stimuli consisted of 76 visual objects (Figure 1). Most of the stimuli were from Snodgrass and Vanderwart [27], while some were designed to resemble these Snodgrass images. These images were used successfully in previous research [23,73,79] (see Supplementary Table 1 for a list of the names of all of these objects). On each trial, two visual objects were presented concurrently in a side-by-side fashion with a fixation cross in between the visual objects (Figure 1). The array of stimuli, which was composed of both visual objects, was presented on the screen with a subtended visual angle of $17.76^{\circ} \times 5.96^{\circ}$ (15 cm × 5 cm). Each object occupied the visual angle of $6.56^{\circ} \times 5.96^{\circ}$ (5.5 cm × 5 cm).

2.3. *Procedures*

All subjects completed 38 trials in this modified version of the RIT. Each image was shown only once. For each trial, whether a given object appeared on the left side of the screen or on the right side of the screen was random. At the beginning of the experimental session, subjects were instructed that, on each trial, they would be shown two objects, with one object appearing on the left, and the other object appearing on the right. Subjects were instructed to not think of the name of any of the objects that were presented. If a subject did happen to think of the name of any of the objects, then the subject was instructed to indicate by button press each time that they happened to think of the name of any of the objects. It was emphasized to subjects that they should respond in this way as quickly as possible (trials in which RTs for a button press were less than or equal to 200 ms were excluded from analysis. This resulted in the loss of the data from only one trial). The presentation duration of the visual objects (6 s) was based on that of Allen et al. [23], with a longer duration allocated for the presentation of two objects (i.e., 50% more time was given from the original 4 second duration). If subjects did not happen to think of the name of any of the objects, then they did not respond in any way. Subjects were told that they could indicate by pressing the "z" key on the keyboard if they happened to think of the name of the object presented on the left of the fixation cross, and the character key "/" on the keyboard if they happened to think of the name of the object presented on the right of the fixation cross. In addition, subjects were informed that the keys correspond to the location of the object presentation (e.g., "z" key which is located on the left side of the keyboard for the objects presented on the left; "/" key which is located on the right side of the keyboard for the objects presented on the right). Both keys were covered with colored paper so that the keys could be easily distinguished from the other, neighboring keys. The "z" and "/" keys were chosen because (a) they are on opposite sides of a standard keyboard, thereby minimizing subjects' confusion; (b) the location of the keys are equidistant in relation to the spacebar. The pairing of keys to either spatial location on the screen were not counterbalanced because this could lead to undesired effects such as the Simon Effect [80].

Once subjects completed the experiment, they completed a set of psychological assessments[7], as well as a series of funneled debriefing questions (following the procedures of Bargh & Chartrand [83]), which included general questions to assess whether subjects (a) were aware of the purpose of the study; (b) had any strategies for completing the task; (c) had anything interfere with their performance on the task; (d) knew the names of all of the presented objects; (e) thought of object names in a language other than English; (f) pressed the buttons in response to thinking of the names in another language. Additionally, subjects were asked questions regarding their performance on the task, to assess whether they (g) often thought of the names of both of the objects when the name of one object came to mind. These questions were included only to assess if a subject's data were acceptable for data analysis. From 52 subjects, data from 45 subjects were included in the analysis. The data for 7 subjects were excluded from analysis because (a) subjects did not follow instructions (e.g., looking away from the screen when stimuli were presented); (b) equipment malfunction (e.g., unexpected quitting of the computer software); (c) subjects did not press the button when they thought of the name of the object in a language other than English.

3. Results

Although the stimulus environment was more complicated than that of previous RITs, an RIT effect still emerged. The RIT effect is quantified as the proportion of trials on which an involuntary subvocalization arises in response to the presentations of the stimuli. The proportion of trials on which subjects had at least one involuntary subvocalization was 0.78 (*SD* = 0.20; *SE* = 0.03), a proportion that was significantly different from zero, $t\ (44) = 26.39$, $p < 0.0001$. This proportion is comparable to the proportions found in previous studies, which involved the presentation of only one stimulus at a time (e.g., 86% in Allen et al. [23]; 87% in Cho et al. [28]; 73% in Merrick et al. [29]). The same significant result was found with arcsine transformations of the proportion data, $t\ (44) = 27.44$, $p < 0.0001$. Arcsine transformations are often used to statistically normalize data that are in the form of proportions. Of the 45 subjects, 16 had an RIT effect on over 90% of the trials; 10 had an RIT effect on 80% to 90% of the trials; 9 had an RIT effect on 60% to 79% of the trials, and the percentages for the remaining 10 subjects were 58%, 58%, 58%, 53%, 53%, 50%, 45%, 37%, 37%, 34%. For trials on which there was an RIT effect, the mean latency of this effect was 2,493.57 ms (*SD* = 694.58, *SE* = 103.54). The latencies were comparable to those of previous studies (e.g., *M* = 1,451.27 ms [*SD* = 611.42] in Allen et al. [23]; *M* = 2,323.91 ms [*SD* = 1,183.01] in Cho et al. [28]; *M* = 1,745.97 ms [*SD* = 620.86] in Merrick et al. [29]).

The RIT effect occurred for both objects on a proportion of 0.35 of the trials (*SD* = 0.31; *SE* = 0.05), which was significantly different from zero, $t\ (44) = 7.43$, $p < 0.0001$, and was comparable to what was found in Merrick et al. [29], the only other RIT study in which two thoughts were triggered into the conscious field by external stimuli. This finding regarding an effect for both objects is also

[7] At the conclusion of the experimental session, subjects completed a series of psychological questionnaires (e.g., Generalized Anxiety Disorder 7-item scale [81]) to assess if inter-individual differences such as high levels of anxiety and depression interact with valence of the stimuli (see discussions of these data in Cho [82]). For present purposes, these data are unrelated to the focus of the current project and have no bearing on the data here under investigation. Hence, they will not be discussed any further. For further information regarding inter-individual measures and the valence of the stimuli, see Cho [82].

found with arcsine transformations of the proportion data, $t\ (44) = 9.35$, $p < 0.0001$.

If subjects experienced multiple stimulus-elicited thoughts during a trial, they then self-reported this by pressing the appropriate button each time that they had such a thought. The mean number of RIT effects per 6s trial (that is, the RIT rate per trial) was 2.13 (*SD* = 3.03; *SE* = 0.45), with a range of 0.37 to 19.66. Whether an object appeared on the left of the screen or on the right of the screen did not affect this rate, $t\ (44) = 0.07$, $p = 0.95$, nor the likelihood of there being any RIT effect, $t\ (44) = 1.12$, $p = 0.27$.

3.1. *Replication*

We replicated our primary findings in a different sample from the same population (San Francisco State University students, $n = 47$). The procedures in this experiment were identical to those of the previous experiment, except that the number of stimuli was 72 instead of 76 and that the size of the stimuli was a bit larger: The array of stimuli, which was composed of both visual objects, was presented on the screen with a subtended visual angle of $34.32^{\circ} \times 11.75^{\circ}$ (21 cm × 7 cm). Each object occupied the visual angle of 16.37° (9.78 cm × 9.78 cm). The proportion of trials on which subjects had at least one involuntary subvocalization was 0.91 (*SD* = 0.16; *SE* = 0.02), a proportion that was significantly different from zero, $t\ (46) = 38.56$, $p < 0.0001$. The RIT effect occurred for both objects on a proportion of 0.63 (*SD* = 0.27; *SE* = 0.04), which was significantly different from zero, $t\ (46) = 15.61$, $p < 0.0001$. If subjects experienced multiple RIT effects during a trial, they then self-reported this by pressing the appropriate button each time that they had such a thought. The mean number of RIT effects per 6 s trial (that is, the RIT rate per trial) was 4.67 (*SD* = 4.22; *SE* = 0.62), with a range of 0.36 to 19.63.

4. Discussion

Can an RIT with more than one (non-focal) stimulus elicit a sequence of involuntary, high-level thoughts? The present data suggest that the answer to this question is yes. An RIT effect (involuntary subvocalization) occurred for both objects on 35% of the trials, which is comparable to what was found in Merrick et al. [29], the only other RIT study in which two thoughts were triggered by external stimuli. The data are noteworthy because this is one of the first demonstrations of more than one thought being triggered through external control. The mean number of RIT effects per 6 s trial was 2.13, with a range of 0.37 to 19.66. These findings were replicated in an experiment having a different sample of subjects. Together, the data suggest that the mechanisms giving rise to involuntary subvocalization can be employed more than once within a short span.

The present experiment is the first RIT study in which more than one stimulus was presented simultaneously to the subject and in which the subject was not directly focusing visually on any of the critical stimuli. The RIT effect survived in such a (relatively) more complicated context, in which the perceptual scene contained more than one object and in which the subject was instructed to not look directly at any of the objects, which is unlike what occurred in previous RITs. On 78% of the 38 trials, subjects had at least one involuntary subvocalization. This percentage is comparable to the proportions found in previous studies, which involved the presentation of only one stimulus at a time (e.g., 86% in Allen et al. [23]; 87% in Cho et al. [28]; and 73% in Merrick et al. [29]). Moreover, the mean latency (~2.5 s) of the first RIT effect per trial was comparable to that found in previous studies (e.g., M = 1,451.27 ms [SD = 611.42] in Allen et al. [23]; M = 2,323.91 ms [SD = 1,183.01] in Cho et al. [28]; M = 1,745.97 ms [SD = 620.86] in Merrick et al. [29]). The data also revealed that the likelihood of an effect seemed not to be influenced by whether an object was presented on the left of the screen or on the right of the screen. In short, our replication of both the latency data and the data regarding the likelihood of an RIT effect provides additional evidence that, even in contexts more complex than those of previous studies, the RIT is a robust and reliable phenomenon.

In line with our theoretical views, N. E. Miller [15] proposes that conscious content is more constrained than appears to be the case and that, under the right conditions, content activation can resemble reflexive, stimulus-to-response mappings. As noted above, elicitations of conscious content can be easier to control and predict than overt action [22]. From this point of view, the unpredictability of conscious contents in everyday life reflects, not the lack of external control, but rather the vagaries of quotidian stimulus scenes. As observed in our experiment, even multiple thoughts can be controlled externally in ways that are systematic and nontrivial. Regarding such constraint, it has been posited that conscious contents should be construed as highly constrained outputs of the nervous system [84]. These outputs are the result of "multiple constraint satisfaction" [5]. In our paradigm, the activation of conscious contents depended on a combination of both set and stimulus conditions. Regarding that which enters consciousness, these two factors could be deemed to be *determinant*, at least in our experimental arrangement. In this way, the RIT effect in our study builds on the important research by Gollwitzer [26] on "implementation intentions" (in which sets lead to automatic, stimulus-triggered behavioral dispositions) by demonstrating that, once certain sets are induced, responses to environmental stimuli can resemble reflex-like processes, even when the responses depend on sophisticated, unconscious mechanisms. Future investigations using the present variant of the RIT may examine the neural correlates of the various events involved during each trial (e.g., induction and maintenance of the task-related action sets and the entry into consciousness of the involuntary subvocalization).

4.1. The nature of the RIT effect

The RIT effect is a rich phenomenon that can be mined experimentally in many ways. We will not pretend to understand all aspects of what occurs in this effect, an effect that involves the involuntary entry into consciousness of high-level contents (see discussion in Allen et al. [23]). At the present stage of understanding, one can conclude the following. First, it seems that, for the involuntary effect to arise, the relevant action set must be activated. This activation stems from the instructions provided by the experimenter [23]. Without such an activation of set, it is unlikely that subjects would experience the phonological representations of the names of the objects that happen to be perceived visually. From at least the beginning of the trial until the onset of the visual object, the action set is then held in memory. During this time, the action set held in mind can be regarded as a case of *imageless thought*. This is because the action set influences behavioral dispositions without being maintained explicitly in consciousness [85] (see recent, relevant research in Scullin et al. [86]) (imageless thought was investigated first by theorists of the Würzburg School of Psychology [87]). During the trial, the final phenomenon of interest occurs when the appearance of a visual object begins the stages of processing that, somehow, leads to the consciousness of the involuntary imagery (e.g., subvocalization of the object name).

4.2. *Implications for theory*

The RIT effect corroborates what can be observed in everyday life—that conscious contents, including high-level, sophisticated contents, often "just happen". In the task, the generation of high-level conscious contents (e.g., subvocalizations) are generated involuntarily. This conclusion is consistent with passive frame theory [10]. In the theory, the mechanisms generating conscious contents are themselves unconscious, and so are the mechanisms responding to the contents (which are mechanisms that are distinct from the systems that generate conscious contents). In short, in a form of "unidirectional communication", conscious contents (e.g., a red apple and an urge) are "sampled" only by action systems, which are themselves unconscious. In the theoretical framework, one conscious content does not, in a sense, "know" of (a) the nature of other conscious contents in the conscious field nor of (b) the nature of ongoing behavior and whether or not the content is relevant to ongoing behavior. It has been proposed that this form of "built-in ignorance" on the part of the cognitive apparatus is actually adaptive (see [88,89]).

4.3. *Limitations of the present approach*

In these kinds of experiments about the occurrence of conscious thought, it is difficult to avoid the technique of self-report. As mentioned above, this technique has well-known limitations. For example, self-reports can be inaccurate as a result of subjects basing their reports on a strategy of how to comport oneself during an experiment (see discussion in Morsella et al. [34]). In addition, inaccurate memories of fleeting conscious contents can lead to incorrect self-reports [33]. Given the robustness and reliability of the RIT phenomenon and the aforementioned data from the RIT including the rhyming task [40], we do not believe that these well known limitations undermine the validity of the present findings.

4.4. *Concluding comments*

While keeping the shortcomings of the RIT in mind, it is important to reiterate that the RIT is the kind of paradigm that, because it builds incrementally on a robust phenomenon, has of recent been encouraged by leading researchers in the field (e.g., [74,75]).

The component processes of the RIT are of interest in disparate subfields of the study of mind and brain, including consciousness, attention, decision making, cognitive control, imagery, psychopathology and action control. Because much is known about the neural correlates of many of the component processes underlying the RIT effect, the paradigm is a rich and fecund experimental approach for hypothesis-testing investigations in the field of neuroscience. The paradigm is also perfectly suited for scanner-based neuroimaging research, because it involves a simple procedure for presenting stimuli, and because the dependent measure does not require complicated movements on the part of the subject. More generally, the RIT reveals that the generation of conscious contents, one of the greatest mysteries in science [3,76,77], can be studied experimentally.

Acknowledgment

This research was supported by the Center for Human Culture and Behavior at San Francisco

State University.

Supplementary table

Table 1. List of visual objects (line drawings).

Ambulance	Knife
Angel	Lightning
Axe	Lion
Ball	Lips
Balloon	Mosquito
Bed	Motorcycle
Bicycle	Necklace
Bird	Noose
Bomb	Paintbrush
Bullet	Pumpkin
Butterfly	Rabbit
Cake	Rainbow
Candy	Ring
Cannon	Snowflake
Cigarette	Snowman
Claws	Star
Cockroach	Sun
Coffin	Swan
Crown	Swing
Devil	Top
Dog	Tree
Dynamite	Trophy
Fire	Wagon
Fireworks	Waterfall
Flower	World
Fly	Poison
Gravestones	Razor
Grenade	Robber
Guillotine	Scorpion
Guitar	Shark
Gun	Snake
Heart	Spider
House	Tank
Jail	Thorn
Jaws	Tiger
Jewel	Tornado
Kite	Volcano
Kitten	Wasp

References

1. Di Lollo V, Enns JT, Rensink RA (2000) Competition for consciousness among visual events: The psychophysics of reentrant visual pathways. *J Exp Psychol Gen* 129: 481–507.
2. Mathewson KE, Gratton G, Fabiani M, et al. (2009) To see or not to see: Prestimulus alpha phase predicts visual awareness. *J Neurosci* 29: 2725–2732.
3. Crick F, Koch C (2003) A framework for consciousness. *Nat Neurosci* 6: 119–126.
4. Most SB, Scholl BJ, Clifford ER, et al. (2005) What you see is what you set: Sustained inattentional blindness and the capture of awareness. *Psychol Rev* 112: 217–242.
5. Merker B (2007) Consciousness without a cerebral cortex: A challenge for neuroscience and medicine. *Behav Brain Sci* 30: 63–134.
6. Freeman WJ (2006) William James on consciousness, revisited. *Chaos Complexity Lett* 1: 17–42.
7. Köhler W (1948) Gestalt psychology: An introduction to new concepts in modern psychology. *Q Rev Biol.*
8. Searle JR (2000) Consciousness. *Annu Rev Neurosci* 23: 557–578.
9. Gazzaley A, D'Esposito M (2007) Unifying prefrontal cortex function: Executive control, neural networks and top-down modulation, In: Miller B, Cummings J (Ed.), *The human frontal lobes: Functions and disorders,* New York: Guilford Press, 187–206.
10. Ezequiel M, Godwin CA, Jantz TK, et al. (2015) Homing in on consciousness in the nervous system: An action-based synthesis. *Behav Brain Sci* 39: 1–17.
11. Ach N (1905/1951) Determining tendencies: Awareness, In: Rapaport D (Ed.), *Organization and pathology of thought*, New York: Columbia University Press, 15–38.
12. Freud S, Brill AA (1938) The basic writings of Sigmund Freud. New York: Modern Library.
13. Helmholtz Hv (1856/1925) Treatise of physiological optics: Concerning the perceptions in general, In: T. Shipley (Ed.), *Classics in psychology,* New York: Philosophy Library, 79–127.
14. James W (1950) The principles of psychology. *Am J Psychol* 2: 761.
15. Miller NE (1959) Liberalization of basic S-R concepts: Extensions to conflict behavior, motivation, and social learning, In: Koch S (Ed.), *Psychology: A study of a science, Vol. 2*, New York: McGraw-Hill, 196–292.
16. Wegner DM (1990) White bears and other unwanted thoughts. *Suppr Obsession Psychol Mental Control.*
17. Lashley KS (1956) Cerebral organization and behavior, In: *Proceedings of the association for research in nervouse and mental diseases,* 36: 1–18.
18. Miller GA (1962) Psychology: The science of mental life. *Pelican Books.*
19. Fodor JA (1983) Modularity of mind: An essay on faculty psychology. Cambridge, MA: The MIT press.
20. Morsella E (2005) The function of phenomenal states: Supramodular interaction theory. *Psychol Rev* 112: 1000–1021.
21. Ohman A, Mineka S (2001) Fears, phobias, and preparedness: Toward an evolved module of fear and fear learning. *Psychol Rev* 108: 483–522.
22. Bargh JA, Morsella E (2008) The unconscious mind. *Perspect Psychol Sci* 3: 73–79.
23. Allen AK, Wilkins K, Gazzaley A, et al. (2013) Conscious thoughts from reflex-like processes: A new experimental paradigm for consciousness research. *Conscious Cognition* 22: 1318–1331.

24. Bhangal S, Cho H, Geisler MW, et al. (2016) The prospective nature of voluntary action: Insights from the reflexive imagery task. *Rev Gen Psychol* 20: 101–117.
25. Stroop JR (1935) Studies of interference in serial verbal reactions. *J Exp Psychol Gen* 121: 15–23.
26. Gollwitzer PM (1999) Implementation intentions: Strong effects of simple plans. *Am Psychol* 54: 493–503.
27. Snodgrass JG, Vanderwart M (1980) A standardized set of 260 pictures: Norms for name agreement, image agreement, familiarity, and visual complexity. *J Exp Psychol Hum Learn Mem* 6: 174–215.
28. Cho H, Godwin CA, Geisler MW, et al. (2014) Internally generated conscious contents: Interactions between sustained mental imagery and involuntary subvocalizations. *Front Psychol* 5: 1445.
29. Merrick C, Farnia M, Jantz TK, et al. (2015) External control of the stream of consciousness: Stimulus-based effects on involuntary thought sequences. *Conscious Cognition* 33: 217–225.
30. Levelt WJM (1989) Speaking: From intention to articulation. Cambridge, MA: The MIT Press.
31. Cho H, Zarolia P, Gazzaley A, et al. (2016) Involuntary symbol manipulation (Pig Latin) from external control: Implications for thought suppression. *Acta Psychol* 166: 37–41.
32. Miller BL, Cummings JL (2007) The human frontal lobes: Functions and disorders, second edition. New York: Guilford Press.
33. Block N (2007) Consciousness, accessibility, and the mesh between psychology and neuroscience. *Behav Brain Sci* 30: 481–548.
34. Morsella E, Wilson LE, Berger CC, et al. (2009) Subjective aspects of cognitive control at different stages of processing. *Atten Percept Psychophysics* 71: 1807–1824.
35. Mason MF, Norton MI, Horn JDV, et al. (2007) Wandering minds: The default network and stimulus-independent thought. *Science* 315: 393–345.
36. Mcvay JC, Kane MJ (2010) Does mind wandering reflect executive function or executive failure? Comment on Smallwood and Schooler (2006) and Watkins (2008). *Psycho Bull* 136: 198–207.
37. Mitchell JP, Heatherton TF, Kelley WM, et al. (2010) Separating sustained from transient aspects of cognitive control during thought suppression. *Psychol Sci* 18: 292–297.
38. Pasley BN, David SV, Mesgarani N, et al. (2012) Reconstructing speech from human auditory cortex. *PLoS Biol* 10: e1001251.
39. Wyland CL, Kelley WM, Macrae CN, et al. (2003) Neural correlates of thought suppression. *Neuropsychologia* 41: 1863–1867.
40. Cushing D, Morsella E (2016) The polymodal role of consciousness in adaptive action selection: A paradigm for neuroimaging, In: Poster presented at the Annual Convention of the Society for Cognitive Neuroscience, New York.
41. Wegner DM (1994) Ironic processes of thought control. *Psychol Rev* 101: 34–52.
42. Bhangal S, Merrick C, Morsella E (2015) Ironic effects as reflexive responses: Evidence from word frequency effects on involuntary subvocalizations. *Acta Psychol* 159: 33–40.
43. Bhangal S, Allen AK, Geisler MW, et al. (2016) Conscious contents as reflexive processes: Evidence from the habituation of high-level cognitions. *Conscious Cognition* 41: 177–188.
44. Merrick C, Cho H, Morsella E (2014) The reflexive imagery task: Unintentional imagery despite extensive training and voluntary set selection. Unpublished Manuscript, San Francisco State University.

45. Allen AK, Krisst L, Montemayor C, et al. (2016) Entry of involuntary conscious contents from ambiguous images. *Psychol Conscious Theory Res Pract* 3: 326–337.
46. Rassin E (2005) Thought suppression. Amsterdam, Netherlands: Elsevier.
47. Miller EK (2000) The prefrontal cortex and cognitive control. *Nat Rev Neurosci* 1: 59–65.
48. Munakata Y, Herd SA, Chatham CH, et al. (2011) A unified framework for inhibitory control. *Trends Cognit Sci* 15: 453–459.
49. Anderson MC, Ochsner KN, Kuhl B, et al. (2004) Neural systems underlying the suppression of unwanted memories. *Science* 303: 232–235.
50. Giuliano RJ, Wicha NY (2010) Why the white bear is still there: Electrophysiological evidence for ironic semantic activation during thought suppression. *Brain Res* 1316: 62–74.
51. Gazzaley A, Nobre AC (2011) Top-down modulation: Bridging selective attention and working memory. *Trends Cognit Sci* 16: 129–135.
52. Cohen JD, Dunbar K, McClelland JL (1990) On the control of automatic processes: A parallel distributed processing account of the Stroop effect. *Psychol Rev* 97: 332–361.
53. Brown JW, Braver TS (2005) Learned predictions of error likelihood in the anterior cingulate cortex. *Science* 307: 1118–1121.
54. Botvinick MM (2007) Conflict monitoring and decision making: Reconciling two perspectives on anterior cingulate function. *Cognit Affective Behav Neurosci* 7: 356–366.
55. Levy BJ, Anderson MC (2002) Inhibitory processes and the control of memory retrieval. *Trends Cognit Sci* 6: 299–305.
56. Levy BJ, Anderson MC (2008) Individual differences in the suppression of unwanted memories: The executive deficit hypothesis. *Acta Psychol* 127: 623–635.
57. Levy BJ, Anderson MC (2012) Purging of memories from conscious awareness tracked in the human brain. *J Neurosci* 32: 16785–16794.
58. Hickok G (2009) Eight problems for the mirror neuron theory of action understanding in monkeys and humans. *J Cognit Neurosci* 21: 1229–1243.
59. Schomers MR, Kirilina E, Weigand A, et al. (2015) Causal influence of articulatory motor cortex on comprehending single spoken words: TMS evidence. *Cereb Cortex* 25: 3894–3902.
60. Buchsbaum BR (2013) The role of consciousness in the phonological loop: Hidden in plain sight. *Front Psychol* 4: 496.
61. Buchsbaum BR, D'Esposito M (2008) The search for the phonological store: From loop to convolution. *J Cognit Neurosci* 20: 762–778.
62. Dewitt I, Rauschecker JP (2012) Phoneme and word recognitionin the auditory ventral stream. *Proc Nat Acad Sci U S A* 109: 505–514.
63. Eggert GH, Wernicke C (1874/1977) Wernicke's works on aphasia: A sourcebook and review. Hague, Netherlands: Mouton.
64. Gazzaniga MS, Ivry RB, Mangun GR (2009) Cognitive neuroscience: The biology of the mind, 3rd edition. New York: W. W. Norton & Company, Inc.
65. Peramunage D, Blumstein SE, Myers EB, et al. (2011) Phonological neighborhood effects in spoken word production: An fMRI study. *J Cognit Neurosci* 23: 593–603.
66. Scott M (2013) Corollary discharge provides the sensory content of inner speech. *Psychol Sci* 24: 1824–1830.

67. Ford JM, Gray M, Faustman WO, et al. (2005) Reduced gamma-band coherence to distorted feedback during speech when what you say is not what you hear. *Int J Psychophysiology* 57: 143–150.
68. Mahon BZ, Caramazza A (2008) A critical look at the embodied cognition hypothesis and a new proposal for grounding conceptual content. *J Physiol Paris* 102: 59–70.
69. Gruber O, Gruber E, Falkai P (2005) Neural correlates of working memory deficits in schizophrenic patients. Ways to establish neurocognitive endophenotypes of psychiatric disorders. *Radiologe* 45: 153–160.
70. Müller NG, Knight RT (2006) The functional neuroanatomy of working memory: Contributions of human brain lesion studies. *Neurosci* 139: 51–58.
71. Sato M, Baciu M, Loevenbruck H, et al. (2004) Multistable representation of speech forms: A functional MRI study of verbal transformations. *NeuroImage* 23: 1143–1151.
72. Vallar G, Corno M, Basso A (1992) Auditory and visual verbal short-term memory in aphasia. *Cortex* 28: 383–389.
73. Pugh SR, Morsella E, Geisler MW (2014) Involuntary cognitions of positive and negative images: Behavioral consequences and EEG correlates. Poster presented at the Graduate Student Showcase at San Francisco State University, San Francisco.
74. Fiedler K (2017) What constitutes strong psychological science? The (neglected) role of diagnosticity and a priori theorizing. *Perspect Psychol Sci* 12: 46–61.
75. Nosek BA, Spies JR, Motyl M (2012) Scientific utopia II: Restructuring incentives and practices to promote truth over publishability. *Perspect Psychol Sci* 7: 615–631.
76. Dehaene S (2014) Consciousness and the brain: Deciphering how the brain codes our thoughts. New York: Viking.
77. Koch C, Massimini M, Boly M, et al. (2016) Neural correlates of consciousness: Progress and problems. *Nat Rev Neurosci* 17: 307–321.
78. Cohen JD, Macwhinney B, Flatt M, et al. (1993) PsyScope: A new graphic interactive environment for designing psychology experiments. *Behav Res Methods Instrum Comput* 25: 257–271.
79. Morsella E, Miozzo M (2002) Evidence for a cascade model of lexical access in speech production. *J Exp Psychol Learn Mem Cognit* 28: 555–563.
80. Simon JR, Hinrichs JV, Craft JL (1970) Auditory S-R compatibility: Reaction time as a function of ear-hand correspondence and ear-response-location correspondence. *J Exp Psychol* 86: 97–102.
81. Spitzer RL, Kroenke K, Williams JBW, et al. (2006) A brief measure for assessing generalized anxiety disorder: The GAD-7. *Arch Intern Med* 166: 1092–1097
82. Cho H (2015) Cognitive bias in involuntary cognitions toward negative-valenced stimuli in highly anxious/depressive groups. Masters Thesis, San Francisco State University.
83. Bargh JA, Chartrand TL (2000) The mind in the middle: A practical guide to priming and automaticity research, In: Reis HT, Judd CM (Eds.), *Handbook of research methods in social and personality psychology,* Cambridge, England: Cambridge University Press, 253–285.
84. Wundt W (1902/1904) Principles of physiological psychology. Translated from the Fifth German Edition (1904) by Titchener EB, London: Swan Sonnenschein.
85. Woodworth RS (1915) A revision of imageless thought. *Psychol Rev* 22: 1–27.

86. Scullin MK, McDaniel MA, Einstein GO (2010) Control of cost in prospective memory: Evidence for spontaneous retrieval processes. *J Exp Psychol Learn Mem Cognit* 36: 190–203.
87. Schultz DP, Schultz SE (1996) A history of modern psychology, sixth edition. San Diego: Harbrace College Publishers.
88. Baumeister RF, Vohs KD, DeWall N, et al. (2007) How emotion shapes behavior: Feedback, anticipation, and reflection, rather than direct causation. *Pers Social Psychol Rev* 11: 167–203.
89. Firestone C, Scholl BJ (2016) Cognition does not affect perception: Evaluating the evidence for "top-down" effects. *Behav Brain Sci* 39: 1–77.

12

Classification of Spike Wave Propagations in a Cultured Neuronal Network: Investigating a Brain Communication Mechanism

Yoshi Nishitani [1,*], **Chie Hosokawa** [2], **Yuko Mizuno-Matsumoto** [3], **Tomomitsu Miyoshi** [4], **and Shinichi Tamura** [5]

[1] Dept. of Radiology, Graduate School of Medicine, Osaka University, Suita 565-0871, Japan;

[2] Biomedical Research Institute, AIST, Ikeda, Osaka 563-8577, Japan;

[3] Graduate School of Applied Informatics, University of Hyogo, Kobe 650-0044, Japan;

[4] Dept. of Integrative Physiology, Graduate School of Medicine, Osaka University, Suita 565-0871, Japan;

[5] NBL Technovator Co., Ltd., 631 Shindachimakino, Sennan 590-0522, Japan

* **Correspondence:** Email: ynishitani1027@gmail.com

Abstract: In brain information science, it is still unclear how multiple data can be stored and transmitted in ambiguously behaving neuronal networks. In the present study, we analyze the spatiotemporal propagation of spike trains in neuronal networks. Recently, spike propagation was observed functioning as a cluster of excitation waves (spike wave propagation) in cultured neuronal networks. We now assume that spike wave propagations are just events of communications in the brain. However, in reality, various spike wave propagations are generated in neuronal networks. Thus, there should be some mechanism to classify these spike wave propagations so that multiple communications in brain can be distinguished. To prove this assumption, we attempt to classify various spike wave propagations generated from different stimulated neurons using our original spatiotemporal pattern matching method for spike temporal patterns at each neuron in spike wave propagation in the cultured neuronal network. Based on the experimental results, it became clear that spike wave propagations have various temporal patterns from stimulated neurons. Therefore these stimulated neurons could be classified at several neurons away from the stimulated neurons. These are the *classifiable neurons*. Moreover, distribution of *classifiable neurons* in a network is also different when stimulated neurons generating spike wave propagations are different. These results suggest that distinct communications occur via multiple communication links and that *classifiable neurons* serve this function.

Keywords: cultured neuronal network; spike wave propagation; spatiotemporal form; classifying; multiple communications

---

1. Introduction

The brain is an intellectual information processing system [1–5]. How a neuronal network of ambiguously behaving neurons establishes a highly reliable information processing system, distinct communication, and organized communication links is an unanswered question. Despite many researchers attempting to solve this question, it remains a mystery.

In previous studies, factors such as spatiotemporal coding, the Synfire chain, and the spatiotemporal form of spike activity were considered the fundamental generators of natural intelligence in the brain [6–11]. However, basic communication functions between neurons have not been elucidated in these studies. Therefore, the abovementioned question still remains unsolved.

Recently, we focused on distinct and different communication to investigate the previously mentioned question [12–15]. In previous work [16], spike propagation as a cluster of excitation waves, termed as spike wave propagation, was observed in cultured neuronal networks. However, in those experiments, it was only observed that various spike wave propagations were generated in neuronal networks. The details of these mechanisms were still unclear.

To investigate these mechanisms, we simulated a 9 × 9 2D mesh neural network consisting of an integrate-and-fire model without leak. Resulting from this method, multiplex communication is possible at a success rate of 99% [17]. This result suggested that distinction of the spike wave propagation spatiotemporal form was the clue to classifying multiple communications in the brain. Here, we assume spike wave propagations are just communication events in the brain and attempt to prove this assumption. However, physiological experiments, analysis, and discussions about these events have yet to be reported [17].

In this study, we attempt to classify various spike wave propagation from different stimulated neurons in cultured neuronal networks, as well as discuss the implications of these classifying results in a view of brain communication. The authors' research group is presently studying the functions of neuronal networks by combining experiments with cultured neuronal networks with artificial neural network simulations. This paper corresponds to previous work on the ability of remote receiving neurons to identify two transmitting neuron groups stimulated in a neuronal network, i.e., 2 to 1 communication [17]. These mechanisms may be the basis of higher cortical functions.

The aim of this study is to investigate the most essential question in our study: to identify what the spatiotemporal form of spike wave propagation suggests in view of communication in brain physiologically.

2. Methods

2.1. Cell cultures

Cell cultures of hippocampal neurons were dissected from Wistar rats on embryonic day 18. The procedure conformed to the protocols approved by the Institutional Animal Care and Use Committee of the National Institute of Advanced Industrial Science and Technology. Hippocampi were dissociated with 0.1% trypsin (Invitrogen; Tokyo, Japan) in Ca^{2+}- and Mg^{2+}-free phosphate-buffered saline at 37°C for 15 min. The dissociated neurons were planted at a density of 3.3 × 105 cells/mm^2 in polyethylentimine-coated microelectrode array (MEA) dishes (MED-P515A, Alpha MED Scientific; Kadoma, Japan) with 8 × 8 planar microelectrodes. The size and spacing of the electrodes were 50 × 50 μm^2 and 150 or 450 μm, respectively. To position the neuronal networks in the central area of each MEA dish, a cloning ring with an inner diameter of 7 mm was used. The ring was removed the following day. Neurons adhered to the substrate of the MEAs, covering all electrodes.

Neurons were maintained at 37°C in a humidified atmosphere of 5% CO_2 and cultured for 21–40 days in Dulbecco's modified Eagle's medium (Invitrogen), which contained 5% horse serum and 5% fetal calf serum with supplements of 100 U/ml penicillin, 100 μg/ml streptomycin, and 5 μg/ml insulin. Half of the culture medium was renewed twice per week. In this study, four cultured cell samples at 22–50 days in vitro were prepared and are referred to as Cultures 1, 2, 3, and 4. Figure 1 shows a micrograph of the cultured neurons in an MEA.

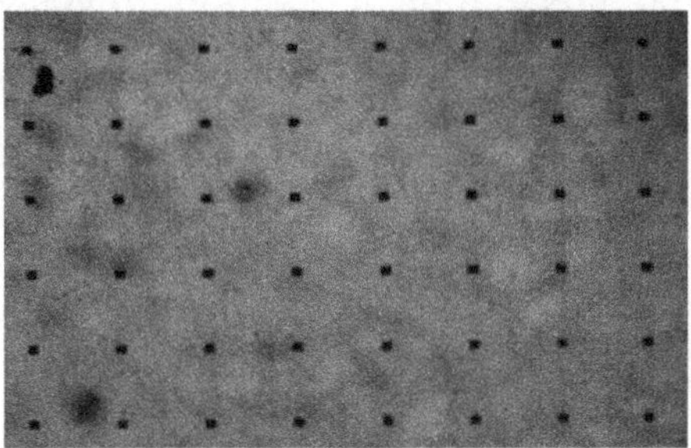

Figure 1. Micrograph of cultured neurons in an MEA (×20).

2.2. Stimulated spike recording

Stimulated spikes were recorded using MED64 (Alpha MED Scientific; Osaka Japan), an extracellular recording system with 64 electrodes (channels). The size of each electrode is approximately the size of a neuron. The recording was performed for 3 s at a sampling rate of 20 kHz.

A selected channel was stimulated at 5 ms after the start of the recording. The stimulation signal was a current-controlled bipolar pulse (positive, then negative) with a strength of 10 uA and a duration of 100 us.

Two to three channels in each culture were selected as the stimulation channels, and they were subjected to 10–15 recordings. In this study, the stimulated channels are referred to as StimA, StimB, and StimC. Incidentally, this study investigates whether the original stimulated channels (StimA, B, or C) can be identified from spike train at each channel (including multi-neurons), rather than by single neurons. Therefore, spike sorting was not performed.

2.3. Coding spike trains

The recorded spike trains were coded as follows: first, raster plots were generated by detecting peaks above a pre-specified threshold on each channel in the recorded spike responses [18]. Then, spike interval trains were calculated from the raster plot data.

2.4. Classifying procedure

Previously [16], effort was made to analyze the differences in the spike spatiotemporal pattern corresponding to the stimulated neuron using the dynamic time warping (DTW) method. This method uses a dynamic programming technique to find the minimum distance by stretching or shrinking the linearly or non-linearly warped time series and is thus useful for finding the optimal alignment between two non-uniform time series [19]. However, the DTW method does not offer an adequate resolution [20]. Therefore, the qualities of the analysis results were not enough to clarify whether multiple spike waves are classifiable.

The brain must have some physiological learning mechanism for classifying spike wave propagations with various temporal patterns. Considering previous experimental results, we used an analytical method with a learning algorithm instead of DTW. In the field of machine learning, back propagation, deep learning, etc. are well known. Though these methods, which imitate the behavior of physiological neuronal networks, are very effective for classifying various and complex data, the learning algorithm seems to be better suited for arranging physiological behavior to fit machine learning. Therefore, in this study, we use a simpler learning algorithm based on the arithmetical average method, which seems to have more compatibility with natural recognition (See Supplementary S-1).

The outline of classifying procedure is as follows.

Repeat for each 64 channel on MED64

(1) Spike train is learned by 5–10 spike temporal patterns with the same stimulated neuron (called neuron *A* temporarily). This spike train form is termed *Learning pattern A*.

(2) *Learning pattern B* (stimulated neuron is neuron *B*) are created by the same method as *Learning pattern A*.

(3) To find *classifiable neurons*, the resemblance of spike train (before learning) on trial (named *Trial Data*) and *learning pattern A or B* was estimated by the procedure described in Supplementary S-2.

3. Results

**To explain the detection method of classifiable neurons, the results of Cultures 1 and 2 are in described in detail.*

3.1. Culture 1

In Culture 1, 15 spike responses were recorded when channel 4 was stimulated. Five spike responses from the 15 were used for *Trial Data* named *Tr401, Tr402, . . . Tr405*, while the other 10 spike responses were used for *Learning Pattern 4*. Next, five *Trial Data* named *Tr2801, Tr2802, . . . Tr2805*, and *Learning Pattern 28* (channel 28 is stimulated) were created by the same procedure as *Tr401-Tr405* and *Learning Pattern 4*.

Figure 2 shows the result of the resemblance test for *Tr2801*. In Fig. 2b, which focused on channel 16, the mean value of *SpsetTrial* was significantly greater than that of *SpsetLocal* (see Supplementary S-2), when the stimulated neuron of the trial was different than that in the learning pattern. No significant difference was observed when the stimulated neuron of *Trial Data* was the same as in learning pattern (Figure 2a). This result suggested that the stimulated neuron of these *Trial Data* was not neuron 4. In other words, these *Trial Data* can be extracted from *Leaning Pattern 4* and the stimulated neuron 28 can be classified successfully as a neuron on channel 16. Therefore, this neuron was a *classifiable neuron*. In this trial, there were 14 *classifiable neurons*. Table 1a shows the number of *classifiable neuron* in each trial in Culture 1.

3.2. Culture 2

In Culture 2, *Tr1301, Tr1302, . . . Tr1305, Learning Pattern 13, Tr3001, Tr3002, . . . Tr3005, Learning Pattern 30, Tr5401, Tr5402, . . . Tr5405*, and *Learning Pattern 54* (the stimulated neurons were channels 13, 30, and 54, respectively) were prepared for experiments and learning patterns were created by 5-spike responses. Figure 3 shows the estimation result of the comparison for *Tr1304*. Sixteen *classifiable neurons* were observed through comparison with *Learning Pattern 54* and 10 through comparison with *Learning Pattern 30*. Table 1b shows the number of *classifiable neurons* for each trial.

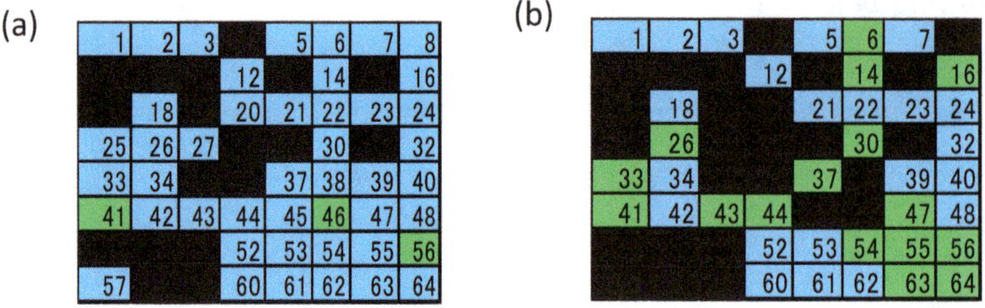

Figure 2. Estimation results of the comparisons for Tr2801. (a) Comparison with *Learning pattern 28* (b) Comparison with *Learning pattern 4*. Green cells indicate that the mean value of *SpsetTrial* was significantly greater than that of *SpsetLocal* (see Supplementary S-2). Blue cells indicate that *SpsetTrial* was not significantly greater than *SpsetLocal*. Gray cells indicate no spikes or that the number of spike was less than eight in the recording.

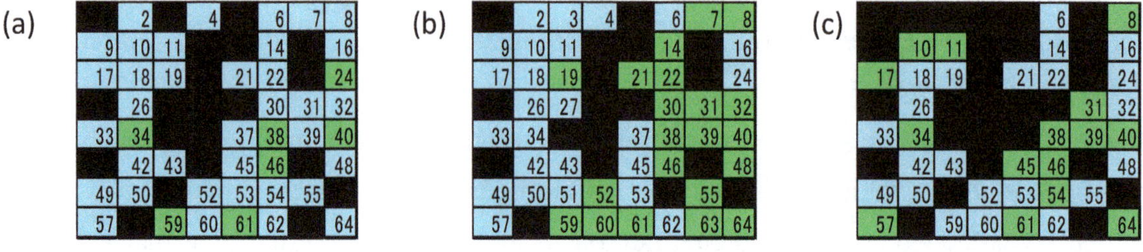

Figure 3. Estimation results of the comparisons for Tr1304. (a) Comparison with *Learning Pattern 13* (b) Comparison with *Learning Pattern 54* (c) Comparison with *Learning Pattern 30*. Green cells indicate the mean value of *SpsetTrial* was significantly greater than that of *SpsetLocal* (see Supplementary S-2). Blue cells indicate that *SpsetTrial* was not significantly greater than *SpsetLocal*. Gray cells indicate no spikes or that the number of spikes was less than eight in this recording.

3.3. Cultures 3 and 4

For Culture 3, channels 4 and 38 were stimulated. For Culture 4, channels 8, 10, and 57 were stimulated. The detection method of *classifiable neurons* in these cultures was similar to Culture 1 and 2. Therefore, in Culture 3 and 4, only the number of *classifiable neurons* for each *Trial Data* in Table 1c and 1d is shown.

3.4. Comparing with Spike Interval Shuffling data

As shown in Figure 2, Figure 3, and Table 1, *classifiable neurons* were observed in particular areas of neuronal networks. However, there was indication that these *classifiable neurons* were detected accidentally and purpose of the number of experiments performed was not to dispel this doubt. Therefore, we attempted to detect *classifiable neurons* from shuffled spike-interval sequence, called *Interval Shuffle* (*Int. Shuf*) [21], in parts of the trial data in Cultures 2 and 3.

The numbers of *classifiable neurons* from *Interval Shuffle* data were less than from original (non-*Interval Shuffle*) spike-interval data. In Culture 2, the difference between the two was significant ($p < 0.05$, as result of t-test). These results show that the detected *classifiable neurons* from the original spike data were not accidental.

Table 1. The number of *classifiable neurons* for each *Trial Data.*

a. Culture 1

Trial	Classification	
	vs ch 4 stim	vs ch 28 stim
Tr401	–	10
Tr402	–	9
Tr403	–	10
Tr404	–	17
Tr405	–	13
Tr2801	14	–
Tr2802	12	–
Tr2803	13	–
Tr2804	14	–
Tr2805	14	–

b. Culture 2

Trial	Classification		
	vs ch 13 stim	vs ch 54 stim	vs ch 30 stim
Tr1301	–	10	10
Tr1302	–	17	19
Tr1303	–	16	15
Tr1304	–	16	10
Tr1305	–	11	6
Tr5401	21	–	3
Tr5402	18	–	7
Tr5403	16	–	2
Tr5404	19	–	5
Tr5405	19	–	6
Tr3001	16	9	–
Tr3002	21	6	–
Tr3003	8	7	–
Tr3004	15	3	–
Tr3005	10	10	–

c. Culture 3

Trial	Classification	
	vs ch4 stim	vs ch 38 stim
Tr401	–	19
Tr402	–	25
Tr403	–	21
Tr404	–	24
Tr405	–	10
Tr3801	18	–
Tr3802	0	–
Tr3803	19	–
Tr3804	20	–
Tr3805	17	–

d. Culture 4

Trial	Classification		
	vs ch57 stim	vs ch08 stim	vs ch 10 stim
Tr5701	–	9	0
Tr5702	–	2	0
Tr5703	–	8	2
Tr0801	0	–	0
Tr0802	0	–	0
Tr0803	0	–	0
Tr1001	10	7	–

e. Culture 2 (*Int. Shuf*)

Trial	Classification		
	vs ch13 stim	vs ch54 stim	vs ch 30 stim
Tr1301	–	0	0
Tr1302	–	5	1
Tr1303	–	0	0
Tr1304	–	0	2
Tr1305	–	0	3
Tr5401	6	–	0
Tr5402	0	–	0
Tr5403	2	–	0
Tr5404	6	–	3
Tr5405	0	–	0

f. Culture 3(*Int. Shuf*)

Trial	Classification	
	vs ch4 stim	vs ch 38 stim
Tr401	–	3
Tr3805	0	–

4. Discussion

4.1. Discussion on the analysis results

Based on the experimental results, several *classifiable neurons* were observed in particular areas of neuronal networks. In detail, multiplexed spike wave propagation share several neurons and some may be used to classify different spike wave propagations. Accordingly, questions arose considering the distribution of *classifiable neurons*: do both *classifiable* and *non-classifiable neurons* exist in the same neuronal network?

The distribution of *classifiable neurons* is influenced by the distribution of synaptic weights in the neuronal network. It is well known that each neuron has an individually specific (intrinsic) synaptic weight and each neuron is considered *classifiable neuron* or not depending on conditions such as synaptic weights. In the physiological experiments, unlike the simulation experiments [17], it is difficult to determine weight distributions intentionally and only a limited number of realized weight distributions were observed. Therefore, distributions of *classifiable neurons* varied between different cultures.

In attempt to understand why *non-classifiable neurons* are intermingled with *classifiable neurons* are intermingled in the same neuronal network, three conditions of spike wave propagation scheme were presumed, as shown in Figure 4. For simplicity, it was assumed that all neurons were connected to neighboring neurons and spike waves spread radially from stimulated neurons. Due to the influence of the synaptic weight distribution in neuronal networks, each spike wave propagates with its own individual spatiotemporal pattern. Therefore, neurons sharing multiple spike wave propagations could be used to classify different spike wave propagations if a spike wave does not spread to neurons stimulated another spike wave each other (Figure 4 a1-2). However, if one spike wave spreads to neurons stimulated by another spike wave, as shown in Figure 4b, some neurons fire the same temporal patterns, even when a different neuron is stimulated. Results shown in Figure 2, Figure 3, and Table 1 suggest that this condition was realized in neuronal network used in these experiments.

Moreover, it was difficult to classify the stimulations of channel 54 and channel 30 in Culture 2, as fewer *classifiable neurons* were observed. The reason for this result was that spike waves spread to neurons that were stimulated by other spike waves, as shown in Figure 4c. Under this condition, some neurons fire the same temporal patterns, even when a different neuron is stimulated. Additionally, although we assume in this discussion that the spike waves spread in a simple radial direction, neurons are connected randomly in reality. Therefore, both *classifiable neurons* and *non-classifiable neurons* observed (Figures 2 and 3).

From Figures 3b and 3c, the distribution of *classifiable neurons* in *Learning Pattern 54* (stimulated neuron was ch54) was different from the distribution of *classifiable neurons* based on *Learning Pattern 30*. This phenomenon provides explanation for how spikes wave spread, as shown in Figure 4. If a pair of naturally stimulated neurons generate two different spike waves, the distribution of these spike waves and the overlap area are different, thus reflecting the distribution of *classifiable neurons*. Consequently, the spatial distribution of *classifiable neuron*s in the network varies when there are multiple targets for spike waves.

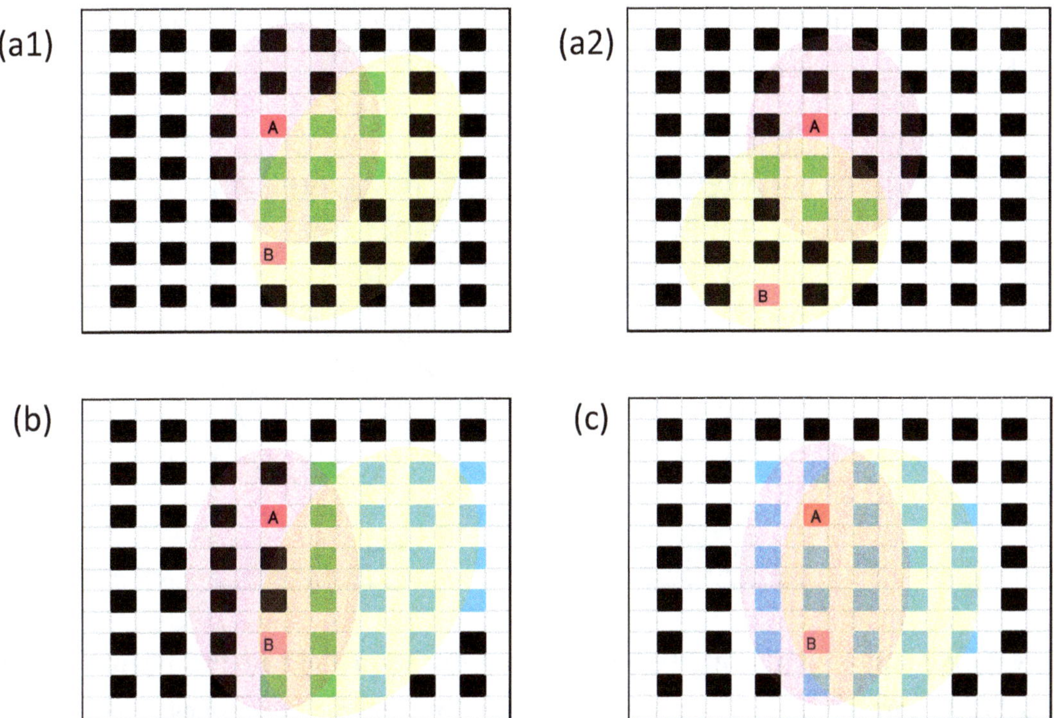

Figure 4 Condition of spike wave propagation scheme. (a1-a2) The spike wave generated from neuron A did not cover neuron B and spike wave generated from neuron B did not cover neuron A. In this condition, each spike wave was generated independently when neuron A or B was stimulated. Neurons overlapping both spike waves (green) generate different temporal patterns when the stimulated neuron was different Therefore, two stimulated neurons were classifiable in this area. If a pair of stimulated neurons generated two different spike waves, the distribution of these spike waves and the overlap area were different, thus reflecting the distribution of *classifiable neurons*. **(a2)** If the location of neuron B was different from **a1**, the spread and distribution of "green neurons," corresponding to the different overlapping areas. **(b)** Spike waves generated from neuron A covered neuron B; neuron B fired and spike wave were generated from neuron B. Under this condition, neurons indicated in blue fired in the same temporal pattern both when neuron A was stimulated and when neuron B was stimulated. Therefore, no difference was observed in the temporal pattern in this area. However, two stimulated neurons were classifiable (green). **(c)** Spike waves generated from neuron A covered neuron B and spike wave generated from neuron B covered neuron A. Both spike wave were generated from either stimulated neuron A or B. Hence, the temporal pattern was observed.

Furthermore, we investigated how multiplexed communication affects the processing of intellectual information in the brain. A simple multiplexed communication in the brain was modeled, as shown in Figure 5. The establishment of a virtual communication link from stimulated neurons to a particular area in the neuronal network was observed. Consequently, specific information was received in a particular area (Figure 5). We consider these processes as the fundamental mechanisms of intelligence in the brain. In fact, we hypothesize that the present model is valid not only for simple situations, but also for more complex similar situations.

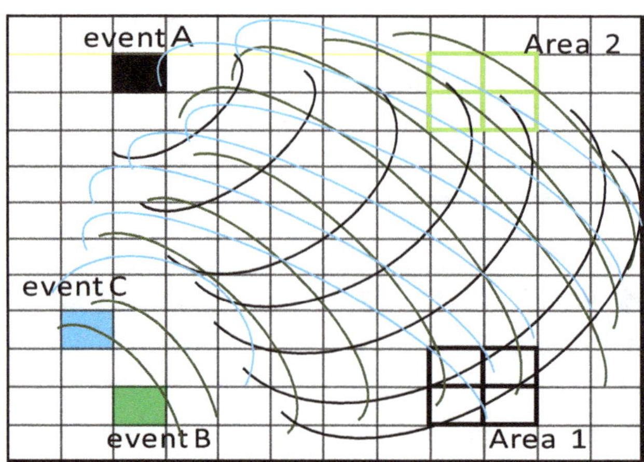

Figure 5. A sample of the multiplexed communication field in the brain. The figure shows events corresponding to stimulated neurons and spike wave propagations. In Area 1, event A was distinguishable from event C and in Area 2, event B was distinguishable from event C because *classifiable neurons* were concentrated in these areas. From a broad perspective, information for event A was receivable in Area 1 and information for event B was receivable in Area 2. Thus, two communication links from event A to Area 1 and from event B to Area 2 were extracted. In this case, event C was the comparison criterion of the spike spatiotemporal pattern of events A and B (if another event, such as event A or B, was the comparison criterion, the communication link for event C could also be extracted).

In contrast, for a few neurons, the mean value of *SpsetTrial* was greater than *SpsetLocal*. The mean value was significantly greater when both the trial pattern and the learning pattern were generated from the same stimulated neurons (Figures 2a and 3a). The results of these experiments suggest the possibility of the incorrect classification of some spike wave propagations. However, such neurons are fewer in number than *classifiable neurons* (when the stimulated neurons are different between the trial and the learning pattern). Therefore, the activities of such neurons may be masked by *classifiable neurons*. In brief, the trials successfully classified the entire neuronal network in a broad way and the experimental results reflect the distribution of synaptic weight in neuronal networks.

4.2. Function of classifiable neurons in the brain

The function of *classifiable neurons* was investigated in the brain. It was considered that *classifiable neurons* may participate in distinguishing different communications in the brain and that multiplexed spike wave propagations correspond to multiplexed communications in the brain. Some communications use the same neurons, as shown in Figure 4. In this case, the function of *classifiable neurons* was to classify multiple communications and recognize individual information. This function is similar to the multiplexed communication mechanism in artificial communication systems, such as mobile phones.

5. Conclusion

In this study, we classified various spike wave propagations individually generated from different stimulated neurons using an original spatiotemporal pattern matching the method of spikes in a cultured neuronal network. Based on the experimental results, *classifiable neurons* were observed in the neuronal network. We also confirmed that the spatial pattern of *classifiable neurons* within the neuronal network depended on stimulated neurons generating different spike wave propagations. These results suggest that distinct communications occur via multiple communication links in the brain and *classifiable neurons* play a significant role in this process.

Moreover, multiplexed communication scheme in the neuronal network were modeled in order to discuss the meaning of the multiplexed communication mechanism with regard to the management of intellectual information in the brain. The results of this study suggest that communication in the neuronal network is the basis of brain activity. This research provides a significant clue to solving one of the deepest mysteries of neuronal networks, namely, how seemingly ambiguous behavior among neurons leads to a reliable information processing system.

In this study, multiplexed communication is only modeled for one simple situation in a neuronal network. Because the comparable spatiotemporal patterns in the present analytical program are limited to two (events A vs B, A vs C, or B vs C), the resulting multiple analyzed spike spatiotemporal pattern includes only a pair of events (events A vs B, A vs C, or B vs C). Thus, the present multiplexed communication scheme is incomplete and further research is required to investigate situations with more than three events. Although the present scheme may be adequate for more complex situations as well, it is necessary to clarify these situations of multiple communications in the brain in future studies.

Lastly, the features of this paper are summarized as follows:

(1) To our current knowledge this study is the first attempt to investigate multiplex communication in a cultured neuronal network.

(2) Experiments and analysis correspond to a simulation experiment in 9×9 2D mesh neural network and sought to identify two transmitting neuron groups stimulated in a simulated

neuronal network, i.e., 2:1 communication [17].

(3) The results of this study show a signal transmission principle in neuronal networks which provides a possible solution to the mystery of the manner of reliable neuronal communication, which is thought to be the basis of brain activity.

Acknowledgements

The authors thank E. Ohnishi and M. Suzuki (AIST) for the cell cultures. This study was partly supported by the Grant-in-Aid for Scientific Research of Exploratory Research JP21656100, JP25630176, JP16K12524, and Scientific Research (A) JP22246054 of the Japan Society for the Promotion of Science. The authors would like to thank Enago (www.enago.jp) for the English language review.

References

1. Bonifazi P, Goldin M, Picardo MA, et al. (2009) GABAergic Hub Neurons Orchestrate Synchrony in Developing Hippocampal Networks. *Science* 326: 1419-1424.
2. Lecerf C (1998) The double loop as a model of a learning neural system. Proceedings World Multiconference on Systemics. *Cybernetics Informatics* 1: 587-594.
3. Choe Y (2003) Analogical Cascade: A Theory on the Role of the Thalamo-Cortical Loop in Brain Function. *Neurocomputing* 1: 52-54.
4. Tamura S, Mizuno-Matsumoto Y, Chen YW, et al. (2009) Association and abstraction on neural circuit loop and coding. *5th Int'l Conf. Intelligent Information Hiding and Multimedia Signal Processing (IIHMSP2009)* 10-07.546 (appears in IEEE Xplore).
5. Thorpre S, Fize D, Marlot C, et al. (1996) Speed of processing in the human visual system. *Nature* 381: 520-522.
6. Shadlen MN, Newsome WT (1998) The variable discharge of cortical neurons: implications for connectivity computation and information coding. *J Neurosci* 18: 3870-3896.
7. Olshausen BA, Field DJ (1996) Emergence of simple-cell receptive field properties by learning a sparse code for natural images. *Letters Nat* 381: 607-609.
8. Bell, Sejnowski T (1997) The independent components of natural scenes are edge filters. *Vision Res* 37: 3327-3338.
9. Klipera, Hornb D, Quene B (2005) The inertial-DNF model: spatiotemporal coding on two time scales. *Neurocomputing* 65-66: 543-548.
10. Takahashi K, Kim S, Coleman TP, et al. (2015) Large-scale spatiotemporal spike patterning consistent with wave propagation in motor cortex. *Nat Commu* 6: 7169. DOI:10.1038/ncomms8169. Available from: http://www.nature.com/ncomms/2015/150521/ncomms8169/full/ncomms8169.html

11. Aviel Y, Horn D, Abeles M (2004) Synfire waves in small balanced networks. *Neural Computation* 58-60: 123-127.
12. Nishitani Y, Hosokawa C, Mizuno-Matsumoto Y, et al. (2012) Detection of M-sequences from spike sequence in neuronal networks. *Comput Intell Neurosci.* Article ID, 862579: 1-9
13. Nishitani Y, Hosokawa C, Mizuno-Matsumoto Y, et al. (2014) Synchronized Code Sequences from Spike Trains in Cultured Neuronal Networks. *Int J Engineer Industries* 5: 13-24.
14. Tamura S, Nishitani Y, Kamimura T, et al. (2013) Multiplexed spatiotemporal communication model in artificial neural networks. *Auto Control Intell Systems* 1: 121-130. DOI: 10.11648/j.acis.20130106.11
15. Tamura S, Nishitani Y, Hosokawa C, et al. (2016) Simulation of code spectrum and code flow of cultured neuronal networks. *Compu Intell Neurosci* 7186092: 1-12.
16. Nishitani Y, Hosokawa C, Mizuno-Matsumoto Y, et al. (2016) Variance of spatiotemporal spiking patterns by different stimulated neurons in cultured neuronal networks. *Int J Acade Res Reflect* 4: 11-19.
17. Shinichi Tamura Yoshi Nishitani, Chie Hosokawa (2016) Feasibility of multiplex communication in 2D mesh asynchronous neural network with fluctuations. *AIMS Neurosci* 3: 385-397.
18. Wagenaar DA, Pine J, Potter SM (2004) Effective parameters for stimulation of dissociated cultures using multi-electrode arrays. *J Neurosci Method* 138: 27-37.
19. Muller M (2007) Dynamic Time Warping. In: Information Retrieval for Music and Motion, Springer.
20. Mei J, Liu M, Wang YF, et al. (2015) Learning a Mahalanobis Distance based Dynamic Time Warping Measure for Multivariate Time Series Classification. *IEEE_cybernetics* Available from: https://www.google.co.jp/?gws_rd=ssl#q=dtw+weakpoint
21. Rivlin-Etzion M, Ritov Y, Heimer G, et al. (2006) Local shuffling of spike trains boosts the accuracy of spike train spectral analysis. *J Neurophysiol* 95: 3245-3256.

13

Effects of glucocorticoids in depression: Role of astrocytes

Pranav Chintamani Joshi and Sugato Benerjee*

Department of Pharmaceutical Sciences and Technology, Birla Institute of Technology, Mesra, Ranchi, India

* **Correspondence:** Email: sbanerjee@bitmesra.ac.in;

Abstract: Astrocytes or astroglia are heterogeneous cells, similar to neurons, that have different properties in different brain regions. The implications of steroid hormones on glial cells and stress-related pathologies have been studied previously. Glucocorticoids (GCs) that are released in response to stress have been shown to be deleterious to neurons in various brain regions. Further, in the light of the effect of GCs on astrocytes, several reports have shown the crucial role of glia. Still, much remains to be done to understand the stress-astrocytes-glucocorticoid interactions associated with the pathological consequences of various CNS disorders. This review is an attempt to summarize the effects of GCs and stress on astrocytes and its implications in depression.

Keywords: anxiety; astrocytes; depression; glucocorticoids; stress

---

1. Introduction

Astrocytes or astroglia are highly heterogeneous glial cells that populate the brain and spinal cord, and are responsible for homeostasis of the central nervous system (CNS). Earlier, it was reported that, about 90% of the cortical tissue volume is made up of astrocytes, whereas the remaining 10% consists of neuronal cell bodies and blood vessels in the rat cerebral cortex [1]. However, the cellular composition of mammalian brain showed that astrocytes are only 20% of its glial cells; the majority (75%) are oligodendrocytes, while microglia amount to only 5% of glial cells in the grey matter [2]. Astrocytes, representing a large glial population in the mammalian brain [3], play a pivotal role in contributing to the brain metabolism [4] and are involved in glutamate clearance from the synapse and cycling of glutamine back into neurons (e.g. Glutamate-glutamine metabolism and transport) [5]. Astrocytes also release gliotransmitters such as glutamate and ATP [6], both onto neurons and other glial cells [6]. In contrast to chemical coupling at the synapse, astrocytes have extensive coupling via gap junctions, forming dynamic networks that passage molecules between astrocytes as well as to other cells in the CNS [7]. This passage includes interactions with the blood-brain barrier (BBB), mainly the vascular endothelial cells, as well as transporting metabolites to supply the energy needs of neurons [7,8].

The adrenal gland which secretes Glucocorticoids (GCs), in response to the signal from the hypothalamus, is responsible for producing a range of effects in response to stress. The release of GCs, a class of steroid hormones, is regulated by the hypothalamic-pituitary-adrenal (HPA) axis [9]. The HPA axis that belongs to neuroendocrine systems is commonly associated with stress signaling and the "fight-or-flight" response [10]. GCs act as potent transcriptional regulators that signal through two types of receptors: The high-affinity mineralocorticoid receptors (MRs) and the lower affinity glucocorticoid receptors (GRs) [11].

The MRs are associated with mechanisms involving lower GC concentrations, while the GRs respond to higher concentrations of GCs, such as levels associated with stressful experiences [12]. Alterations in the GC signaling are thought to contribute to disorders like Major Depression (MD) [13], Alzheimer's disease [14], and Cushing's syndrome [15], etc. A recent study on MD, showed that reduced levels of glial fibrillary acidic protein (GFAP) immunoreactive astrocytes [16] while the release of GCs in response to chronic stress leading to MD has been widely reported [17]. However, the role of stress hormones on astrocytic gene expression patterns, remain largely uncharacterized. Astrocytes are involved in primary biochemical processes and are one of the primary cell types in the brain [18]. An attempt is being made to explore the role of astrocytes in neuropsychiatric disorder like depression [19]. In this review, we primarily focus on the effects of the stress-induced GCs on the astrocytes and their implications in depression.

2. Astrocytes and depression

Initially, depression was viewed as a neuron-based disorder. This "neuron-centric" view of depression is at least partially supported by the known actions of commonly used antidepressants that modulate levels of the neurotransmitters in the brain (e.g. Serotonin by SSRIs) [20]. However, antidepressants target proteins expressed in multiple brain cell types (e.g. astrocytes express NMDA receptors and serotonin receptors [21]), thus distinct mechanisms and cells involved in antidepressant action remain largely unknown. A series of studies in the late 1990s and early 2000s made unexpected associations between depression and changes in cell density of specific cell types in the brain. Rajkowska and colleagues used cell counting approach to investigate how depression impacted cell density and morphology across various brain regions. Based on previous models, they suspected that depression would lead to cell death and decreased cell density in brain regions associated with mood disorders. They found that there were indeed decreases in cell density in areas such as the prefrontal cortex (PFC) [22] and hippocampus [23]. But, their findings were surprising regarding the cell type; the decreases in cell density were associated with morphologies consistent with both neurons and glial cells [24].

Psychiatric disorders like schizophrenia, bipolar disorder and MD involve reduced astrocytes and astroglial atrophy [25]. Postmortem studies of depressed patients showed reduced glial cell densities in the PFC, amygdala and hippocampus [24]. Banasr and Duman demonstrated that the depressive behavior can be induced by chemical astrocytes ablation in the PFC of rat [26]. Moreover, hippocampal astrocytic loss is associated with chronic stress [27] and also chronic stress interferes with glial cell metabolism via glutamatergic mechanisms [28]. It remains unclear as to how dysregulated GCs may be involved in the loss of astrocytes after stress.

These findings inspired biochemical studies that explored specific depression-linked decrease in astrocyte density based on reduced protein expression of GFAP (a biomarker for mature astrocytes). GFAP has shown its significant role in pathogenesis of various CNS pathologies [29]. The GFAP expression studies, showed a 15% loss of total astrocyte volume and decrease in expression in the brains of depressed individuals [24,30], while expression in patients increased after treatment with antidepressants. A different investigation on postmortem amygdale tissue from depressed patients showed reduction in nissl positive astrocytes [31]. Another astroglial marker, the calcium binding protein S100β was reported to be a marker of minor depression [32]. S100β was found to be reduced in the ventral PFC of depressed suicide victims (Figure 1A). The screening of 36 biological markers in 30 inbred mouse strains [33] showed that GFAP, S100β , glyoxalase 1 and histone deacetylase 5 responded to chronic treatment with fluoxetine. Similarly, reduction in the astroglial GFAP-positive cells and its overall immunoreactivity were detected in several animal models of chronic stress [24]. In situ hybridization and RT-qPCR gene expression studies with human brain samples allowed the detection and quantification of the mRNA present in brain sections and showed alterations in several transcripts for astrocyte proteins with depression in the locus coeruleus [24,34]. They include astrocytic markers like S100β, GFAP (Figure 1B), gap junction proteins (gap junction protein alpha 1 and 6 (Gja1 and Gja6)), and membrane channels proteins (Aquaporin-4 (AQP4)). It was also found that the reduction of glutamate transporter (GLT-1), glutamate aspartate transporter (GLAST), glutamine synthetase (GS), connexins (Cx43 and Cx30) [35,36] (Figure 1C). Similarly, the reports show a decrease in the mRNA expression of GLT-1, GLAST, and GS in the anterior cingulate and dorsolateral PFC [37], while some of these transcripts were reduced in other brain areas. This suggests that the astroglial cells may contribute towards altered neuroglial networks in different forms of depression.

In animal models, selective ablation of astroglial cells (L-a-aminoadipic acid, which envenoms astrocytes) triggered depressive behavior [24]. Pharmacological inhibition of astroglial gap junction connectivity [38] or astroglial plasmalemma glutamate transporters resulted in anhedonia [39] (Figure 1F), one of the key symptoms of depression. All these findings in animals subjected to depression models indicate astrocytic abnormality. After chronic exposure to chronic unpredictable stress (CUS), it was found an increase in glutamate release and reduced uptake in the hippocampus [40]. In the learned helplessness model, a similar trend of reduced glutamate uptake was also observed in the PFC, striatum and hippocampus [41]. Studies in rats also showed blockage of astroglial glutamate uptake and was sufficient to induce anhedonic state marked by decreased sucrose consumption [42]. Ketamine and riluzole, which acts as glutamate modulators, have shown antidepressant effects in patients and animal models [43].

Concurrent pathophysiology showed aberrant glutamatergic neurotransmission as a primary mechanism for major psychiatric disorders, including MD [44]. Astrocytes are fundamental elements in glutamatergic and GABAergic neurotransmission being the hubs for glutamate—glutamine and glutamine—GABA shuttles [45]. In the brains of MD patients, expression of astrocyte-specific glutamate transporters GLT-1, GLAST as well as glutamine synthase (GS) (Figure 1D, E) are reduced [24], indicating compromised astrocytic uptake of glutamate, as well as decreased glutamine production.

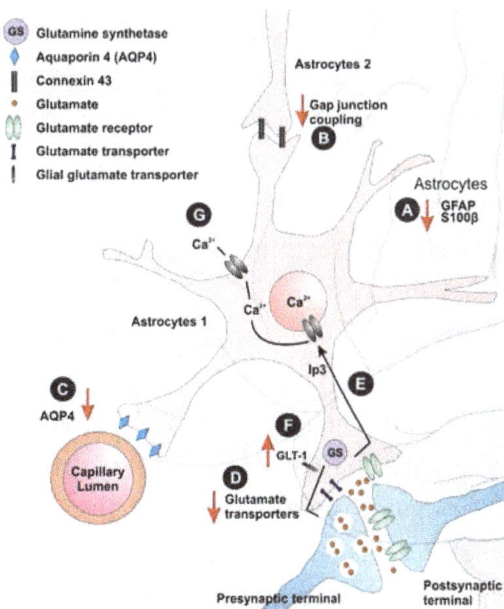

Figure 1. Astrocytic changes in the depressed brain. The crosstalk between the astrocytes and neurons is mediated at the tripartite synapse: A) Astrocyte marker GFAP and cytoplasmic protein S100β expression may alter with depression. B) Astrocyte-specific gap junction protein (Cx43) may alter during stress and depression. C) The water channel marker, AQP4 protein levels is found to reduce in depression. D and E) The expression of certain astrocyte glutamate transporters, as well as glutamine synthase may reduce in MD patients. F) There may be up-regulation of the hippocampal glial glutamate transporter (GLT-1) after chronic stress. G) Astrocytes may also coordinate their function through Ca^{2+} excitability and its downstream signaling in depression.

Interactions between glial and neuronal cells may be impaired at synaptic level in depression-like conditions. Purines may modulate glia-neuron communication bi-directionally, restoring the synaptic efficacy and reversing depression-like behavior [46]. Another possible trigger for depressive episodes was the cytokine signaling in astrocytes [47]. Recent research focused on an alternative form of neuro-glial signaling, namely, secreted extracellular vesicles (EVS) [48]. The EVS, such as ectosomes and exosomes, capable of carrying mRNA and microRNAs (miRNA) have shown a role in intercellular signaling, and may also underlie depressive behavior. The transfer of exosomes to neurons is mediated through oligodendrocytes, microglia and astrocytes, which may either support neurons or promulgate the disease [48]. Thus neuroglia communication at the synaptic level is far from clear and warrants further research.

The mechanism underlying antidepressants action of fluoxetin is mediated by regulating astrocytic AQP4 levels that affects astrocyte morphology and further restore the functional glia-vasculature interface [48]. The decreased astrocyte-specific Cx43 levels, as stated earlier, appear to be related to antidepressant and anxiolytic phenotypes [49]. In accordance, the antidepressants show an intricate pattern linking astrocytes and connexins to address the mechanisms of action of these compounds [50]. Thus the role of astrocytes in depression is far from clear and needs further work.

3. Mechanisms associating stress, GCs, and astrocytic functions

The postmortem studies on humans and animals showed reduction in astrocyte density and function in the limbic regions of the brain suggest probable mechanism contributing to pathology of stress and GCs overproduction [51]. Indeed, a selective volume reduction of hippocampus and PFC was observed following chronic stress [51]. The neuronal proliferation in the dentate gyrus (DG) [52] was decreased after corticosterone treatment and psychosocial stress while the postmortem studies in patients with a history of high-dose steroid treatment. However, there was no reduction in the number of neurons [53]. This suggests that the volume reduction cannot be entirely due to stress-induced reduction of neurogenesis. The increased GCs immunoreactivity was observed in astrocytes of amygdala in depressed patients compared to healthy controls or bipolar disorder patients [54], suggesting that astrocytes may respond to changes in stress hormone levels.

Studies on chronic stress may result in reduced gliogenesis in the hippocampus and PFC [23,28] while *in-vitro* studies showed the dexamethasone (a synthetic glucocorticoid) blocking astrogliogenesis from neural precursor cells. These findings suggest that, the perturbed astroglial cells in stress is likely to contribute in region-specific volume changes commonly observed in stress-related pathologies [55].

The role of astrocytes in neurodegenerative diseases and inflammatory processes is well documented [56]. It is well reported that human postmortem tissue in major depressive disorders (MDD) have shown alterations in the expression of mRNA and protein for astrocyte markers such as GFAP, Cx40, Cx43, AQP4, S100β and glutamatergic markers including GLT-1, GLAST, and GS [53]. When the brain gets injured, astrocytes become activated. This is characterized by changes in the gene expression profiles and high levels of GFAP [57]. In addition to this, exposure to corticosterone for short (6–24 h) and prolonged (3 weeks) period in astrocytic cultures show an increase in GFAP mRNA levels and a decrease when astrocytes were co-cultured with neurons [57]. This supports the findings that GCs may also regulate the synthesis of GFAP. Further, it also suggests the crosstalk between neuron and astrocytes to withstand deleterious effects of corticosterone. Initial *in-vivo* studies on rats have shown decreased hippocampal and cortical GFAP mRNA levels [58] while immunohistochemical studies have shown increased GFAP immunoreactivity in a dose and brain-region specific manner following chronic corticosterone treatment [59]. The complex nature of corticosteroids regulating GFAP during stress can be understood wherein 6 days of stressful activity leads to 30% increase in hippocampal GFAP-immunoreactive astrocytes [60] and at the same instance, the studies on adult rats exposed to early-life stress showed reduced density of GFAP-immunoreactive astrocytes in various limbic regions of brain [61]. This GFAP binary response may suggest a primary astrocyte-mediated neural protection, which may subsequently turn neurotoxic depending on the dose, which will affect the brain region as well as the time of exposure to stress.

Astrocytes express most of the receptors and additionally, ion channels found in neurons are involved in recycling and eliminating glutamate from synapses, thereby contributing to glutamatergic synaptic transmission [62]. The glial transporters help glutamate uptake and conversion to glutamine with the help of enzyme glutamine synthase (GS), which is responsive towards GCs [63]. A current hypothesis states that excessive extra synaptic glutamate leads to the atrophy of apical dendrites seen in hippocampal pyramidal neurons in stressed rats [64]. Studies aiming to understand the regulation of GS have shown glucocorticoid-mediated regulations of glial GS during stress [63]. Likewise, chronic stress showed up-regulation of the hippocampal glial glutamate transporter (GLT-1) (Figure 1F) [65]. This suggests that glutamate cycling is regulated by corticosteroids by induction of GS and GLT-1 expression in a time-dependent manner in distinct subpopulation of astrocytes. The hypothesis that GCs inhibit glucose uptake was substantially evidenced by a study in which it was shown that chronic mild stress exacerbates the consequences of chronic cerebral hypoperfusion [66]. This results in a lack of energy to neurons and astrocytes for high-affinity glutamate reuptake and thus an increase in vulnerability of the brain [67].

Astrocytes lie in proximity of BBB and play an important role in its maintenance by interacting with endothelial cells. On this regard, it would be important to emphasize that modulation of the barrier “tightness” is a result of complex interaction between GCs and cells of neurovascular units including astrocytes [68].

As stated earlier, S100β found primarily in the cytoplasm of astrocytes, and is involved in glia-neuron signaling [69]. The S100β regulates a variety of intra and extracellular functions such as cell growth, metabolism, calcium homeostasis and synaptic plasticity [69]. This suggests the possible role of astrocytes in regulating neuronal synaptic plasticity. Furthermore, reports suggest that S100β concentration was reduced after maternal administration of betamethasone (a synthetic glucocorticoid) in the hippocampus and serum of the neonate rat [70]. This suggests that increased GCs or chronic stress may reduce the expression or function of S100β. In an another study, stress exposure increased S100β concentration in cerebrospinal fluid (CSF) after acute predator stress [71] and chronic restraint stress [72]. These findings reveal the biphasic response of S100β to stress. This observation was also supported by another study where the astrocyte cultures were exposed to dexamethasone (Table 1)[73].

Table 1. Different markers that are expressed in Astrocytes in response to GCs stimuli.

Name of the marker	Function	References
Glial Fibrillary Acidic Protein (GFAP)	Cytoskeletal protein	[58]
S100β	astroglia-specific neurotrophic factor	[82,83]
Nerve growth factor (NGF)	Neurotrophic factor	[73]
Basic fibroblast growth factor (bFGF)	Neurotrophic factor	[73]
N-myc downstream- regulated Gene (Ndrg2)	Cell differentiation factor	[84]
Glutamine synthetase (GS)	Recycling of the glutamate	[37,53,63]
Glial glutamate transporter (GLT-1)	Recycling of the glutamate	[37,53,63]

Astrocytes may coordinate their function through Ca^{2+} excitability and subsequent signaling that have also been implicated in depressive disorders [74]. Surprisingly, astrocytic calcium signaling is regulated by GCs [75]. This apparently suggests the role of GCs in the modulation of glial calcium cell signaling during depression and anxiety. Additionally, the GCs are critical regulators of brain development and brain aging. Rat astrocyte primary culture study showed that dexamethasone increases intracellular and membrane-associated lipocortin-1 (annexin-1) [76] while it increased and reduced expression of nerve growth factor (NGF) in cultured neurons and astrocytes respectively [77].

Recent work focused on how the astrocytes intervene in the GC-induced stress and its probable mechanism. It has been shown that 5' AMP-activated protein kinase (AMPK) may mediate down regulation of GRs in astrocytes of rat PFC [78]. Also, GRs in astrocytes, as a critical stress-responding transcriptional factor, may mediate stress-induced adaptation via regulating the expression of astrocyte-derived neurotrophic factors. Researchers also found that the chronic mild stress-induced decrease in brain-derived neurotrophic factor (BDNF) and Cx43 causing astrocytic dysfunction by forming abnormality in gap junctions in the PFC of rats [79,80]. Some recent studies in emotional processing show astrocytes' crucial role, along with neurons, in the hippocampus, PFC, and amygdala [81]. Thus current astrobiology research suggests an evolving role of neuro-astroglial communication in the modulation of depression, opening new avenues of therapies against depressive disorders.

4. Conclusion

The studies over recent years have started unveiling the role of astrocytes in stress and their response to GCs release thus shifting our understanding from neuron-centric theories towards the role of these glial cells in the neurobiology of stress. However, the role of released GCs in response to stress and its effects on astrocytes need to be explored further in for a better understanding of stress- or glucocorticoid- related brain disorders.

Acknowledgement

The authors sincerely thank Mr. Michael Klug, Department of Mathematics, UC Berkeley, USA, for his diligent proof-reading of this manuscript.

References

1. Volterra A, Magistretti PJ, Haydon PG (2002) The tripartite synapse: Glia in synaptic transmission. New York: Oxford University Press.
2. Pelvig DP, Pakkenberg H, Stark AK, et al. (2008) Neocortical glial cell numbers in human brains. *Neurobiol Aging* 29: 1754–1762.
3. Ge WP, Jia JM (2016) Local production of astrocytes in the cerebral cortex. *Neuroscience* 323: 3–9.
4. Hertz L (2008) Bioenergetics of cerebral ischemia: A cellular perspective. *Neuropharmacology* 55: 289–309.
5. Bröer S, Brookes N (2001) Transfer of glutamine between astrocytes and neurons. *J Neurochem* 77: 705–719.
6. Halassa MM, Fellin T, Haydon PG (2007) The tripartite synapse: Roles for gliotransmission in health and disease. *Trends Mol Med* 13: 54–63.
7. Nualart-Marti A, Solsona C, Fields RD (2013) Gap junction communication in myelinating glia. *Biochim Biophys Acta* 1828: 69–78.
8. Cabezas R, Avila M, Gonzalez J, et al. (2014) Astrocytic modulation of blood brain barrier: Perspectives on Parkinson's disease. *Front Cell Neurosci* 8: 211.
9. Sapolsky RM, Romero LM, Munck AU (2000) How do glucocorticoids influence stress responses? Integrating permissive, suppressive, stimulatory, and preparative actions. *Endocr Rev* 21: 55–89.
10. Chrousos GP (2009) Stress and disorders of the stress system. *Nat Rev Endocrinol* 5: 374–381.
11. De Kloet ER, Van Acker SA, Sibug RM, et al. (2000) Brain mineralocorticoid receptors and centrally regulated functions. *Kidney Int* 57: 1329–1336.

12. Carter BS, Meng F, Thompson RC (2012) Glucocorticoid treatment of astrocytes results in temporally dynamic transcriptome regulation and astrocyte-enriched mRNA changes in vitro. *Physiol Genomics* 44: 1188–1200.
13. Mcewen BS (2005) Glucocorticoids, depression, and mood disorders: Structural remodeling in the brain. *Metabolism* 54: 20–23.
14. Green KN, Billings LM, Roozendaal B, et al. (2006) Glucocorticoids increase amyloid-beta and tau pathology in a mouse model of Alzheimer's disease. *J Neurosci* 26: 9047–9056.
15. Newell-Price J, Bertagna X, Grossman AB, et al. (2006) Cushing's syndrome. *Lancet* 367: 1605–1617.
16. Cobb J, O'Neill K, Milner J, et al. (2016) Density of GFAP-immunoreactive astrocytes is decreased in left hippocampi in major depressive disorder. *Neuroscience* 316: 209–220.
17. Vyas S, Rodrigues AJ, Silva JM, et al. (2016) Chronic stress and glucocorticoids: From neuronal plasticity to neurodegeneration. *Neural Plast* 2016: 6391686.
18. Volterra A, Meldolesi J (2005) Astrocytes, from brain glue to communication elements: The revolution continues. *Nat Rev Neurosci* 6: 626–640.
19. Koyama Y (2015) Functional alterations of astrocytes in mental disorders: Pharmacological significance as a drug target. *Front Cell Neurosci* 9: 261.
20. Carter BS (2013) Glucocorticoid regulation of the astrocyte transcriptome in vitro and in vivo. University of Michigan.
21. Conti F, Debiasi S, Minelli A, et al. (1996) Expression of NR1 and NR2A/B subunits of the NMDA receptor in cortical astrocytes. *Glia* 17: 254–258.
22. Rajkowska G, Miguel-Hidalgo JJ, Wei J, et al. (1999) Morphometric evidence for neuronal and glial prefrontal cell pathology in major depression. *Biol Psychiatry* 45: 1085–1098.
23. Stockmeier CA, Mahajan GJ, Konick LC, et al. (2004) Cellular changes in the postmortem hippocampus in major depression. *Biol Psychiatry* 56: 640–650.
24. Rajkowska G, Stockmeier CA (2013) Astrocyte pathology in major depressive disorder: Insights from human postmortem brain tissue. *Curr Drug Targets* 14: 1225–1236.
25. Verkhratsky A, Rodriguez JJ, Parpura V (2013) Astroglia in neurological diseases. *Future Neurol* 8: 149–158.
26. Banasr M, Duman RS (2008) Glial Loss in the prefrontal cortex is sufficient to induce depressive-like behaviors. *Biol Psychiatry* 64: 863–870.
27. Czeh B, Simon M, Schmelting B, et al. (2005) Astroglial plasticity in the hippocampus is affected by chronic psychosocial stress and concomitant fluoxetine treatment. *Neuropsychopharmacology* 31: 1616–1626.
28. Banasr M, Chowdhury GMI, Terwilliger R, et al. (2010) Glial pathology in an animal model of depression: Reversal of stress-induced cellular, metabolic and behavioral deficits by the glutamate-modulating drug riluzole. *Mol Psychiatry* 15: 501–511.
29. Messing A, Brenner M (2003) GFAP: Functional implications gleaned from studies of genetically engineered mice. *Glia* 43: 87–90.
30. Miguel-Hidalgo JJ, Baucom C, Dilley G, et al. (2000) Glial fibrillary acidic protein immunoreactivity in the prefrontal cortex distinguishes younger from older adults in major depressive disorder. *Biol Psychiatry* 48: 861–873.
31. Bowley MP, Drevets WC, Ongur D, et al. (2002) Low glial numbers in the amygdala in major depressive disorder. *Biol Psychiatry* 52: 404–412.

32. Polyakova M, Sander C, Arelin K, et al. (2015) First evidence for glial pathology in late life minor depression: S100B is increased in males with minor depression. *Front Cell Neurosci* 9: 406.
33. Benton CS, Miller BH, Skwerer S, et al. (2012) Evaluating genetic markers and neurobiochemical analytes for fluoxetine response using a panel of mouse inbred strains. *Psychopharmacology* 221: 297–315.
34. Chandley MJ, Szebeni K, Szebeni A, et al. (2013) Gene expression deficits in pontine locus coeruleus astrocytes in men with major depressive disorder. *J Psychiatry Neurosci* 38: 276–284.
35. Bernard R, Kerman IA, Thompson RC, et al. (2011) Altered expression of glutamate signaling, growth factor, and glia genes in the locus coeruleus of patients with major depression. *Mol Psychiatry* 16: 634–646.
36. Seifert G, Schilling K, Steinhäuser C (2006) Astrocyte dysfunction in neurological disorders: A molecular perspective. *Nat Rev Neurosci* 7: 194.
37. Choudary P, Molnar M, Evans S, et al. (2005) Altered cortical glutamatergic and GABAergic signal transmission with glial involvement in depression. *Proc Natl Acad Sci* 102: 15653–15658.
38. Sun JD, Liu Y, Yuan YH, et al. (2012) Gap junction dysfunction in the prefrontal cortex induces depressive-like behaviors in rats. *Neuropsychopharmacology* 37: 1305–1320.
39. Bechtholt-Gompf AJ, Walther HV, Adams MA, et al. (2010) Blockade of astrocytic glutamate uptake in rats induces signs of anhedonia and impaired spatial memory. *Neuropsychopharmacology* 35: 2049–2059.
40. de Vasconcellos-Bittencourt AP, Vendite DA, Nassif M, et al. (2011) Chronic stress and lithium treatments alter hippocampal glutamate uptake and release in the rat and potentiate necrotic cellular death after oxygen and glucose deprivation. *Neurochem Res* 36: 793–800.
41. Almeida RF, Thomazi AP, Godinho GF, et al. (2010) Effects of depressive-like behavior of rats on brain glutamate uptake. *Neurochem Res* 35: 1164–1171.
42. Bechtholt-Gompf AJ, Walther HV, Adams MA, et al. (2010) Blockade of astrocytic glutamate uptake in rats induces signs of anhedonia and impaired spatial memory. *Neuropsychopharmacology* 35: 2049–2059.
43. Lapidus KA, Soleimani L, Murrough JW (2013) Novel glutamatergic drugs for the treatment of mood disorders. *Neuropsychiatr Dis Treat* 9: 1101–1112.
44. Sanacora G, Treccani G, Popoli M (2012) Towards a glutamate hypothesis of depression: An emerging frontier of neuropsychopharmacology for mood disorders. *Neuropharmacology* 62: 63–77.
45. Paslakis G, Gass P, Deuschle M (2011) [The role of the glutamatergic system in pathophysiology and pharmacotherapy for depression: Preclinical and clinical data]. *Fortschr Neurol Psychiatr* 79: 204–212.
46. Rial D, Lemos C, Pinheiro H, et al. (2015) Depression as a glial-based synaptic dysfunction. *Front Cell Neurosci* 9: 521.
47. Jo WK, Zhang Y, Emrich HM, et al. (2015) Glia in the cytokine-mediated onset of depression: fine tuning the immune response. *Front Cell Neurosci* 9: 268.
48. Brites D, Fernandes A (2015) Neuroinflammation and Depression: Microglia Activation, Extracellular Microvesicles and microRNA Dysregulation. *Front Cell Neurosci* 9: 476.
49. Quesseveur G, Portal B, Basile JA, et al. (2015) Attenuated Levels of Hippocampal Connexin 43 and its Phosphorylation Correlate with Antidepressant- and Anxiolytic-Like Activities in Mice. *Front Cell Neurosci* 9: 490.

50. Jeanson T, Pondaven A, Ezan P, et al. (2015) Antidepressants Impact Connexin 43 Channel Functions in Astrocytes. *Front Cell Neurosci* 9: 495.
51. Fuchs E, Flugge G (2003) Chronic social stress: Effects on limbic brain structures. *Physiol Behav* 79: 417–427.
52. Gould E, Tanapat P (1999) Stress and hippocampal neurogenesis. *Biol Psychiatry* 46: 1472–1479.
53. Rajkowska G, Miguel-Hidalgo JJ (2007) Gliogenesis and glial pathology in depression. *CNS Neurol Disord Drug Targets* 6: 219–233.
54. Wang Q, Verweij EW, Krugers HJ, et al. (2014) Distribution of the glucocorticoid receptor in the human amygdala; changes in mood disorder patients. *Brain Struct Funct* 219: 1615–1626.
55. Czeh B, Muller-Keuker JI, Rygula R, et al. (2007) Chronic social stress inhibits cell proliferation in the adult medial prefrontal cortex: Hemispheric asymmetry and reversal by fluoxetine treatment. *Neuropsychopharmacology* 32: 1490–1503.
56. Pekny M, Nilsson M (2005) Astrocyte activation and reactive gliosis. *Glia* 50: 427–434.
57. Rozovsky I, Laping NJ, Krohn K, et al. (1995) Transcriptional regulation of glial fibrillary acidic protein by corticosterone in rat astrocytes in vitro is influenced by the duration of time in culture and by astrocyte-neuron interactions. *Endocrinology* 136: 2066–2073.
58. O'Callaghan JP, Brinton RE, Mcewen BS (1991) Glucocorticoids regulate the synthesis of glial fibrillary acidic protein in intact and adrenalectomized rats but do not affect its expression following brain injury. *J Neurochem* 57: 860–869.
59. Bridges N, Slais K, Sykova E (2008) The effects of chronic corticosterone on hippocampal astrocyte numbers: A comparison of male and female Wistar rats. *Acta Neurobiol Exp* 68: 131–138.
60. Lambert KG, Gerecke KM, Quadros PS, et al. (2000) Activity-stress increases density of GFAP-immunoreactive astrocytes in the rat hippocampus. *Stress* 3: 275–284.
61. Leventopoulos M, Ruedi-Bettschen D, Knuesel I, et al. (2007) Long-term effects of early life deprivation on brain glia in Fischer rats. *Brain Res* 1142: 119–126.
62. Fields RD, Stevens-Graham B (2002) New insights into neuron-glia communication. *Science* 298: 556–562.
63. Vardimon L, Ben-Dror I, Avisar N, et al. (1999) Glucocorticoid control of glial gene expression. *J Neurobiol* 40: 513–527.
64. Conrad CD (2006) What is the functional significance of chronic stress-induced CA3 dendritic retraction within the hippocampus? *Behav Cogn Neurosci Rev* 5: 41–60.
65. Autry AE, Grillo CA, Piroli GG, et al. (2006) Glucocorticoid regulation of GLT-1 glutamate transporter isoform expression in the rat hippocampus. *Neuroendocrinology* 83: 371–379.
66. Horner HC, Packan DR, Sapolsky RM (1990) Glucocorticoids inhibit glucose transport in cultured hippocampal neurons and glia. *Neuroendocrinology* 52: 57–64.
67. Ritchie LJ, De Butte M, Pappas BA (2004) Chronic mild stress exacerbates the effects of permanent bilateral common carotid artery occlusion on CA1 neurons. *Brain Res* 1014: 228–235.
68. Kroll S, El-Gindi J, Thanabalasundaram G, et al. (2009) Control of the blood-brain barrier by glucocorticoids and the cells of the neurovascular unit. *Ann N Y Acad Sci* 1165: 228–239.
69. Donato R (2001) S100: A multigenic family of calcium-modulated proteins of the EF-hand type with intracellular and extracellular functional roles. *Int J Biochem Cell Biol* 33: 637–668.
70. Bruschettini M, van den Hove DL, Gazzolo D, et al. (2005) A single course of antenatal betamethasone reduces neurotrophic factor S100B concentration in the hippocampus and serum in the neonatal rat. *Brain Res Dev Brain Res* 159: 113–118.

71. Margis R, Zanatto VC, Tramontina F, et al. (2004) Changes in S100B cerebrospinal fluid levels of rats subjected to predator stress. *Brain Res* 1028: 213–218.
72. Scaccianoce S, Del BP, Pannitteri G, et al. (2004) Relationship between stress and circulating levels of S100B protein. *Brain Res* 1004: 208–211.
73. Niu H, Hinkle DA, Wise PM (1997) Dexamethasone regulates basic fibroblast growth factor, nerve growth factor and S100beta expression in cultured hippocampal astrocytes. *Brain Res Mol Brain Res* 51: 97–105.
74. Bazargani N, Attwell D (2016) Astrocyte calcium signaling: the third wave. *Nat Neurosci* 19: 182–189.
75. Simard M, Couldwell WT, Zhang W, et al. (1999) Glucocorticoids-potent modulators of astrocytic calcium signaling. *Glia* 28: 1–12.
76. Mcleod JD, Bolton C (1995) Dexamethasone induces an increase in intracellular and membrane-associated lipocortin-1 (annexin-1) in rat astrocyte primary cultures. *Cell Mol Neurobiol* 15: 193–205.
77. Lindholm D, Castren E, Hengerer B, et al. (1992) Differential Regulation of Nerve Growth Factor (NGF) Synthesis in Neurons and Astrocytes by Glucocorticoid Hormones. *Eur J Neurosci* 4: 404–410.
78. Yuan SY, Liu J, Zhou J, et al. (2016) AMPK Mediates Glucocorticoids Stress-Induced Downregulation of the Glucocorticoid Receptor in Cultured Rat Prefrontal Cortical Astrocytes. *PLoS One* 11: e0159513.
79. Chen J, Wang ZZ, Zuo W, et al. (2016) Effects of chronic mild stress on behavioral and neurobiological parameters—Role of glucocorticoid. *Horm Behav* 78: 150–159.
80. Karisetty BC, Joshi PC, Kumar A, et al. (2017) Sex differences in the effect of chronic mild stress on mouse prefrontal cortical BDNF levels: A role of major ovarian hormones. *Neuroscience* 356: 89–101.
81. Bender CL, Calfa GD, Molina VA (2016) Astrocyte plasticity induced by emotional stress: A new partner in psychiatric physiopathology? *Prog Neuropsychopharmacol Biol Psychiatry* 65: 68–77.
82. Anacker C, Cattaneo A, Luoni A, et al. (2013) Glucocorticoid-related molecular signaling pathways regulating hippocampal neurogenesis. *Neuropsychopharmacology* 38: 872–883.
83. Van DL, Steinbusch HW, Bruschettini M, et al. (2006) Prenatal stress reduces S100B in the neonatal rat hippocampus. *Neuroreport* 17: 1077–1080.
84. Nichols NR, Agolley D, Zieba M, et al. (2005) Glucocorticoid regulation of glial responses during hippocampal neurodegeneration and regeneration. *Brain Res Rev* 48: 287–301.

Permissions

All chapters in this book were first published in NEUROSCIENCE, by AIMS Press; hereby published with permission under the Creative Commons Attribution License or equivalent. Every chapter published in this book has been scrutinized by our experts. Their significance has been extensively debated. The topics covered herein carry significant findings which will fuel the growth of the discipline. They may even be implemented as practical applications or may be referred to as a beginning point for another development.

The contributors of this book come from diverse backgrounds, making this book a truly international effort. This book will bring forth new frontiers with its revolutionizing research information and detailed analysis of the nascent developments around the world.

We would like to thank all the contributing authors for lending their expertise to make the book truly unique. They have played a crucial role in the development of this book. Without their invaluable contributions this book wouldn't have been possible. They have made vital efforts to compile up to date information on the varied aspects of this subject to make this book a valuable addition to the collection of many professionals and students.

This book was conceptualized with the vision of imparting up-to-date information and advanced data in this field. To ensure the same, a matchless editorial board was set up. Every individual on the board went through rigorous rounds of assessment to prove their worth. After which they invested a large part of their time researching and compiling the most relevant data for our readers.

The editorial board has been involved in producing this book since its inception. They have spent rigorous hours researching and exploring the diverse topics which have resulted in the successful publishing of this book. They have passed on their knowledge of decades through this book. To expedite this challenging task, the publisher supported the team at every step. A small team of assistant editors was also appointed to further simplify the editing procedure and attain best results for the readers.

Apart from the editorial board, the designing team has also invested a significant amount of their time in understanding the subject and creating the most relevant covers. They scrutinized every image to scout for the most suitable representation of the subject and create an appropriate cover for the book.

The publishing team has been an ardent support to the editorial, designing and production team. Their endless efforts to recruit the best for this project, has resulted in the accomplishment of this book. They are a veteran in the field of academics and their pool of knowledge is as vast as their experience in printing. Their expertise and guidance has proved useful at every step. Their uncompromising quality standards have made this book an exceptional effort. Their encouragement from time to time has been an inspiration for everyone.

The publisher and the editorial board hope that this book will prove to be a valuable piece of knowledge for researchers, students, practitioners and scholars across the globe.

List of Contributors

Shu Hui Yau, Paul F Sowman and Jon Brock
ARC Centre of Excellence in Cognition and its Disorders, Australia

Shu Hui Yau, Paul F Sowman and Jon Brock
Department of Cognitive Science, Macquarie University, NSW, Australia

Shu Hui Yau
Graduate School of Education, University of Bristol, United Kingdom

Fabrice Bardy
HEARing Co-operative Research Centre, VIC, Australia
National Acoustic Laboratories, NSW, Australia

Jon Brock
Department of Psychology, Macquarie University, NSW, Australia

Lucia P. Pavlova
Department of Higher Nervous Activity and Psychophysiology, Faculty of Biology, St. Petersburg State University, St.-Petersburg, Russia

Dmitrii N. Berlov
Department of Anatomy and Physiology of Humans and Animals, Herzen State Pedagogical University of Russia, St.-Petersburg, Russia
International Research Center of the Functional Materials and Devices of Optoelectronics and Electronics, ITMO University, Saint Petersburg, Russia

Andres Kurismaa
Department of History and Philosophy of Science, Faculty of Science, Charles University in Prague, Czech Republic

Diana C. Oviedo and Ambar R. Perez
Universidad Católica Santa María La Antigua (USMA), Panamá

Hector Lezcano
Facultad de Medicina, Universidad de Panamá, Panamá

Ambar R. Perez, Alcibiades E. Villarreal, Maria B. Carreira, Shantal A. Grajales and Gabrielle B. Britton
Centro de Neurociencias y Unidad de Investigación Clínica, Instituto de Investigaciones Científicas y Servicios de Alta Tecnología (INDICASAT AIP), Panamá

Baltasar Isaza and Lavinia Wesley
Servicio de Radiología, Complejo Hospitalario Arnulfo Arias Madrid, Caja del Seguro Social, Panamá

Sara Fernandez
Departmento de Psicología Básica II (Procesos Cognitivos), Facultad de Psicología, Universidad Complutense de Madrid, Madrid, España

Ana Frank
Servicio de Neurología, Hospital Universitario La Paz, Madrid, España

Galina V. Portnova and Michael S. Atanov
Institute of Higher Nervous Activity and Neurophysiology of RAS, 5A Butlerova St., Moscow 117485, Russia

Galina V. Portnova
The Pushkin State Russian Language Institute

Yoshi Nishitani
Department of Radiology, Graduate School of Medicine, Osaka University, Suita 565-0871, Japan

Chie Hosokawa
Biomedical Research Institute and Advanced Photonics and Biosensing Open Innovation Laboratory, AIST, Ikeda, Osaka 563-8577, Japan

Yuko Mizuno-Matsumoto
Graduate School of Applied Informatics, University of Hyogo, Kobe 650-0044, Japan

Tomomitsu Miyoshi
Department of Integrative Physiology, Graduate School of Medicine, Osaka University, Suita 565-0871, Japan

Shinichi Tamura
NBL Technovator Co., Ltd., Sennan 590-0522, Japan

Chiyoko Kobayashi Frank
School of Psychology, Fielding Graduate University, Santa Barbara, CA, USA
Center for Cognition and Communication, New York, NY, USA

Muh Anshar
Social, Cognitive Robotics and Advanced Artificial Intelligent Research Centre, Department of Electrical Engineering, Universitas Hasanuddin UNHAS Makassar Indonesia

Mary-Anne Williams
Innovation and Enterprise Research Lab, Centre for Artificial Intelligence, University of Technology Sydney UTS Australia

Jonathan R. Emerson, Jack A. Binks, Matthew W. Scott, Ryan P. W. Kenny and Daniel L. Eaves
School of Health and Social Care, Teesside University, Middlesbrough, UK

Khue Vu Nguyen
Department of Medicine, Biochemical Genetics and Metabolism, The Mitochondrial and Metabolic Disease Center, School of Medicine, University of California, San Diego, Building CTF, Room C-103, 214 Dickinson Street, San Diego, CA 92103-8467, USA
Department of Pediatrics, University of California, San Diego, School of Medicine, San Diego, La Jolla, CA 92093, USA

Matthew S. Sherwood and Subhashini Ganapathy
Department of Biomedical, Industrial & Human Factors Engineering, Wright State University, Dayton, OH, USA

Jason G. Parker and Emily E. Diller
Department of Radiology and Imaging Sciences, Indiana University School of Medicine, Indiana University, IN, USA

Emily E. Diller
School of Health Sciences, Purdue University, West Lafayette, IN, USA

Subhashini Ganapathy
Department of Trauma Care, Boonshoft School of Medicine, Wright State University, Dayton, OH, USA

Kevin Bennett
Department of Psychology, Wright State University, Dayton, OH, USA

Jeremy T. Nelson
Department of Defense Hearing Center of Excellence, JBSA-Lackland, USA

Hyein Cho, Wei Dou, Zaviera Reyes, Mark W. Geisler and Ezequiel Morsella
Department of Psychology, San Francisco State University, CA, USA

Ezequiel Morsella
Department of Neurology, University of California, San Francisco, CA, USA

Yoshi Nishitani
Dept. of Radiology, Graduate School of Medicine, Osaka University, Suita 565-0871, Japan

Chie Hosokawa
Biomedical Research Institute, AIST, Ikeda, Osaka 563-8577, Japan

Yuko Mizuno-Matsumoto
Graduate School of Applied Informatics, University of Hyogo, Kobe 650-0044, Japan

Tomomitsu Miyoshi
Dept. of Integrative Physiology, Graduate School of Medicine, Osaka University, Suita 565-0871, Japan

Shinichi Tamura
NBL Technovator Co., Ltd., 631 Shindachimakino, Sennan 590-0522, Japan

Pranav Chintamani Joshi and Sugato Benerjee
Department of Pharmaceutical Sciences and Technology, Birla Institute of Technology, Mesra, Ranchi, India

Index

www.ingramcontent.com/pod-product-compliance
Lightning Source LLC
Chambersburg PA
CBHW050436200326
41458CB00014B/4970
9781632427151